71.⁰⁰

Dietary Fibre, Fibre-Depleted Foods and Disease

Contributors

SHEILA BINGHAM

NORMAN BLACKLOCK

W. GORDON BRYDON

DENIS BURKITT

JOHN CUMMINGS

MARTIN EASTWOOD

HANS ENGLYST

NATHAN FISHER

BARBARA HARLAND

RICHARD F. HARVEY

KENNETH HEATON

PHILIP JAMES

DAVID KRITCHEVSKY

JIM MANN

JEAN MARR

NEIL PAINTER

LEON PROSKY

ISIDOR SEGAL

ALAN SILMAN

DAVID SOUTHGATE

HARRY STEIN

ALISON STEPHEN

FRANK TOVEY

HUGH TROWELL

ALEXANDER WALKER

Dietary Fibre, Fibre-Depleted Foods and Disease

Edited by

HUGH TROWELL
Formerly Consultant
Physician, Uganda

DENIS BURKITT
Formerly Medical Research Council
External Scientific Staff
London, United Kingdom

Both formerly of Makerere University and Mulago Hospital,
Kampala, Uganda

KENNETH HEATON
Reader in Medicine
Bristol Royal Infirmary
Bristol, United Kingdom

Foreword by
Sir **RICHARD DOLL**
Emeritus Regius Professor of Medicine
University of Oxford
Oxford, United Kingdom

1985

ACADEMIC PRESS
(Harcourt Brace Jovanovich, Publishers)
LONDON ORLANDO SAN DIEGO NEW YORK
TORONTO MONTREAL SYDNEY TOKYO

ACADEMIC PRESS INC. (LONDON) LTD.
24–28 Oval Road
LONDON NW1 7DX

United States Edition published by
ACADEMIC PRESS, INC.
Orlando, Florida 32887

British Library Cataloguing in Publication Data

Dietary fibre, fibre-depleted foods and disease.
   1. Fibre in human nutrition
   I. Trowell, H. C. II. Burkitt, D. P.
   III. Heaton, K. W.
   613.2'8   TX553.F53

Library of Congress Cataloging in Publication Data
Main entry under title:

Dietary fibre, fibre-depleted foods and disease.

   Includes bibliographies and index.
   1. Fiber deficiency diseases. 2. High-fiber diet.
I. Trowell, H. C. (Hubert Carey) II. Burkitt, D. P.
(Denis P.) III. Heaton, K. W. (Kenneth Willoughby)
[DNLM: 1. Cardiovascular Diseases—etiology. 2. Diet—
adverse effects. 3. Dietary Fiber. 4. Gastrointestinal
Diseases—etiology. 5. Metabolic Diseases—etiology.
WB 427 D5657]
RC627.F5D55 1985   616.3'96   84-24335
ISBN 0-12-701160-9 (alk. paper)

Dedicated to Sir Frances Avery Jones, C. B. E., Doyen of British gastrologists in the 1970s. He encouraged dietary fibre research at the MRC Gastroenterological Unit of the Central Middlesex Hospital, London, and others elsewhere.

Contents

Contributors

Numbers in parentheses indicate the pages on which the authors' contributions begin.

SHEILA BINGHAM (77), Dunn Clinical Nutrition Centre, Addenbrooke's Hospital, Cambridge CB2 1QE, United Kingdom

NORMAN BLACKLOCK (345), Department of Urological Surgery, University of South Manchester, West Didsbury, Manchester M20 8LR, United Kingdom

W. GORDON BRYDON (105), Wolfson Gastrointestinal Laboratories, Department of Medicine, Western General Hospital, Edinburgh EH4 2XU, Scotland

DENIS BURKITT (21, 191, 317, 419), The Old House, Bussage, Stroud, Gloucestershire GL6 8AX, United Kingdom. *Formerly:* Medical Research Council External Scientific Staff, London, and Surgeon, Uganda Government and Department of Surgery, Makerere University, Kampala, Uganda

JOHN CUMMINGS (161), Medical Research Council, Dunn Clinical Nutrition Centre, Addenbrooke's Hospital, Cambridge, CB2 1QE, United Kingdom

MARTIN EASTWOOD (105), Wolfson Gastrointestinal Laboratories, Department of Medicine, Western General Hospital, Edinburgh EH4 2XU, Scotland

HANS ENGLYST (31), Cand. Agro., Medical Research Council, Dunn Nutritional Laboratory, Cambridge CB2 1QE, United Kingdom

NATHAN FISHER (377), Flour Milling and Baking Research Association, Chorley Wood WD3 5SH, United Kingdom

BARBARA HARLAND* (57), Division of Nutrition, U.S. Food and Drug Administration, Washington, D.C. 20204, USA

RICHARD F. HARVEY (217), Department of Medicine, Frenchay Hospital, Bristol BS16 1LE, United Kingdom

KENNETH HEATON (21, 205, 289, 391, 419), University Department of Medicine, Bristol Royal Infirmary, Bristol BS2 8HW, United Kingdom

PHILIP JAMES (249), The Rowett Research Institute, Bucksburn, Aberdeen AB2 9SB, Scotland

DAVID KRITCHEVSKY (305), The Wistar Institute, Philadelphia, Pennsylvania 19104, USA

*Present address: School of Human Ecology, Howard University, Washington, D.C. 20059, USA.

ix

Jim Mann (263), Department of Community Medicine and General Practice, Radcliffe Infirmary, Oxford OX2 6HE, United Kingdom

Jean Marr (403), Department of Clinical Epidemiology and General Practice, The Royal Free Hospital School of Medicine, London NW3 2PF, United Kingdom

Neil Painter (145), Manor House Hospital, London NW11 7HX, United Kingdom

Leon Prosky (57), Division of Nutrition, U.S. Food and Drug Administration, Washington, D.C. 20204, USA

Isidor Segal (241), Gastroenterology Unit, Baragwanath Hospital, University of Witwatersrand, Johannesburg 2013, South Africa

Alan Silman (403), London Hospital Medical College, London E1 2AD, United Kingdom

David Southgate (31), Agricultural and Food Research Council, Food Research Institute, Norwich NR4 7UA, United Kingdom

Harry Stein (331), Department of Pediatrics, Baragwanath Hospital, University of Witwatersrand, Johannesburg 2013, South Africa

Alison Stephen (133), Department of Environment and Preventive Medicine, Medical College of St. Bartholomew's Hospital, London EC1M 6BQ, United Kingdom

Frank Tovey (229), Basingstoke District Hospital, Basingstoke, Hants RG24 9NA, United Kingdom

Hugh Trowell (1, 21, 419), Windover, Woodgreen, Fordingbridge Hampshire SP6 2AZ, United Kingdom. *Formerly:* Physician, Uganda Government and Department of Medicine, Makerere University, Kampala, Uganda

Alexander Walker (191, 331, 361), Human Biochemistry Research Unit, South African Institute for Medical Research, Johannesburg, South Africa

Foreword

Ideas, like living organisms, have their natural history, growing from conception through a more or less tumultuous adolescence and a reproductive maturity to an old age, when they act as a bar to further progress. During this time they may become so modified that their origin is obscured. Interest in dietary fibre is, however, so recent that we can still recognize its origin in Peter Cleave's concept of "the saccharine disease". Under this title Cleave brought together a variety of conditions characteristic of industrial society which, he thought, were due to overconsumption of carbohydrates, made easy to absorb and unsatisfying to the appetite by the refinement that they had undergone in the course of their preparation for the Western market. Stimulating though this idea was, it did not attract much support, because it failed to provide a comprehensible explanation for the pathogenesis of many of the diseases concerned. When, however, Trowell and Burkitt inverted the idea by suggesting that the dietary fibre that had been removed in the course of the refinement of carbohydrate was a specific nutrient and that many pathological effects could be attributed to a deficiency of it, a whole new vista of possible mechanisms was revealed.

The validity of this idea was so easily demonstrated by personal experience, insofar as it related to the easy and regular passage of stools, and the corollary that we should return to a more natural diet corresponded so well with the ecological spirit of the times, that the idea was widely accepted and national diets began to be modified, while the scientific evidence lagged behind. Now, however, the biochemical and physiological facts are beginning to emerge; dietary fibre has been broken down to numerous component parts, and sufficient background information is available to formulate and test hypotheses about the role of the different components of fibre in the pathogenesis of individual diseases. With the publication of Trowell, Burkitt, and Heaton's book, the ideas that Cleave, Burkitt, and Trowell so imaginatively conceived seem to have come of age, and the way is now open for those solid scientific advances that will permit the permanent control of another section of unnecessary and avoidable disease. To have been invited to write a foreword to a book which marks such an important step forward in the development of biological knowledge is a privilege for which I am deeply indebted to the authors.

Sir Richard Doll, F.R.S.

Preface

A medical book may be considered successful if its sales justify the subsequent publication of a second edition. On the other hand, a few pioneer books may be so seminal that there should never be any question of a second edition of the same book. In our previous book "Refined Carbohydrate Foods and Disease: Some Implications of Dietary Fibre," edited by D. P. Burkitt and H. C. Trowell (1975), Sir Richard Doll wrote "Once every 10 years or so a new idea emerges about the cause of disease. . . . vitamin deficiency . . . auto-immunity. . . . To these we may now add a deficiency of dietary fibre. But whether it will be as seminal an idea as that of vitamin deficiency or as sterile as that of stress, we shall probably not know for another 10 years."

Ten years have passed. In 1975 no food tables published data concerning the dietary fibre content of foods; almost no book on nutrition, gastroenterology or medicine even mentioned dietary fibre or named its constituents. Many regarded fibre as a gastrointestinal irritant, and called it roughage. Medical recommendations to the millers had always been to remove as much fibre as possible from the flour. Others regarded fibre merely as cellulose and had added this to chemically defined diets in animal nutritional experiments of dubious validity. All this has completely changed. For instance the (British) Committee on Medical Aspects of Food Policy (1981) reported much evidence that dietary fibre was an important health-promoting component of the diet; it advocated increased consumption of bread, especially brown and wholemeal varieties, as well as vegetables and fruit.

Recently the (British) Health Education Council (1983) recommended multiple changes in the national diet. It recommended that dietary fibre intake should increase some 50%, the largest single recommended change of one component of the present diet.

In 1982, the editors asked the publishers to refrain from any reprinting of their original book. In this they had contributed some two-thirds of the chapters: these should be handed over as far as possible to those conducting research in some disease or aspect of a complex nutritional problem. First it was essential to enlist the help of a younger editor. They were indeed fortunate to receive an acceptance from Dr. K. W. Heaton. He had been the secretary of the Royal College of Physicians report "Medical Aspects of Dietary Fibre" (1980). Our new book follows largely the pattern of the chapters of that book. It omits, however, a chapter on dental caries, since there is widespread agreement that sucrose, a fibre-depleted food, is a major causative factor. Many chapters of the present book conclude with the author's own summary. The final chapter of the book summarises briefly all the chapters.

We thank Sir Richard Doll for most kindly writing the Foreword to the present book. Others who have helped us by careful secretarial work are Mrs. Jennifer Masefield, Mrs. Priscilla Tippet, and Mrs. Natalie Adams; also, as librarian Mrs. Jenny Allen. There are others who wish to remain unnamed.

Hugh Trowell
Denis Burkitt
Kenneth Heaton

References

BURKITT, D. P. and TROWELL, H. S. (1975). "Refined Carbohydrate Foods and Disease: Some Implications of Dietary Fibre." Academic Press, London and New York.

Committee on Medical Aspects of Food Policy (1981). "Nutritional Aspects of Bread and Flour." HM Stationery Office, London.

Health Education Council (1983). "Proposals for Nutritional Guidelines for Health Education in Britain." London. Summarised in *Lancet,* 1983, **2,** 719–721, 782–785, 835–837, 902–905.

Royal College of Physicians of London (1980). "Medical Aspects of Dietary Fibre." Pitman Medical, London.

Dietary Fibre, Fibre-Depleted Foods and Disease

Chapter 1

Dietary fibre: a paradigm

HUGH TROWELL

I. Introduction

Before unravelling the tangled story of dietary fibre it will be helpful to define the meaning of a term that did not occur as a subject category in the Index Medicus until 1982.

All constituents of the diet can be named and defined in terms of their chemical composition, even if the group of substances that comprise dietary fibre presents different aspects to food analysts, botanists, cereal chemists, nutritionists and gastroenterologists. Dietary fibre has been defined *chemically* as "the sum of the polysaccharides and lignin which are not digested by the endogenous secretions of the human gastrointestinal tract; this fraction has a variable composition and is made up of different types of polysaccharides (cellulose, hemicelluloses and pectic substances and the noncarbohydrate lignin)" (Paul and Southgate, 1978). *Dr. D.A.T. Southgate* pioneered

1

the analysis of dietary fibre more than 15 years ago. This provided the scientific basis of knowledge concerning this complex group of substances.

II. New concept, new paradigm

The paradigm forces scientists to investigate some part of nature in detail and depth that would otherwise be unimaginable (Kuhn, 1970).

The importance of dietary fibre as a constituent of the diet was increasingly recognised in Britain following the Report of the Royal College of Physicians of London (1980), hereafter called the RCP Report (1980). Official recognition came in the report of the Panel on Bread, Flour and Other Cereal Products (1981). Only a few years previously, Van Soest (1978), speaking at the U.S. National Institutes of Health Symposium on the Role of Dietary Fibre in Health, protested that terms such as fibre, cellulose and roughage were still rarely found in textbooks of human nutrition and when they did occur the information was usually inaccurate. A brief account of the concept of dietary fibre in human nutrition was given to open the symposium (Trowell, 1978a).

Dietary fibre previously had been called roughage and was considered a gastrointestinal irritant; this is now known to be incorrect. Dietary fibre had also been called unavailable carbohydrates by food analysts in Britain; this is now known to be incorrect because bacterial fermentation of dietary fibre in the colon contributes a small amount of absorbable energy.

In this chapter I will describe how a small *group* of doctors (named in *italics*) aided the recognition during the 1970s. But the story of fibre winds back long before those years. This was not a group of doctors who were working together in one place. It was a widely dispersed group who were eventually attracted to a new concept, that of dietary fibre. Similar groups have been described by Kuhn (1970), Professor of Philosophy and Science at Massachusetts Institute of Technology, in his seminal study "The Structure of Scientific Revolutions." He discussed how a new concept, which he called a paradigm, emerges. Two characteristics mark all new paradigms: first "the achievement was sufficiently unprecedented to attract an enduring group of adherents"; second "it was sufficiently open-ended to leave all sorts of problems for the redefined group" to investigate (Kuhn, 1970, p. 10). He repeatedly emphasised a *group*. He described in great detail the pattern of events that always precedes the birth of a new paradigm. There is the anomaly that arrests attention, then the crisis in the minds of the observers, followed by the confusion at the birth of the new concept, then the conflicts that inevitably occur. There can be small revolutions due to small paradigms, as well as large ones (Kuhn, 1970, p. 49).

A new paradigm is always born out of awareness of an anomaly (Kuhn, 1970, pp. 52–65). The rarity of many diseases of civilization among developing African peasants was the anomaly. These peasants had often been poorly fed, they had many infections, but they rarely developed the cardiovascular, alimentary and degenerative diseases of civilization (Walker, 1956, 1982). This was indeed an anomaly. A tension and a crisis occurred in the minds of those who observed it (Kuhn, 1970, pp. 77–91).

New paradigms "are tradition-shattering complements to the tradition-bound activity of normal science" (Kuhn, 1970, p. 6). With great discernment, this book pointed out that discoveries had previously been described in a naive manner. A discovery is not "a single simple act . . . attributable to an individual and to a moment in time . . . [it is] a new sort of phenomenon [which] is a necessarily complex event, one which involves recognizing both *that* something is and *what* it is (author's italics) . . . discovery is a process and must take time" (Kuhn, 1970, p. 55).

With regard to dietary fibre, first, it was realised *that* a group of substances existed in all natural plant foods of man, since it occurred in plant cell walls [and cell wall material present in bran] and, second, *what* this group actually is had been poorly defined, rarely analysed and seldom investigated. I therefore defined this group of substances as

> that portion of food which is derived from the cellular walls of plants which is digested very poorly by human beings . . . Fibre is composed largely of cellulose . . . one of the most diverse molecules in nature . . . arranged in long chains, which may form a lattice-work. Mingled with the fine fibrils of cellulose are other substances which are poorly digested: hemicelluloses, pentosans, pectins and lignin and traces of gummy materials . . . Fibre is not merely cellulose; it is quite different from chemically pure cellulose, but on more than one occasion has been regarded as identical (Trowell, 1972a).

This definition was shortened but basically unaltered in other communications that stressed the difference between crude fibre (p. 14) and dietary fibre (Trowell, 1972b, 1973). Derived from plant cell walls and not digested by human alimentary enzymes, starch was excluded from all these definitions and was never named at that time or subsequently as a constituent of dietary fibre. Complete indigestibility by human alimentary enzymes is one, but only one, of the characteristic features of all the polysaccharide constituents of dietary fibre. This explains why it *survives* as latticework to package and surround digestible nutrients in the upper alimentary tract and thus delays and alters digestion; it also explains why it is usually the main group of dietary constituents to enter the large bowel and profoundly alter colonic function.

This process of the recognition first that dietary fibre exists, and second what dietary fibre is, took place slowly in my mind during 1970 and 1971 as I conferred with other members of the dietary fibre group (p. 11) and studied books on botany, plant cell walls (Preston, 1974) and the milling of cereals.

III.   Many tributaries, one stream

At least six tributaries eventually combined to form the large river of dietary fibre. Some explorers, moving downstream along one tributary, were surprised, even upset, to meet others who had been travelling, even much longer, down another.

A.   Bran: United States and Britain (1920s–1940s)

The first tributary arose from the investigation of the fibre-rich bran in the United States from 1920 to 1943; this emphasised its laxative action. Eventually bran was condemned by conservative medical opinion (American Medical Association, 1936). Thereafter publications soon ceased. In Britain, Dimock (1937) was the first doctor to investigate in detail the laxative action of prepared bran in constipation; he used it also in the treatment of other colonic disorders. His publications were succeeded by those of Cleave (1941) and others early in the 1940s, all of whom used bran as a laxative.

B.   British National flour (1941–1953)

The second tributary started in Britain during World War II (1939–1945). Shortages of wheat imports necessitated the milling of high-extraction, high-fibre National flour, voluntary in 1941, mandatory from 1942 until 1953. Medical advisers asked that the fibre, considered indigestible and an irritant, should be kept as low as possible. The crude fibre (p. 14) content of the flour was consequently reported frequently in medical journals (Trowell, 1979). Eventually British cereal chemists began to estimate by direct analysis the cellulose, hemicelluloses and lignin, at the present time called dietary fibre, of the flour (Fraser and Holmes, 1959). These total figures were about three times higher than those of crude fibre and demonstrated the inadequacy of the latter definition.

C.   South African blacks: westernization of diets

The third tributary arose in South Africa. In that country, more clearly than in any other part of Africa, blacks in the rural homelands eat much high-fibre, lightly processed complex carbohydrate foods (starch). When they move into urban areas they begin to eat smaller amounts of low-fibre, highly processed complex carbohydrate foods and more fibre-free fat and sugar and few vegetables. They change from very high cereal-fibre diets to relatively lower cereal-fibre diets during westernization.

   Dr. A. R. P. Walker, the doyen of fibre research in Africa, had trained as a biochemist in Britain and then emigrated to South Africa in 1938. He has always acknowledged his debt to McCarrison (1921, 1940), who in India had praised the excellent physiques of people in north Indian communities, who ate mainly whole cereals, fruit and vegetables. During World War II, South Africa also experienced wheat shortages; these necessitated the milling of high-extraction, high-fibre flour. It was feared that this would lead to decreased absorption of calcium, but observations on both whites and blacks demonstrated that calcium balance was fairly soon achieved (Walker *et al.*, 1948).

In 1947 I visited South Africa and met Dr. Walker, who had begun to study bowel motility in South African blacks (Walker, 1947). He amazed me by stating that cereal fibre was *not* a gastrointestinal irritant: this challenged existing teaching. It also contradicted a notion that the intractable diarrhoea of kwashiorkor was due to roughage in the maize meal diet of black children. Data were being collected for a book on kwashiorkor (Trowell *et al.*, 1952). Slowly the complex aetiology of this disease was explored; now it is called protein–energy malnutrition (PEM). Four years later this disease began to be described in standard medical textbooks. It is the most common, severe malnutritional disease in the world. In 1975 the Nutrition Foundations of Europe, North America and other countries began to sponsor the republication of a few selected classic works on nutrition. They reprinted "Kwashiorkor" (Trowell, *et al.*, 1982) as the fourth selected nutrition classic, the only one at present from the twentieth century.

Soon Walker and his colleagues began to relate the *whole* unusual pattern of metabolic disease in South African blacks to the *whole* pattern of their diet, emphasising, but not exclusively, the role of fibre. They were the first to suggest that high intake of fibre (cellulose) might be a protective factor against coronary heart disease (Bersohn *et al.*, 1956). Gallstones and appendicitis were also recognised to be rare in blacks (Walker, 1956). In rural areas, blacks rarely developed either obesity or diabetes; their diets contained small amounts of risk factors such as fat, cholesterol and animal protein, but more protective factors such as a high intake of lightly processed, high-fibre cereals. Blacks also were very physically active and smoked fewer cigarettes than whites. Almost every year for the past 35 years, Walker and his colleagues have published several articles on the different patterns of disease and the different diets of black, white, Indian, and coloured populations in South Africa (Walker, 1982).

D. Diseases of civilization

1. A challenging anomaly

The fourth tributary concerns the attempt to define and explain the diseases of civilization and merits a detailed consideration. These diseases are those which have high incidences in almost all affluent technological Western communities but are rare in developing poor peasant communities of the Third World. At one time they were regarded as due to the stress of modern life.

This explanation has been rejected: blacks in Africa suffer much stress. Subsequently it was surmised that an explanation lay in the small number of blacks that survived into middle age. This too has been shown to be erroneous. In South Africa many thousands of blacks live to middle age and at 50 years of age their expectation of life exceeds that of South African whites (Walker, 1974). Many considered that the diet, housing and medical care of the blacks were inferior to that of the whites, but middle-aged blacks lived longer than the whites. This was the anomaly. It had distressed everyone who, like myself, has taught medicine or surgery at a medical school in sub-Saharan Africa; it has puzzled those who sailed the seven seas like Captain T. L. Cleave (p. 8); it has intrigued those who travelled to many continents like D. P. Burkitt (p. 13).

2.   *List of diseases*

Table 1.1 summarises briefly the main epidemiological data concerning the alleged diseases of civilization listed in books from 1937 to 1981. Donnison (1937) and Gelfand (1944) considered that the apparent absence of these diseases in African blacks was due to the absence of mental stress. The former had worked for nearly 3 years among primitive tribes in the Kenya highlands; the latter had treated urban Zimbabwe blacks for 6 years. After teaching medicine for 29 years in what have become the university medical schools of Kenya and Uganda, my study of non-infective diseases in sub-Saharan blacks contained a longer list and gave over 500 citations from six sub-Saharan medical journals of Africa (Trowell, 1960).

3.   *Colonic diseases*

"Non-Infective Disease in Africa" (Trowell, 1960) was written after all the data has been assembled during another visit to South Africa in 1958. In the chapter that discusses alimentary diseases, but in *no* other chapter, it is stated that *all* the relatively common non-infective diseases of the large bowel were rare in sub-Saharan blacks

> who pass a bulky soft stool two or three times in a day . . . Natural [Black] African diets are high in their fibre content . . . In towns . . . refined flours, sugar and fats form a large part of the diet, which may contain little fibre . . . Faeces [therefore] pass sluggishly along the colon and are evacuated as small desiccated masses rather than the bulky soft pultaceous stool of the peasant . . . It would be fanciful to ascribe the pattern of colonic diseases entirely [to this] . . . yet it is an interesting hypothesis (Trowell, 1960 pp. 217–222).

It was suggested that a high consumption of fibre-rich, lightly processed complex carbohydrate (starch) foods were a protective factor in the *whole* group of eight non-infective diseases of the large bowel. Possibly this is the first publication to report, with supporting clinical and necropsy data and 23 literature citations and personal communications, the rarity of diverticular

TABLE 1.1. Diseases of civilization listed in books from 1937 to 1981[a]

Investigators:	Donnison	Trowell	Cleave and Campbell	Burkitt and Trowell	Trowell and Burkitt
Year:	1937[b]	1960[c]	1966[d]	1975[c]	1981[c,e]
Countries:	Kenya	Africa	Africa, India	—	Five continents
Dental caries	No	+	+	+	+
Constipation	AD	+	+	+	+
Appendicitis	+	+	+	+	+
Diverticular disease	AD	+	+	+	+
Haemorrhoids	AD	+	+	+	+
Colo-rectal cancer	AD	+	AD	+	+
Obesity	+	+	+	+	+
Diabetes type II	+	+	+	+	+
Coronary heart	+	+	+	+	+
Gallstones	+	+	+	+	+
Varicose veins, DVT[f]	+	+	+	+	+
Hypertension[g]	+	?	AD	AD	+
Thyrotoxicosis	+	+	AD	+	+
Pernicious anaemia	+	+	AD	+	+
Rheumatoid arthritis	AD	+	AD	+	+
Renal stone	+	+	+	+	+
Duodenal ulcer	+	?	+	?	No

[a] +, Agrees; no, disagrees; AD, absent data; ?, doubtful.

[b] Gelfand (1944) in Zimbabwe largely concurred.

[c] Also irritable bowel syndrome, polyp of colon, ulcerative colitis, Crohn's disease, hiatal hernia, multiple sclerosis, myxoedema, Hashimoto's thyroiditis, hypoparathyroidism, myasthenia gravis, Paget's disease, gout and pulmonary embolism.

[d] Also hiatal hernia, pyelonephritis and eclampsia.

[e] Also many autoimmune and endocrine diseases, likewise cancer of the breast, corpus uteri, prostate and lung (Doll and Armstrong, 1981).

[f] Deep vein thrombosis.

[g] Absent until salt is added to food.

disease, irritable bowel syndrome, colo-rectal cancer and polyp, ulcerative colitis and Crohn's disease in African blacks, and to ascribe this rarity to the protective action of fibre. Others had reported previously, with supporting data, its protective role in constipation, appendicitis and haemorrhoids. This view was formulated after visiting Johannesburg for the second time in 1958. There Dr. J. Higginson and Dr. A. G. Oettlé had already recorded the data of their then unpublished report on colo-rectal cancer necropsies in Johannesburg Bantu 1953-1955. Blacks had one-eighth of the number of colo-rectal cancers compared with U.S. blacks of comparable number, sex and age (Trowell, 1960 pp. 217–222).

Subsequently Higginson and Oettlé (1957, cited in Trowell, 1960-p. 219) published their necropsy data concerning colo-rectal cancer in South African blacks. They reported that its rarity was associated with eating a "natural diet in which the relevant features remain to be discovered", but they suggested that the large amount of roughage in their diet and the rarity of constipation should be noted. They did not mention the bulkiness of the African stools, or the rapid intestinal transit, or the rarity of the other non-infective colonic diseases in the blacks. In their subsequent publications on cancer (Oettlé, 1964; Higginson, 1966), neither mentioned fibre nor roughage as a possible protective factor in colo-rectal cancer. It is submitted that the suggestion that fibre might be a protective factor in colo-rectal cancer and other disorders of the large bowel had been more clearly stated by myself (Trowell, 1960 pp. 217–222).

4. Diabetes

It was also postulated that the African rural peasant diet of large amounts of lightly processed, fibre-rich "high-carbohydrate [starch] low-fat diets possibly contributed to a lower fasting blood-sugar and a flatter tolerance curve [in African Blacks] and among such persons less might eventually evolve into frank diabetes" (Trowell, 1960 p. 308). This hypothesis was strengthened subsequently by new data that reported both increased glucose tolerance and fat tolerance in South African black children (Walker et al., 1970a). A formal hypothesis "that fibre-depleted starchy foods are conducive to the development of diabetes in susceptible human genotypes" (Trowell, 1975a) was eventually proposed.

E. Saccharine disease

1. The hypothesis

The bold and comprehensive hypothesis that *all* the diseases of civilization were really manifestations of a single overall so-called saccharine disease has done much in England to focus attention on refined carbohydrates. It put emphasis on sugar, as in the book's title, but recognised the role of fibre in some colonic disorders (Cleave, 1956). The basic concept was couched in terms of evolution. It was considered that the biggest change in the food during recent centuries concerned the manufacture by machinery of concentrated carbohydrates, refined sugar and refined white flour. Sugar had been concentrated more because 90% had been removed in the fibrous pith (bagasse) and consumption had risen considerably. White flour had been concentrated less, for only 30% had been removed with the bran. Sugar was therefore more unnatural, more concentrated, and more harmful than white flour. It was submitted that overconsumption would inevitably occur because these two carbohydrates had been concentrated. The outlining of this far-reaching hypothesis appeared to some doctors to be based on logical reasoning, but lacked supporting epidemiological and experimental data.

For many years *Surgeon Captain T. L. Cleave,* after his retirement from the Royal Navy, collected in a voluminous correspondence much supporting data concerning the incidence of these diseases in many countries, especially those of Africa. He did not appear to have read, and he never cited data from, any book or medical journal in Africa except the journals of South Africa, and he did not mention the previous epidemiological studies in Africa listed in Table 1.1.

Subsequently he contacted Dr. D. G. Campbell, a physician in Durban, South Africa; together they produced "Diabetes, Coronary Thrombosis and the Saccharine Disease" (Cleave and Campbell, 1966), which discussed the diseases listed in Table 1.1

The second edition incorporated *Mr. N. S. Painter's* study of diverticular disease. Their summary divided their list of the diseases of civilization into three groups.

1. Overconsumption caused diabetes, obesity and coronary thrombosis. It also encouraged *Escherichia coli* infections such as cholecystitis, appendicitis, diverticulitis and pyelonephritis.

2. Removal of fibre caused colonic stasis, with its complications of diverticular disease, haemorrhoids and varicose veins; also dental caries and parodontal disease.

3. Removal of the protein [during the refining of the foods] caused peptic ulcer (Cleave *et al.*, 1969).

The third book had the postulated mechanisms and list of diseases almost unchanged, but cancer of the colon due to fibre deficiency appeared for the first time (Cleave, 1974).

2. *Sugar*

Certain doctors received very considerable stimulus from the saccharine disease hypothesis (Burkitt, 1973; Heaton, 1980). The neologism saccharine, signifying related to sugar, perhaps tied the whole hypothesis too much to the postulated role of sugar as the major aetiological factor in obesity, diabetes, gallstones and coronary heart disease. This was achieved largely through "overnutrition", another new term, which again was never clearly defined. For several years there has been a consensus of opinion among the majority of nutritionists that present levels of sucrose consumption have not been proved to be a risk factor in these diseases.

3. *Fibre*

Too little attention was paid by many to the second part of the overall saccharine disease hypothesis, that of fibre deficiency; this causes not only constipation and haemorrhoids, as others had postulated, but also diverticular disease and varicose veins. This acted as a stimulus to surgeons to consider its role not only in these diseases (p. 9) but also in appendicitis (p. 13), colo-rectal cancer (p. 13) and hiatal hernia (p. 14).

4. A critique

No detailed critique of the basic concepts of the overall hypothesis has been traced. Three manufactured foods, refined sugar, white flour and white rice, were postulated to have caused all the diseases of civilization. They were called refined carbohydrates. Sugar was mostly blamed: it had been concentrated by machinery eight times; it was consumed no longer as in the natural state and consumption had risen considerably in recent centuries. White flour was also blamed but was less injurious for it had been concentrated less. Actually white flour has only 6% more energy than wholemeal: this cannot be deemed concentration. Recent analysis has reported that white flour has only one-third of the dietary fibre of wholemeal. Probably more attention should have been paid to this, rather than to the alleged concentration, especially because white bread consumption had fallen considerably in many Western countries in recent years. How could decreased consumption of an alleged injurious food accompany the increased incidence of coronary heart and other diseases? Finally, no definition of refined carbohydrate foods was given apart from the statement that they had been "altered from the natural state"; they were not defined in terms of fibre depletion. It was not stated whether rye crispbread, oatmeal and maize meal were unrefined or refined foods. Strange to relate, no clear definition of refined carbohydrate foods has been traced in any book, article or in the RCP Report (1980), until proposed recently by Trowell (1983). (See further discussion of definitions in Chapter 2).

Refined means purified and freed from impurities. Sugar has indeed been refined by the removal of irritant indigestible bagasse pith. White flour, however, has not been purified, that is refined, by the removal of much dietary fibre, which is not an irritant but promotes health. Other desirable nutrients, protein, vitamins and minerals are reduced by the milling. Possibly it is inappropriate to create a new artificial group of foods, called refined carbohydrates, out of much concentrated fibre-free water-soluble refined sugar and little concentrated low-fibre water-insoluble, highly processed complex carbohydrates (starch) in white flour.

Plant foods are also processed to produce concentrated fibre-free vegetable oils, fats and margarine. Milk has been concentrated to produce butter. These concentrated fatty foods were not considered to be risk factors in any disease. These foods are expensive for poor Third World peasants, the poorest of whom eat 11% fat energy, about 9% being present as unseparated fibre-associated fat in the plant foods. Affluent modern Western men eat 40% fat energy and only 1–2% is unseparated fibre-associated fat present in plant foods. The remainder of the fat is present in meat, milk and various processed fats, butter and oils (Périssé et al., 1969). As poverty gave way to affluence in recent centuries, the 30% increase in fibre-free fat energy was a much larger dietary change than the 15% rise in fibre-free sugar energy. The saccharine disease hypothesis concentrated its attention too exclusively on the increased consumption of sugar to explain increased incidence of the diseases of civilization. It denied that high fat consumption was a risk factor in coronary heart disease or any other disorder. This seriously limited the scope of the enquiry concerning the causes of the many diseases of civilization to the carbohydrate-rich foods, but westernization of the diets involves multiple dietary changes.

Little information was offered concerning fibre (Cleave, 1974). The term "dietary fibre" was never mentioned, its main constituents were not named, its origin in plant cell walls was not described and its indigestibility by human alimentary enzymes was not specifically stated. Nevertheless, the hypothesis stimulated much thought and research. Without this hypothesis as a spur, our books (Burkitt and Trowell, 1975; Trowell and Burkitt, 1981, and the present volume) would never have been attempted.

F. Western diseases: recent data

The term "diseases of civilization" stigmatised Asians and Africans, who seldom get these diseases, as uncivilized, so that the term "Western diseases" has slowly replaced it (Burkitt, 1973; Trowell and Burkitt, 1981). These are the diseases of *uncertain aetiology* which appear to be characteristic of modern affluent technological Western communities. (Diseases related to cigarette smoking and others such as industrial accidents and hazards have a known aetiology. They are truly Western diseases, but have been excluded from the present investigation). The first step was to relate the reported incidence of these diseases (Table 1.1), in Africa and parts of Asia, to multiple dietary changes (Burkitt and Trowell, 1975). This study emphasised the protective role of dietary fibre more than the postulated injurious role of sugar and fibre-depleted complex carbohydrates in all the colonic disorders.

Subsequently it appeared desirable to establish the *validity* of this list of Western diseases irrespective of any postulated hypotheses concerning the diet. A provisional list of Western diseases was compiled. It included all those listed in Table 1.1, but excluded duodenal ulcer (p. 229). This list was sent to 34 contributors working at various university medical schools in five continents. Replies from these investigators manifested a very strong consensus of opinion that these 17 diseases were rare in hunter–gatherers, uncommon in developing peasant communities, but became common during westernization of the diets and changes in lifestyle such as decreased physical activity and increased cigarette smoking (Trowell and Burkitt, 1981).

G. Other pioneers: the dietary fibre group

Mr. N. S. Painter (personal communication, 1977), a London consultant surgeon, still remembers that the British wartime high-fibre National bread was laxative. In 1960 at Oxford he used three open-ended water-filled tubes, coupled with ciné-radiology, to study intracolonic pressures in diverticular disease. This raised speculations as to whether the standard low-residue diet treatment was appropriate. In 1967 he began to treat diverticular disease with bran and he contacted Surgeon Captain T. L. Cleave. His monograph (Painter, 1975) on diverticular disease presented much evidence that this disease was due to fibre deficiency and that it was characteristic of modern Western civilization. He initiated the revolution in the treatment of diverticular disease with bran as a part of a high-fibre diet. This stimulated him, and other gastroenterologists, to investigate the action of dietary fibre on the alimentary tract in health and in other colonic diseases.

Dr. M. A. Eastwood (personal communication, 1982), presently conducting research at the Wolfson Gastrointestinal Laboratories, University of Edinburgh, became interested during 1961 in the distribution of bile salts in the small intestine of rats fed a fibre-free diet (Eastwood and Boyd, 1967). While giving first-aid lectures at a brewery, he noticed that bran, left in the mash, looked similar to the intestinal contents of rats fed a fibre-rich chow. Eastwood and his colleagues continued to research the physical and biological properties of fibre within the gastrointestinal tract. He arranged a Nutrition Society symposium on fibre at Edinburgh in 1972.

Dr. K. W. Heaton (personal communication, 1982), Reader in Medicine of Bristol University, became interested in the early 1960s in reports that coronary heart disease was associated with high intakes of sucrose (Yudkin, 1957). His research on the enterohepatic circulation of bile salts revealed papers that reported that diets rich in sucrose or glucose, when fed to rats, impaired the synthesis of bile salts and reduced the bile salt pool. Adding cellulose to the diet largely corrected these abnormalities. In 1968 he heard from M. A. Eastwood that lignin bound bile salts. By chance in 1969 he read the second edition of *The Saccharine Disease* (p. 8) and he entered into a long correspondence with Surgeon Captain T. L. Cleave. He became impressed with the basic concept that refined carbohydrate foods were artificial and had much potential for causing disease. In 1970 reports from the United States stated that gallstone patients had a reduced bile salt pool. This led Heaton (1972) to propose a comprehensive hypothesis for the aetiology of cholesterol gallstones. His subsequent research has tested this hypothesis and examined the fibre–obesity connection. He was Secretary of the Royal College of Physicians of London Working Party on dietary fibre which reported on this in 1980 (p. 2).

Dr. S. L. Malhotra, an Indian physician, has published many papers during the past 20 years relating the different diets, based on either whole wheat of northern India or white rice of southern India, to numerous diseases, such as peptic ulcer (Malhotra, 1967) and coronary heart disease (Malhotra, 1968).

Mr. F. I. Tovey, a consultant surgeon presently at Basingstoke General

Hospital, England, had formerly practised in India for many years. During the 1960s and 1970s he conducted extensive surveys of duodenal ulcer throughout India and parts of Pakistan, also in most sub-Saharan countries in Africa (p. 229). The geographical distribution of duodenal ulcer was found not to correlate, as formerly supposed, with the consumption of refined carbohydrate foods. For instance, an area of extremely high incidence has been found in the Nile-Congo watershed among undeveloped tribes that eat almost no refined carbohydrate foods (p. 233). Duodenal ulcer must therefore not be considered to be exclusively a disease of modern Western civilization (Table 1.1). Unidentified protective factors, not dietary fibre, are present in certain foods but not in others (p. 238).

IV.   The mainstream: dietary fibre (1970s)

A.   The emergence of the concept

Mr. D. P. Burkitt came as a young surgeon to what is now Makerere University Medical School Hospital, Uganda, early in 1948. In 1957 when I was in charge of the paediatric ward I called him for consultation on a child with a puzzling lesion involving his jaws. It was this patient who started Burkitt's investigation of the tumour that now bears his name. At present this tumour seems most likely to become the first human cancer that is causally associated with a virus, the Epstein-Barr virus, first isolated from it.

Subsequently, Burkitt travelled widely in Africa to establish the peculiar geographical distribution of this cancer. He became increasingly puzzled by the apparent rarity of many surgical and medical diseases in African blacks, although these disorders were common in Europe, and in whites in Africa. In 1966 he returned to England to continue his cancer work at the Medical Research Council (MRC). In 1967 *Sir Richard Doll* introduced him to *Surgeon Captain T. L. Cleave.* This was the first of several extremely stimulating meetings. Burkitt, therefore, sent monthly questionnaires for 2 years to over 200 hospitals, mostly in rural areas, in over 20 countries in Africa and Asia. This confirmed the rarity of all these diseases in many rural peasant communities.

Soon Burkitt started to diverge from the major portion of Cleave's hypothesis. For instance, he related appendicitis to low fibre intakes rather than high sugar consumption (Burkitt, 1971a). He wrote his first major paper that provided evidence that dietary fibre might be protective against colo-rectal cancer (Burkitt, 1971b). As a result, he has been credited by some with this proposal. He considers that the concept came to him through the work of Walker and his colleagues in Johannesburg (Walker *et al.,* 1970b). In the 1970s, Burkitt became the focal point of the *group* of English doctors who had been stimulated by Cleave's saccharine disease hypothesis. He has continued to collect epidemiological and experimental data and to lecture frequently in all five continents. He has contributed papers on transit times, faecal weights and constipation. He has postulated that the raised intra-abdominal pressures generated by straining to pass firm, small-volume stools, contribute to the pathogenesis of varicose veins, deep vein thrombosis, pulmonary embolism, pelvic phleboliths, haemorrhoids (Chapter 19) and hiatal hernia (Chapter 14).

In 1970 I retired from an interlude of 11 years in a country vicarage and returned to Uganda to deliver a lecture on the history of PEM. Unexpectedly I heard Burkitt lecture on diseases of the colon and fibre. On returning from Uganda he read "Non-Infective Disease in Africa" (Trowell, 1960), then out of print, and he introduced me to the saccharine disease hypothesis (Cleave *et al.*, 1969). Before long we thought we might edit a book together on diseases related to refined carbohydrate foods; he had background in surgical diseases, while I had experience in medical disorders.

B.   New definition: change of view

Kuhn (1970, p. 111) wrote "Led by a new paradigm scientists . . . look in new places, . . . during revolutions scientists see new and different things when looking with familiar instruments in places they have looked before".

1.   Fibre: not present in the textbooks, but in the plant foods

In an early draft of our proposed book on refined carbohydrates, Burkitt wrote and asked me to "define fibre". Quite simple, I thought, but in 1971 words such as fibre, cellulose or roughage could not be found in any textbook of nutrition, medicine, surgery, gastro-enterology, or in any medical journal, or in the Index Medicus or in British Food Tables. Actually, the term "fibre" had been in the *botanical* literature for nearly 300 years, ever since Nehemiah Grew gave a demonstration of plant cell walls to the Royal Society in 1671 and subsequently wrote: "In the pith of . . . plants not only the threads of which the bladders [cells]; may sometimes with the help of a good Glass [microscope], be distinctly seen. Yet one of these Fibres . . . " (Preston, 1974, p. 4).

2.   Crude fibre

One British Food Table was eventually found which reported the *crude* fibre content of tropical foods but did not define the term (Platt, 1962). The Weende method to analyse the crude fibre of animal forages is of uncertain origin, but has been used for over 150 years and in the United States it has been approved by the Association of Official Analytical Chemists. Crude fibre is the residue left after extraction with hot dilute acid followed by dilute alkali. However, up to 50% of cellulose and 85% of hemicelluloses are lost during the extraction (Van Soest, 1978). In Britain, the MRC's "Composi-

tion of Foods" (McCance and Widdowson, 1969) published data on unavailable carbohydrates for fruit and vegetables, but not for cereals; and it did not
define this term among the other defined dietary constituents. Later in that
volume, Widdowson (1969) stated that "the so-called unavailable carbohydrates . . . are made up of hemicelluloses and fibre", but there was no definition of fibre. Polysaccharide chemists referred disdainfully to "the so-called
hemicelluloses", and advocated abolishing the term because "classification is
more satisfactorily based on chemical structure" (Aspinall, 1970). Clearly no
generic name had been given for all the undigested non-starch polysaccharides (NSP) in the plant foods of man. It was essential to propose a new term
for this group of substances.

3. Confusion

Confusion reigned over this disordered field of fibre in the 1960s and early
1970s. Dietary surveys had reported, on rare occasions, crude fibre intakes;
usually these data were omitted. Fibre had been regarded usually as cellulose,
an inert substance in the human alimentary tract. Laboratory experiments
had reported data from animals fed chemically defined diets that sometimes
contained no cellulose, at other times purified wood cellulose had been added. This did not package the complex carbohydrates as do plant cell walls.
Consequently it differs markedly from natural cellulose in its physical and
biological properties (Van Soest, 1978). In other experiments designed to
produce diseases, such as hyperlipidaemia or diabetes, in animals that were
fed diets containing a variety of cereal foodstuffs, the crude fibre content had
rarely been reported. I realised that I could obtain the omitted crude fibre
figures from the manufacturer of the laboratory feed, and insert these figures
in the existing published articles.

4. Seeing new and different things

Therein lay a situation possibly never to be repeated in the long history of
medical science. One disease after another in these diseased animals and in
man could be studied, and the crude fibre figures could be inserted, since they
had almost *invariably* been omitted (Trowell, 1978a). The results were
amazing. It proved possible to write a series of communications that reported
that fibre-rich laboratory chows and foods, also constituents of dietary fibre
such as cellulose and pectin, prevented or reduced hyperlipidaemia (Trowell,
1972b, c), coronary heart disease (Trowell, 1976b), diabetes mellitus
(Trowell, 1974b, 1975a), obesity (Trowell, 1975b) and certain forms of
venous and cardiac thrombosis (Trowell, 1976a) in human and animal
experiments.

5. Redefining fibre

During 1971, consultations with younger colleagues, notably *Dr. M. A. Eastwood, Dr. D. A. T. Southgate* and *Dr. K. W. Heaton,* led to a decision to

redefine the term "crude fibre", which was in common and approved use for over 150 years, as "dietary fibre". This changed the inappropriate adjective but retained the time-honoured noun. Dietary fibre was defined in terms of the plant cell *walls* as "the skeletal remains that are resistant to digestion by the enzymes of man" (Trowell, 1972c) (p. 3). Subsequently it was found that Hipsley (1953) had used the term "dietary fibre" in the title of an article on pregnancy toxaemia. A footnote stated that this was cellulose, hemicelluloses and lignin. Nevertheless, the figures reported in the article referred to, and accepted, the crude fibre content of the various foods.

C.   Recent definitions and developments

1.   Enlarging the definition

It was slowly realised that the indigestible plant polysaccharides in cereal grains and leguminous seeds were not confined to the plant cell *walls*. A presentation of the original definition to the U.S. Nutrition Study Section of the National Institutes of Health Workshop in January 1974 elicited criticisms that a chemical definition and analysis of dietary fibre could not be confined to the undigested polysaccharide remnants of plant cell *walls* but must include undigested storage polysaccharides of comparable chemical composition, which are present within the body of the cell. This was accepted in the second enlarged definition (Trowell, 1974a) and subsequently confirmed during a discussion at a meeting of the Oxford Nutrition Society (Trowell *et al.*, 1976). *Dr. D. A. T. Southgate* participated in this second enlarged definition. He subsequently pointed out that present analytic methods did not distinguish indigestible plant cell-wall polysaccharides from those coming from indigestible storage polysaccharides present within the plant cells (Southgate, 1977). The Association of Official Analytic Chemists (AOAC) adopted this definition of dietary fibre in 1980 (p. 60).

This second, enlarged definition includes also indigestible mucilages and algal polysaccharides. It was also suggested that undigested fibre-associated substances, which are not polysaccharides, such as indigestible cell-wall protein, silica, waxes and cutins, must be considered (Cummings, 1976). It was proposed that dietary fibre and these other associated undigested substances together should be called the dietary fibre complex (Trowell, 1976b). At the present time there is considerable international agreement concerning the principal constituents of dietary fibre. They are all polysaccharides, mainly cellulose, hemicelluloses and pectic substances, conveniently designated non-starch polysaccharides (NSP). The human digestive tract secretes only α-glucosidase emzymes; they can usually digest well fine-ruptured, cooked starch granules, but they cannot digest at all any of the polysaccharides of dietary fibre (Southgate, 1977; Spiller and Briggs, 1979). Therein lies a clear point of distinction from starch.

2. *Dietary fibre and other edible fibres*

The development of pharmaceutical polysaccharide preparations had necessitated the introduction of a new terminological umbrella, that of edible fibre (Godding, 1976). Discussions in California elicited a joint statement by four people (Trowell, *et al.*, 1978). We suggested that edible fibre should contain four groups of undigested polysaccharides: (1) dietary fibre, its definition was not changed and its main constituents were named, but starch was not included; (2) partially synthetic polysaccharides; (3) pharmaceutical polysaccharides; (4) animal fibre-like materials such as aminopolysaccharides. These four groups together were referred to as edible fibre, meaning "safe to be eaten". This aided the retrieval of information derived from different fields. A bibliography was published for the year 1978; it contained some 451 citations on dietary fibre and edible fibre (Avenell *et al.*, 1982a). This is followed by 528 citations for 1979 (Avenell *et al.*, 1982b) and 480 for 1980 (Avenell *et al.*, 1983), many more than previously (Trowell, 1979).

3. *Fibre research*

Medical history, however, will surely record that these budding ideas concerning dietary fibre would never have blossomed in Britain if not strongly supported by *Sir Francis Avery Jones*. He was the doyen of British gastroenterologists in the 1970s. He had noted the apparent absence of diverticular disease in China during a visit in 1957. The preface to "Management of Constipation" (Jones and Godding, 1972) stated that "the immediate adverse effect of low-fibre diets is constipation, the long, time-lapse adverse effects include diverticular disease and in all probability malignancy".

Sir Francis wrote that "my mother and indeed other members of the family were Allinson fans, and I have always had brown bread" (personal communication, 1973). He strongly encouraged *Dr. E. N. Rowlands,* the Director of the MRC Gastroenterology Unit, Central Middlesex Hospital, London, to build a research programme on dietary fibre. There, *Dr. J. H. Cummings, Dr. A. R. Leeds and Dr. D. J. Jenkins* started their work, assisted by *Dr. G. Metz, Dr. M. Gassull and Dr. B. Cochet.* It was a pleasure for me to meet and talk to this group about fibre, with special emphasis on diabetes, in March 1973. Subsequently these workers dispersed to various units in Cambridge, London and Oxford, Melbourne, Barcelona and Geneva. They continued research on dietary fibre and fibre-rich foods in colonic function, in diabetes mellitus, and in the pathogenesis of bowel disorders. Sir Francis advocated the appointment of the Royal College of Physicians Working Party on Dietary Fibre in 1977. It subsequently issued the RCP Report *Medical Aspects of Dietary Fibre* (1980).

V.   A critique of dietary fibre hypotheses

The RCP Report (1980, p. iii) criticised the overall dietary fibre hypothesis as too generalised and vague so that it could not be falsified. Karl Popper, the philosopher, regarded such failings to be characteristic of pseudo-science. But the so-called fibre hypothesis is not a single hypothesis. It contains a number of hypotheses, each supported by epidemiological and experimental data, concerning the aetiology of specified diseases, all of which have an unknown cause, even if some risk factors in certain diseases have been identified. These individual hypotheses will be verified, modified or disproved, when eventually the causes of these individual diseases have been discovered.

In broad terms these dietary fibre hypotheses postulate that a high consumption of lightly processed complex carbohydrate foods, which contain much dietary fibre, protects ethnic groups, whose ancestors ate a comparable diet for many millennia, from a wide variety of Western diseases which are characteristics of modern affluent Western communities. The ancient traditional diet of man differed from the modern diet; the former diet was also low-fat, low-sucrose, low-animal protein, low-cholesterol, even low-salt, and it differed in other respects from the modern diet; moreover, formerly physical activity was high and other factors, such as cigarette smoking, were absent.

In certain diseases such as constipation, a low intake of dietary fibre, especially that derived from cereals, will probably be accepted to be the major causative factor. In other diseases the dietary fibre intakes may prove to be more a marker of certain other features of the diet; an example is the very low-fat intake in African blacks that accompanies the low incidence of coronary heart disease. In every specified Western disease, it should be possible to verify or falsify its own dietary fibre hypothesis.

Meanwhile, the list of Western diseases stands valid, even after more than 45 years since its initial publication (Table 1.1). *Only one disease has been removed from the list;* duodenal ulcer is very common in some of the least developed black communities of the remote Nile-Congo watershed (p. 233). Research therefore, is trying to identify substances present in some plant foods but not in others, which in minute amounts will aid healing (p. 238). These substances are not present in dietary fibre.

It should be easy to disprove other members of the list. *This has not occurred.* It raises an enormous problem. The list contains many of the most common causes of death, disease and disability in aging Western man. The problem will not go away. It will call other people for its solution: an old paradigm that is forever new.

Acknowledgements

I thank Dr. David Bloor, Science Studies Unit of the University of Edinburgh, for reading an early draft of this chapter; he advised me to study what Kuhn had written about the role of paradigms in scientific revolutions.

References

American Medical Association Council on Foods (1936). *J. Am. Med. Assoc.* 107, 874–877.
ASPINALL, G. A. (1970). "Polysaccharides", pp. 43, 105. Pergamon, Oxford.
AVENELL, A., LEEDS, A. R. and TROWELL, H. C. (1982a). *J. Plant Foods* 4, 145–177.
AVENELL, A., LEEDS, A. R. and TROWELL, H. C. (1982b). *J. Plant Foods* 4, 199–232.
AVENELL, A., LEEDS, A. R. and TROWELL, H. C. (1983). *J. Plant Foods* 5, 81–113.
BERSOHN, I., WALKER, A. R. and HIGGINSON, J. (1956). *S. Afr. Med. J.* 30, 411–412.
BURKITT, D. P. (1971a). *Br. J. Surg.* 58, 695–699.
BURKITT, D. P. (1971b). *Cancer* 28, 3–13.
BURKITT, D. P. (1973). *Br. Med. J.* 1, 274–278.
BURKITT, D. P. and TROWELL, H. C. (1975). "Refined Carbohydrate Foods and Disease: Some Implications of Dietary Fibre." Academic Press, London and New York.
CLEAVE, T. L. (1941). *Br. Med. J.* 2, 790–791.
CLEAVE, T. L. (1956). *J. R. Nav. Med. Serv.* 42, 55–83.
CLEAVE, T. L. (1974). "The Saccharine Disease." John Wright, Bristol.
CLEAVE, T. L. and CAMPBELL, G. D. (1966). "Diabetes, Coronary Thrombosis and the Saccharine Disease." John Wright, Bristol.
CLEAVE, T. L., CAMPBELL, G. D. and PAINTER, N. S. (1969). "Diabetes, Coronary Heart Disease and the Saccharine Disease." John Wright, Bristol.
CUMMINGS, J. H. (1976). *In* "Fiber in Human Nutrition" (G. A. Spiller and R. J. Amen, eds), pp. 1–30. Plenum, New York.
DIMOCK, E. M. (1937). *Br. Med. J.* 1, 960–909.
DOLL, R. and ARMSTRONG, B. (1981). *In* "Western Diseases: Their Emergence and Prevention" (H. C. Trowell and D. P. Burkitt, eds), pp. 93–110. Edward Arnold, London.
DONNISON, C. P. (1937). "Civilization and Disease." Baillière, London.
EASTWOOD, M. A. and BOYD, G. S. (1967). *Biochim. Biophys. Acta* 137, 393–396.
FRASER, J. R. and HOLMES, D. C. (1959). *J. Sci. Food Agric.* 10, 506–512.
GELFAND, M. (1944). "The Sick African." Stewart Publishing, Cape Town.
GODDING, E. W. (1976). *Lancet* 1, 1129.
HEATON. K. W. (1972). "Bile Salts in Health and Disease." Churchill-Livingstone, Edinburgh and London.
HEATON, K. W. (1980). *J. R. Nav. Med. Serv.* 66, 5–10.
HIGGINSON, J. (1966). *J. Natl. Cancer Inst. (U. S.)* 37, 527–545.
HIGGINSON, J. and OETTLÉ, A. G. (1960). *J. Natl. Cancer Inst. (U. S.)* 24, 589–671.
HIPSLEY, E. H. (1953). *Br. Med. J.* 2, 420–422.
JONES, F. A. and GODDING, E. W. (1972). "Management of Constipation", p. ix. Blackwell, Oxford.
KUHN, T. S. (1970). "The Structure of Scientific Revolutions", 2nd edition, p. 24. University of Chicago Press, Chicago.
MCCANCE, R. A. and WIDDOWSON, E. M. (1969). "The Composition of Foods." HM Stationery Office, London.
MCCARRISON, R. (1921). "Studies in Deficiency Disease." Frowde, Hodder & Stoughton, London.
MCCARRISON, R. (1940) *Br. Med. J.* 1, 984–987.
MALHOTRA, S. L. (1967). *Gut* 8, 180–188.
MALHOTRA, S. L. (1968). *Br. Heart J.* 29, 895–905.
OETTLÉ, A. G. (1964). *J. Natl. Cancer Inst.* 33, 383–436.
PAINTER, N. S. (1975). "Diverticular Disease of the Colon: A Deficiency Disease of Western Civilization." Heinemann, London.
Panel on Bread, Flour and Other Cereal Products (1981). "Nutritional Aspects of Bread and Flour." HM Stationery Office, London.

20   H. TROWELL

PAUL, A. A. and SOUTHGATE, D. A., eds. (1978). *In* "McCance and Widdowson's The Composition of Foods". 4th edition, pp. 8–9. HM Stationery Office, London.

PÉRISSÉ, J., SIZARET, F. and FRANÇOISE, P. (1969). *FAO Nutr. Newsl.* **7**, 1–9.

PLATT, B. S. (1962). "Tables of Representative Values of Foods Used in Tropical Countries." HM Stationery Office, London.

PRESTON, R. D. (1974). "The Physical Biology of Plant Cell Walls." Chapman & Hall, London.

Royal College of Physicians of London (1980). "Medical Aspects of Dietary Fibre." London.

SOUTHGATE, D. A. (1977). *Nutr. Rev.* **35**, 31–37.

SPILLER, G. A. and BRIGGS, G. (1979). *Am. J. Clin. Nutr.* **32**, 2374–2375.

TROWELL, H. C. (1960). "Non-Infective Disease in Africa." Edward Arnold, London.

TROWELL, H. (1972a). *Rev. Eur. Etud. Clin. Biol.* **17**, 345–349.

TROWELL, H. (1972b). *Am. J. Clin. Nutr.* **25**, 926–932.

TROWELL, H. (1972c). *Atherosclerosis* **16**, 138–140.

TROWELL, H. (1973). *Proc. Nutr. Soc.* **32**, 151–157.

TROWELL, H. (1974a). *Lancet* **1**, 503.

TROWELL, H. (1974b). *Lancet* **2**, 998–1002.

TROWELL, H. (1975a). *Diabetes* **24**, 762–765.

TROWELL, H. (1975b). *Plant Foods Man* **1**, 157–168.

TROWELL, H. (1976a). *Thromb. Haemostasis* **36**, 489–492.

TROWELL, H. (1976b). *Am. J. Clin. Nutr.* **29**, 417—427.

TROWELL, H. (1978a). *Am. J. Clin. Nutr.* **31**, S3-S11.

TROWELL, H. (1978b). *Am. J. Clin. Nutr.* **31**, S53–S57.

TROWELL, H. C. (1979). "Dietary Fibre in Human Nutrition: A Bibliography." Libbey, London.

TROWELL, H. C. (1983). *Hum. Nutr. Clin. Nutr.* **37C**, 236, 312, 314.

TROWELL, H. C. and BURKITT, D. P. (eds) (1981). "Western Diseases: Their Emergence and Prevention." Edward Arnold, London.

TROWELL, H. C., DAVIES, J. N. and DEAN, R. F. (1952). "Kwashiorkor." Edward Arnold, London.

TROWELL, H., SOUTHGATE, D. A., WOLEVER, T. M., LEEDS, A. R., GASSULL, M. A. and JENKINS, D. J. (1976). *Lancet* **1**, 967.

TROWELL, H., GODDING, E., SPILLER, G. and BRIGGS, G. (1978). *Am. J. Clin. Nutr.* **31**, 1489–1490.

TROWELL, H. C., DAVIES, J. N. P. and DEAN, R. F. A. (1982). "Kwashiorkor." Academic Press, New York.

VAN SOEST, P. J. (1978). *Am. J. Clin. Nutr.* **31**, S12–S20.

WALKER, A. R. (1947). *S. Afr. Med. J.* **21**, 590–596.

WALKER, A. R. (1956). *Nutr. Rev.* **14**, 321–324.

WALKER, A. R. (1974). *Postgrad. Med. J.* **50**, 29–32.

WALKER, A. R. (1982). *S. Afr. Med. J.* **61**, 126–129.

WALKER, A. R., FOX, F. W. and IRVING, J. T. (1948). *Biochem. J.* **42**, 452–462.

WALKER, A. R., WALKER, B. F. and RICHARDSON, B. D. (1970a). *Lancet* **2**, 51–52.

WALKER, A. R. P., WALKER, B. F. and RICHARDSON, B. D. (1970b). *Br. Med. J.* **3**, 48–49.

WIDDOWSON, E. M. (1969). *In* "The Composition of Foods" (R. A. McCance and E. M. Widdowson, eds), 3rd edition, p. 171. HM Stationery Office, London.

YUDKIN, J. (1957). *Am. J. Clin. Nutr.* **20**, 108–115.

Chapter 2

Definitions of dietary fibre and fibre-depleted foods

HUGH TROWELL, DENIS BURKITT and KENNETH HEATON

This chapter discusses exclusively two basic interrelated concepts in human nutrition, dietary fibre and fibre-depleted foods. The remainder of the book discusses possible relationships between these two factors to certain medical and surgical diseases, the former recently reviewed by Heaton (1983), the latter by Burkitt (1983). Additional information about other possible implications are discussed by Dr. Kenneth Heaton in Chapter 24.

I. Defining dietary fibre

A. A botanical concept

Preston (1974) has reviewed the introduction of the term "fibre" into botany by Malpighi and Grew in the 1670s in England. Grew, using only a primitive type of microscope, became convinced that the solid framework of plants, now called the cell walls, consisted of fine threads, called fibres. About 160 years ago, animal feeds began to be analysed for fibre by a crude test; thus the product was called crude fibre. It is the residue that remains after sequential extraction by hot dilute acid followed by dilute alkali. Eventually it was realised that most of the hemicelluloses and cellulose had been lost and never recorded in the estimation.

B.   Available and unavailable carbohydrates

Nutritionists have struggled for nearly 100 years with the problem of calculating how much of the food is digested and becomes available for metabolism or storage. Widdowson (1960) reviewed the work of Rubner towards the end of the last century concerning "cell-wall membranes"; these are the basis of dietary fibre. She also reviewed the work of Atwater in the early years of this century concerning the availability of the nutrients, or how much is "digestible" as he called it. Actually he preferred the new term "available"; the remainder was "unavailable". The unavailable carbohydrates are celluloses and hemicelluloses; these are the main constituents of what is now called dietary fibre.

C.   Analysis of unavailable carbohydrates

It has always proved difficult to analyse the various carbohydrates. In fact, until recently the carbohydrate content of a plant food was assessed and reported "by difference". That is to say all the other recognised major constituents of a carbohydrate-containing food, its water, ash, fat and protein were individually analysed and the sum of these fractions was deducted from the total weight, then reported as total carbohydrate "by difference".

This unsatisfactory state of affairs was severely criticised by the Food and Agriculture Organisation which stated that "the correct approach is by extension of analytical work to include all substances covered by 'carbohydrates by difference'" (Widdowson, 1960). Successive editions of McCance and Widdowson's *Composition of Foods* from 1940 to 1960 began to report first, the direct analysis of the available carbohydrates, starch, sugars and dextrin, and second, but only recently, the direct analysis of the unavailable carbohydrates, defining these "for all practical purposes . . . as the sum of the polysaccharides and lignin which are not digested by the endogenous secretions of the gastro-intestinal tract . . . made up of several different types of polysaccharide (pectic substances, hemicelluloses and cellulose) and the non-carbohydrate lignin". These were then called dietary fibre (Paul and Southgate, 1978). The term "unavailable carbohydrate" has fallen into disuse because it has become apparent that bacterial fermentation of these polysaccharides in the large bowel contributes a small amount of absorbed energy.

D.   Dietary fibre

The botanical term "fibre" slowly came into usage in relation to animal forages in the nineteenth century and a crude method of analysis employing easily obtained reagents was used to measure a residue called crude fibre. Few food tables in human nutrition reported the crude fibre content of the plant foods. Nutritionists equated fibre with cellulose and, in animal experiments, they added chemically pure cellulose to chemically defined diets. Trowell (1972a) suggested the term "dietary fibre", preserving the time-honoured noun "fibre" but changing the adjective "crude" because he desired to show both the inadequacy of crude fibre figures and the necessity of analysing *all* the unavailable carbohydrates, (duly named as cellulose, hemicelluloses, pectin, gums) and lignin in the *diet* (Trowell, 1972b, c).

The hallmark of all the substances included in the term "dietary fibre" was that they were not digested *at all* by the alimentary enzymes of man: this preserved the link with Atwater and indigestibility, also with McCance and unavailability. At first it was considered that all these substances came from plant cell walls; then helpful criticism by carbohydrate chemists led to the inclusion of all undigested polysaccharides, such as the storage polysaccharides present in large amounts in leguminous seeds (Trowell, 1974). Probably few foods are completely digested and particles can be identified in the faeces. Starch is often digested poorly, especially if poorly cooked and if the cell walls have not been ruptured by milling; however, starch was never listed as a possible component of dietary fibre (Trowell *et al.*, 1978).

Cummings (1983) reviewed data on the digestion of starch in the small intestine. It is technically possible by an intubation technique to measure the passage of dietary starch into the colon and such a study has been reported in seven normal subjects after eating meals containing 20 g or 60 g starch (Stephen *et al.*, 1983). Between 2 and 20% of starch escaped digestion and absorption in the small bowel. This agrees with previous indirect measurements using breath tests. People in developing communities consume a high intake of starch foods, sometimes poorly processed and cooked, and this has been said to increase indigestibility. They also consume a high intake of the associated dietary fibre in their lightly processed farinaceous food. Both undigested starch and the dietary fibre provide available substrate for the growth in the colon of anaerobic microflora; these contribute between 40 and 55% of the solids in the colon and the faeces.

The poor digestion of starch has two important aspects. First high intakes of starch, often both poorly processed and cooked, at least in poor developing communities, together with dietary fibre affect colonic function and disease. Second, in the analysis of dietary fibre it has proved difficult to separate "resistant starch", as it is called, from dietary fibre, thereby inflating erroneously the reported values of the latter (Southgate and Englyst, p. 46). In the present state of knowledge, resistant starch should not be regarded the same as starch undigested in the small intestine.

Plant cell walls also contain cell-wall protein, glycoproteins, and hydroxyproline; these are firmly bound to the structural polysaccharides (Preston, 1974, pp. 59–65). Inorganic materials, calcium, potassium, and magnesium, even silica, are also present; all of these may influence the action of the structural polysaccharides (Southgate and Englyst, pp. 37–38.)

E.   Criticisms of terminology and definition

An early but often repeated criticism of the term dietary fibre is that only cellulose is fibrous in the sense of being filamentous (Royal College of Physicians, 1980). This is correct if fibre is viewed through a microscope, but modern biophysical studies of plant cell walls have employed X-ray analysis during the past two decades; these report not only cellulose microfibrils but they describe "fibre bundles" and even measure the "fibre axis" of the hemicelluloses (Preston, 1975).

Uncertainties about the enzyme indigestibility of certain polysaccharides, previously mentioned, have encouraged some research workers to suggest that non-starch polysaccharides (NSP) is a better term and might even replace that of dietary fibre (Cummings, 1981). This definition, however, would probably include dextrins, inulin and glycogen present in liver, pharmaceutical polysaccharides and certain food additives. Some consider that lignin should be excluded from any definition of dietary fibre; only small amounts are present in food.

It is the fate of many new concepts in medicine to receive initially an inappropriate name so that rival terms are subsequently suggested. Vitamins soon turned out not to be vital amines and hemicelluloses are not the precursors of cellulose. Increasing knowledge usually modifies and clarifies the definition; it has seldom replaced the time-worn terminology. Fibre is a very old botanical term. One decisive test for any new terminology, or new definition, is how many persons recognise its superiority and start to employ it. Actually this is the only test of acceptability. Thus far the term "dietary fibre" and its definition, naming its main chemical constituents, remains unrivalled in popularity.

It has been stated that there are three definitions or conceptions of dietary fibre (Royal College of Physicians, 1980, p. 8). The (first) botanical description limits the term to cell-wall material; it does not include the undigested storage polysaccharides, present in large amount in leguminous seeds. There is no way in which only the undigested cell-wall polysaccharides can be estimated or the degree of which disruption of plant cell walls during milling, cooking or mastication can be measured. The (second) so-called physiological definition of Trowell (1974, 1976) is almost the same as the (third) chemical definition of the unavailable carbohydrates and lignin (Paul and Southgate, 1978). When the U.S. Association of Official Analytic Chemists (AOAC) began work on an acceptable definition and method for the analysis of dietary fibre, they circulated U.S. scientists and "more than one hundred responses were received . . most respondents preferred the definition of Trowell (1974) of 'remnants of plant cells resistant to hydrolysis by the alimentary enzymes of man'" and its main chemical constituents were named to include hemicelluloses, celluloses, lignin, oligosaccharides, pectins, gums and waxes (p. 60).

Those who compile a bibliography of dietary fibre in human nutrition are forced to define the term and name its components (Trowell *et al.*, 1978). This communication employed the term "edible fibre", which signified "safe to be eaten", to include dietary fibre and its components as previously mentioned, also undigested animal polysaccharides present in connective tissues and undigested pharmaceutical polysaccharide preparations, such as ispaghula. Bibliographies have been published on dietary fibre in human nutrition for 1978 and 1979, (Avenell *et al.*, 1982a, b, 1983), which use this definition.

II.   Defining fibre-depleted plant foods

A.   Concentrated refined carbohydrates

Graham (1837) was among the first in the United States to praise the ancient wholemeal bread and to condemn the more modern white bread as "unnatural" and "concentrated". Cleave (1974) developed this concept considerably in various publications. He suggested that refined sugar, white flour and white rice were the common refined carbohydrates and that they caused many diseases of modern civilisation. He considered that concentration was the hallmark of refined carbohydrates. He offered no formal definition of refined carbohydrates but stated that "removal of fibre has formed the basis of the . . . conception since it was first presented in 1956".

Trowell (1975a) accepted Cleave's list of refined carbohydrate foods and also added low-fibre cornflour, pearled barley and fine millet meal. Nevertheless, no formal definition of refined carbohydrate foods was offered. He too considered that reduction of the dietary fibre during modern food processing was the hallmark of refined carbohydrate foods. Slowly the term "fibre-depleted foods" began to creep into the literature (Heaton, 1973; Trowell, 1973, 1975b).

B.   Objections to the terminology

There are serious objections to the use of the undefined term "refined carbohydrates". Many of these foods contain protein and fat; they are not merely carbohydrate. Strictly speaking, sugar (sucrose) is the only common refined carbohydrate in the diet: it is a refined, i.e. purified, fibre-free carbohydrate. During manufacture its indigestible bagasse fibres and other impurities are removed and no one can eat, but only chew and suck, sugar cane. Nevertheless it is possible to eat sugar beet, but few eat this variety of beetroot. It is indeed unfortunate that sugar manufacturers call certain varieties of brown sugar unrefined sugar, but no dietary fibre is present.

On the other hand, white flour has not been refined, i.e. purified, by removing health-promoting fibre, vitamins and minerals. If it is incorrect to call white flour refined, it is doubtful if wheat wholemeal can be called unrefined. Let it be called by its own name; therefore let wheat wholemeal, oatmeal, maize meal any cereal meal (as that term is used in Britain but not in the United States), and brown rice, which are the ancient traditional foods of man, all be regarded as full-fibre foods irrespective of their varying contents of dietary fibre (Table 2.1). In the United States, wheat wholemeal is called by a wide variety of names, such as wholewheat flour or wheat flour, to distinguish it from white flour (see p. 65). The different names can cause much confusion. Graham bread is genuine wheat wholemeal, 100% extraction. In all these cereal products it is assumed that the indigestible chaff or husk has been removed from the grain, for man has never eaten these tough outer coats. This is a development of Cleave's hypothesis, based on evolution, that man had adapted well to his "natural" foods (Cleave, 1974, p. 1). Perhaps it would be more accurate to say that man was well adapted to his "ancient traditional foods". Opinions differ concerning the definition of the natural foods of man because he is almost the only creature who, throughout his long history, has altered considerably the structure and form and, equally important, the amounts eaten of many foods (Southgate, 1984).

C.   Fibre-depleted fats and oils

Vegetable fats and oils also have been processed and concentrated; consumption has risen considerably during the present century in the Western world. These are all concentrated fibre-depleted foods prepared from groundnuts, soya beans, cotton seed, sunflower and rape seeds (Trowell, 1983). There is also olive oil; this latter is one of the traditional foods of man and it has been used for many centuries in Mediterranean countries. These concentrated vegetable fats include margarine and vegetable oils used in cooking. Probably, like sugar, they also may inflate energy intakes because they increase palatability. Nutritionists now advise a reduced intake of fat, oils and sugar in all slimming diets.

D.   Interaction of undigested dietary fibre and digestible nutrients

It is important to remember that the undigested dietary fibre differs radically from the digestible nutrients (starch, sugar, protein and fats), but the pres-

TABLE 2.1. Common full-fibre and fibre-depleted plant foods of man [dietary fibre (g/100 g)]

Full-fibre		Lightly depleted		Heavily depleted		Fibre-free
Wheat wholemeal	9.6	Brown flour	7.5	White flour	3.0	Sugar, white or brown
Brown rice	4.3			White rice	2.4	Syrups[d]
Oatmeal, rolled oats	7.0					Vegetable fat and oils
Maize meal[a]		Maize meal		Tapioca[a]		Margarine
Barley, raw	6.5	(refined)[a]		Cornflour[a]		Beer
Peas, dried	16.7			Barley, pearled[a]		Cider, sweet
Beans, haricot	25.4			Sago[a]		Liqueurs, sweet
Soya flour	14.3			Arrowroot[a]		Wine, sweet
Peanuts	8.1					Honey
Potatoes	2.1[b]					Fruit juice, sweet
Fruit and vegetables[c]						

[a] Assessed from estimates of crude fibre (Platt, 1962).
[b] Water 75%; multiply by four for comparison with other drier foods.
[c] Also other lightly processed cereals, leguminous seeds, oil seeds and nuts.
[d] Glucose syrups and modified glucose/fructose syrups.

ence of the former alters the digestion of the latter, and this also affects the whole gastrointestinal tract. New concepts are needed for the evaluation of a complex interplay of these two different components of the diet. Botanists and biophysicists emphasise the complex structure of dietary fibre derived largely, but not exclusively, from plant cell walls; it also includes all the cell-wall material such as that present in the bran layers of wheat, and there are also undigested storage polysaccharides. In the upper part of the alimentary tract, dietary fibre remains as partially intact wrappings or as viscous packing material that surrounds and mingles with the digestible carbohydrates, (starch and sugars), protein and fat and slows down their digestion and absorption. Digestion of these nutrients is facilitated by rupturing of some of the plant cell walls during mastication and also during the milling of cereals. Heat also bursts the starch granules and increases digestibility. Man seldom eats much raw starch; this is always difficult to digest. Anaerobic bacterial fermentation of the dietary fibre polysaccharides may start in the small intestine but only proceeds apace in the large bowel. This fermentation provides energy for the growth of faecal bacteria which provide bulk for the stool, also some absorbed short-chain fatty acids, and these provide a little energy for the host.

E. A new chapter in human nutrition

A new chapter in human nutrition is therefore beginning and will evolve its own terminology and concepts. In this new field many questions remain unanswered. For instance, how much depletion or even disruption of the plant cell wall must occur for the food to be classified as fibre-depleted? Some consider that all fruit juices, wines and beer, which contain various sugars but almost no fibre, should be regarded as fibre-depleted. Others object and point out that mankind has used the teeth to crush fruit to form juices in the mouth while any fibrous matter was spat out in the pith. This occurs, for instance, when segments of an orange are sucked. Fibre-depleted olive oil has been consumed for centuries in the Mediterranean countries, and is not listed in Table 2.1

F. Overall dietary fibre hypothesis

The essence of the dietary fibre hypothesis as we see it is that man has not adapted well to certain highly processed *modern* foods. The effects of this maladaptation are most evident with foods whose consumption has risen rapidly during the last one or two centuries. This concerns specially sugar, fat and oils. White flour is also involved, but consumption of all cereal products has fallen considerably during the past two centuries.

It is certain that the ancient diet of almost all mankind was based on a high consumption of plant foods. Cereals and starch staples, such as potatoes, still provide most of the food for poor peasants who grow their own food or buy what is cheap and stores well. Cereals and starch staples by themselves are not appetizing, so that milk, fat and oil have been added for thousands of years, but sugar combined also with fat has been added in the Western world only in recent centuries.

Neither sugar nor fats are often consumed by themselves; sugar is usually diluted in liquids or foods. Refined sugar is rarely eaten by itself, or even stolen from a spoon by children, but sugar lumps are often sucked, as are sweets and all forms of confectionery. Toffee and fudge, a mixture of sugar and fat, however, are very palatable. In the United States, and probably in other Western countries, three-quarters of the refined sugar consumption is taken in manufactured food products or beverages; direct consumer use accounts for only about one-quarter. Fats and oils are often added to other foods to render them palatable. Thus, slices of bread are rarely consumed without butter or margarine. Added fats and oils are an essential part of many cooking recipes; foods such as meat or fish, even fatty fish such as herrings, mackerel and salmon (fat 12–19%) are often fried, as are fatty meats such as bacon and sausages.

Mixed with starch-containing foods, fats, oils and sugar inflate energy intakes in certain persons and, in our opinion, often produce obesity and overweight in susceptible phenotypes in Western communities, but rarely in peasants of the Third World. This suggestion, relying mostly on sugar, was set forth by Cleave (1974), p. 13, while food intake regulation by fibre was discussed by Heaton (1980). All slimming diets recommend a reduction of sugar and fat; food such as cakes, biscuits and puddings; and drinks that contain these ingredients.

Table 2.1 lists the common full-fibre (unrefined) and fibre-depleted (refined) foods of man. The lists are not comprehensive or universally applicable. Consideration must be given to the amount of food or drink that is taken. For instance, beer is included because it contains maltose but no fibre, and large amounts are often drunk; it can be fattening. Sweet cider, sweet wines and sweet liqueurs contain much sugar but no fibre and are therefore listed. Honey, although a natural food, contains various sugars, but no fibre; small amounts are probably harmless, but it is listed lest those who are prohibited sugar (sucrose) think that they may take honey *ad libitum*. Sweetened fruit juices contain added sugar (sucrose) and syrups are therefore listed. Unsweetened fruit juices are not listed although there are arguments for doing so (p. 397). Any *sweet* alcoholic drink and sweet beverages such as drinking chocolate contain much sucrose; they could be added to the list, in addition to certain coffee and chicory essences. On the other hand, most dry table wines contain no sucrose but only very small amounts of glucose and fructose; these wines are therefore not listed in Table 2.1. These data concerning the various sugars in food and drink are derived from the review of Southgate *et al.*, 1978).

Finally, we propose that the term fibre-depleted food should be used in place of refined carbohydrate. Similarly, the term unrefined carbohydrate should be replaced by full-fibre or fibre-intact food.

References

AVENELL, A., LEEDS, A. R. and TROWELL, H. C. (1982a). *Plant Foods Man* **4**, 145–177.
AVENELL, A., LEEDS, A. R. and TROWELL, H. C. (1982b). *Plant Foods Man* **4**, 199–232.
AVENELL, A., LEEDS, A. R. AND TROWELL, H. C. (1983). *J. Plant Foods* **5**, 81–112.
BURKITT, D. P. (1983). *Postgrad. Med. J.* **59**, 232–235.
CLEAVE, T. L. (1974). "The Saccharine Disease", p. 9. John Wright, Bristol.
CUMMINGS, J. H. (1981). *Br. Med. Bull.* **37**, 65–70.
CUMMINGS, J. H. (1983). *Lancet* **1**, 1206–1209.
GRAHAM, S. (1837). "A Treatise on Bread and Bread Making". Light and Stearns, Boston.
HEATON, K. W. (1973). *Lancet* **2**, 1418–1421.
HEATON, K. W. (1980). *In* "Medical Aspects of Dietary Fiber" (G. A. Spiller and R. M. Kay, eds), pp. 223–238. Plenum, New York.
HEATON, K. W. (1983). *Hum. Nutr. Clin. Nutr.* 37C, 151–170.
PAUL, A. A. and SOUTHGATE, D. A. T. (1978). *In* "McCance and Widdowson's The Composition of Foods", 4th edition, pp. 8–9, HM Stationery Office, London.
PLATT, B. S. (1962). "Tables of Representative Values of Foods Commonly used in Tropical Countries." HM Stationery Office, London.
PRESTON, R. D. (1974). "The Physical Biology of Plant Cell Walls", pp. 4, 5. Chapman & Hall, London.
PRESTON, R. D. (1975). "X-ray Analysis and the Structure of the Components of Plant Cell Walls", pp. 200–210. North-Holland Pub. Amsterdam.
Royal College of Physicians (1980). "Medical Aspects of Dietary Fibre", p. 9. Pitman Medical, London.
SOUTHGATE, D. A. T. (1984). *Br. Med. J.* **288**, 881–882.

SOUTHGATE, D. A. T., PAUL, A. A., DEAN, A. C. and CHRISTIE, A. A. (1978). *J. Hum. Nutr.* **32,** 335–347.

STEPHEN, A. M., HADDAH, A. C. and PHILLIPS, A. (1983). *Gastroenterology,* **85,** 589–595.

TROWELL, H. (1972a). *Rev. Eur. Etud. Clin. Biol.* **17,** 345–349.

TROWELL, H. (1972b). *Am. J. Clin. Nutr.* **25,** 926–932.

TROWELL, H. (1972c). *Atherosclerosis* **16,** 138–140.

TROWELL, H. (1973). *Proc. Nutr. Soc.* **32,** 151–157.

TROWELL, H. (1974). *Lancet* **1,** 503.

TROWELL, H. C. (1975a). *In* "Refined Carbohydrate Foods and Disease, Some Implications of Dietary Fibre" (D. P. Burkitt and H. C. Trowell, eds), p. 31. Academic Press, London.

TROWELL, H. C. (1975b). *Diabetes* **24,** 762–765.

TROWELL, H. (1976). *Am. J. Clin. Nutr.* **29,** 417–427.

TROWELL, H. C. (1983). *Hum. Nutr. Clin. Nutr.* **37C,** 236, 312.

TROWELL, H. GODDING, E., SPILLER, G. and BRIGGS, G. (1978). *Am. J. Clin. Nutr.* **31,** 1489–1490.

WIDDOWSON, E. M. (1960). *In* (R. A. McCance and E. M. Widdowson, eds), "The Composition of Foods" 2nd edition, pp. 171–175. HM Stationery Office, London.

Chapter 3

Dietary fibre: chemistry, physical properties and analysis

DAVID SOUTHGATE and HANS ENGLYST

I. Introduction: definition of dietary fibre

In the original conception of the term, "dietary fibre" (Hipsley, 1953; Trowell, 1972) was seen as comprising the materials in the diet derived from the plant cell walls in the foods that make up the diet (Southgate, 1982). The term is unsatisfactory in many respects: first, because it is difficult to define in precise chemical terms; second, because it has been confused with the fibre (crude fibre) of the classical Weende proximate system of food analysis; and third, because many of the components of the plant cell wall which are part of dietary fibre as originally conceived are not fibrous in the generally accepted sense of the word. If, however, dietary fibre is accepted as a name that is

Dietary Fibre, Fibre-Depleted Foods
and Disease

being used to describe the complex and variable mixture of substances found in a diet that contains plant cell walls, it is possible to discuss its chemistry and physical properties. It is more difficult to produce a completely satisfactory analytical method for measuring dietary fibre. A definition of the kind proposed by Trowell *et al.* (1976) provides a basis for an analytical method. The use of the term "non-starch polysaccharides" (Englyst *et al.*, 1982) is an evolutionary development of the principles first enunciated by McCance and Lawrence (1929) when they separated the carbohydrates in foods into "available" (free sugars, starches and dextrin) and "unavailable" (all the remainder, together with the non-carbohydrate lignin). The ideas of McCance and Lawrence (1929) were used by McCance *et al.* (1936) when they devised methods for measuring starch and dextrins in foods so that their "unavailable carbohydrates" were, in essence, the non-starch fraction.

In the diets that formed the basis of the original hypothesis relating to dietary fibre (Burkitt and Trowell, 1975), dietary fibre was derived almost completely from plant cell walls in foods—in diets that include processed foods, other polysaccharides are present which are structurally related to components of the plant cell walls. These might reasonably be expected to exhibit some of the properties of cell-wall components and they have accordingly been used as models in studies of the mode of action of dietary fibre (Cummings *et al.*, 1979; Prynne and Southgate, 1979).

Working precepts

The following precepts will be used as the basis for the contents of this chapter.

1. Dietary fibre is the term used for the mixture of substances in a food or diet that is derived primarily from the plant cell walls.

2. The components of dietary fibre are principally complex polysaccharides and, in addition to polysaccharides derived directly from the plant cell walls, include non-starch storage polysaccharides and any chemically related polysaccharides that may be present in a food or diet.

3. The non-carbohydrate components of plant cell walls, for example, lignin, cutin, suberin, protein and inorganic constituents are quantitatively minor constituents but may modify the properties and physiological behaviour of the polysaccharides.

4. The polysaccharide components share a common feature in that they do not contain α-glucosidic linkages and therefore can be measured as the non α-glucan polysaccharides, i.e. the non-starch polysaccharides (NSP).

5. The measurement of the non α-glucan polysaccharides thus provides a good index of the dietary fibre in a food or diet. In foods rich in lignin, the values obtained will be lower than dietary fibre in the strict sense, but for many foods and diets the contribution of the non-carbohydrate components

is quantitatively small. The role of these non-carbohydrates in modifying the behaviour of dietary fibre may, however, be significant but can only be assessed by measuring them independently of the major carbohydrate components. For example, a value for NSP gives an indication of the amount of this material available for fermentation by the microflora in the large bowel and a value for lignin gives an indicator of the extent to which this material will be fermented.

This chapter therefore reviews first the chemistry of the components in foods derived from the plant cell wall, and then those components that are not directly present in the cell wall when consumed (but that may have been derived from cell walls originally).

Their physical properties are discussed in Section III; Section IV outlines the amounts of dietary fibre in foods, and Section V deals with the use of food composition tables to estimate intakes of dietary fibre.

II. Chemistry

A.   Material derived from plant cell walls

The components of dietary fibre are derived principally from the plant cell walls in foods and are therefore consumed in the form of cell-wall material. In this the various components are organised into a range of complex structures. The details of the actual organisation of the components has been the subject of considerable research and a number of models have been proposed that attempt to account for the known properties of the wall (Albersheim, 1977).

In some of these models, the polysaccharides are visualised as being covalently linked in a "supramolecular" structure; in others, the covalent linking is not assumed to be present.

The models share the common features in which the microfibrils of cellulose are imbedded in a matrix of non-cellulosic polysaccharides and proteins. As the cell wall matures, the non-carbohydrate polymer lignin is formed in the matrix. Protein appears to be an essential element of the wall structure and may play a role in the determination of the organisation of the polysaccharide components. The wall frequently contains inorganic materials; in some cell walls there is evidence that these inorganic materials are an integral part of the wall structure (Jones, 1978).

In cereals such as wheat, the thick outer layers of the threshed grain are composed of cell-wall material. These are the bran layers that surround the endosperm; the latter contains thin-walled endosperm cells that contain starch granules. The whole grain is milled to produce high-fibre wholemeal; most of the bran layers are removed during the milling of low-fibre white flour (see Chapter 23).

Table 3.1. Composition of typical plant cell walls
(percentage of dry cell wall)[a]

	Immature	Mature
Cellulose	24.8	38.3
Non-cellulosic polysaccharides	51.0	43.4
Lignin	Trace	16.7
Waxes, etc.	4.2	Trace
Protein	9.4	3.2
Ash	Trace	1.4

[a] After Siegel, 1968.

The relation between the detailed organisation of the components of the cell wall and the physiological properties of dietary fibre when it is consumed are not clearly established, but it is essential to recognise that, in food and the diet, dietary fibre cannot be regarded as merely the sum of its components; these components are organised into discrete structures and this organisation in itself confers other properties on the mixture.

B.   Structural polysaccharides

The composition of cell-wall material from some typical cell walls is given in Table 3.1 This shows that the polysaccharides comprise the major part of the wall and the discussion of the chemistry of dietary fibre involves, firstly, a review of the polysaccharide components.

There have been a number of extensive recent reviews on this topic and these should be consulted for details (Selvendran, 1983); the following account is a summary of the main features.

It is convenient to consider the cell-wall polysaccharides as falling into two major classes; *cellulose* and the matrix or *non-cellulosic polysaccharides* (NCP) (Albersheim, 1965).

1.   Cellulose

The cellulosic polysaccharides are characterised as linear, $\beta 1 \rightarrow 4$-D glucans of high molecular weight. In the cell wall, the polysaccharide is present in the form of microfibrils composed of several molecular chains. The configuration of the $\beta 1 \rightarrow 4$-D glucan chain is such that close packing can occur, permitting strong hydrogen bonding between the parallel chains. The regular molecular arrangement in the fibril confers a degree of crystallinity and native cellulose gives a defined X-ray diffraction pattern. Regions of less-ordered patterns and non-crystallinity are found at intervals. The structural features of cellulose are responsible for the characteristic physical properties of cellulose fibres and the low chemical reactivity of the cellulose molecule. The regular molecular arrangement must be disrupted (as, for example, by swelling in alkali or strong acid) before hydrolysis or other reactions will occur at a significant rate. The non-crystalline regions of the molecule appear to be the most reactive. In the cell wall, the cellulose fibrils are imbedded in a matrix of NCP and lignin and the fibrils appear to be sheathed in xylan or xyloglucan polysaccharides.

Although the degree of polymerisation of cellulose is always high, isolated cellulose preparations exhibit a range of molecular size. It is probable that in the native cellulose some variation in chain length occurs. Nevertheless, some depolymerisation does occur during the isolation of cellulose, particularly from woody (lignified) tissues because of the vigorous oxidative conditions necessary for the solubilisation of lignin.

Isolated cellulose preparations usually have some functional groups introduced during the isolation. Depolymerisation can take place when cellulose is ball-milled and, after prolonged treatment, colloidal (apparently water-soluble) and depolymerised preparations are produced.

2.   *Non-cellulosic polysaccharides (NCP)*

The matrix of the cell wall contains a range of polysaccharides that may contain several different monosaccharides and uronic acids. In the classical schemes for the classification of cell-wall polysaccharides based on sequential extraction, the NCP include pectic substances and the hemicelluloses. The sequential extraction procedures did not produce structurally homogeneous fractions, and there is considerable evidence that some of the fractions were artefacts of the extraction procedure. Albersheim (1965) suggested that it was preferable to group them under the descriptive term *"non-cellulosic polysac-charides"* for the spectrum of polymers ranging from those rich in uronic acids (the pectic fraction) to those poor in uronic acids (the hemicelluloses).

The NCP include water-soluble and water-insoluble polysaccharides. The solubility in water depends on pH, more being extracted at higher pH. Some of the hemicellulosic members of the group, which are initially insoluble in water but can be extracted with dilute alkali, become water soluble once extracted. The NCP can be classified according to the major monosaccharide present, which usually forms the backbone chain of the molecule. Table 3.2 summarises the major classes of NCP on this basis.

(*a*) *Rhamnogalacturonans.* These form the major component of the pectic fraction soluble in hot water or hot ammonium oxalate solution. The backbone of the molecule is largely galacturonic acid residues with rhamnose insertions at intervals. The backbone typically bears galactose and arabinose side chains. These side chains are more easily hydrolysed than the main chain and commerical samples of pectin have usually lost the majority of them. The uronic acid groups are partially esterified with methoxyl groups.

TABLE 3.2. Principal types of non-cellulosic polysaccharides of the plant cell wall

Classical nomenclature	Polysaccharide type	Main structural features	Distribution and properties
Pectic substances	Rhamnogalacturonans	$\alpha_{1\rightarrow4}$-D-galacturonans with rhamnosyl insertions Variable proportion of carboxyl groups carry methoxyl groups	Found in all plant tissues—important components of immature cell walls. Water-soluble, forms gels and combines with divalent ions. Methoxyl groups on uronic acid residues affect gelling properties.
	Arabinogalactans	$\beta_{1\rightarrow4}$ or $_{1\rightarrow3}$-D-galactopyranosides with *arabino*-side chains	Found in most plant tissues; water-soluble.
Glucans	β-glucans	$\beta_{1\rightarrow3}$, $_{1\rightarrow4}$-D-glucopyranosides	Widely distributed (especially in cereals) water-soluble, forming gummy solutions.
Hemicelluloses	Galactomannans	$\beta_{1\rightarrow4}$-D-mannopyranosides with *galacto*-side chains	Found in small amounts in many cell walls. These polysaccharides are the storage form in many seeds (including leguminosea); they may be deposited in the wall or within the cell.
	Xylans	$\beta_{1\rightarrow4}$-D-xylopyranosyl chains with branching $(1\rightarrow3)$ and with *arabino*- and 4-O methyl *glucurono*-side chains	Found in virtually all cell walls. Insoluble in native state, but many are water-soluble after extraction. Solubility increases with extent of substituent side chains.
	Xyloglucans	$\beta_{1\rightarrow4}$-D-glucans with *xylo*-side chains	Found in virtually all cell walls, water-insoluble until extracted.

(b) *Arabinogalactans.* These are water-soluble, highly branched structures with galactose forming the main backbone and branches of the molecule with short arabinosyl branches. Rhamnogalacturonans and arabinogalactans are the typical matrix polysaccharides of the cell walls of immature parenchymatous tissues that make up the bulk of the tissue in fruits and vegetables.

(c) β-*glucans.* Cereals contain variable amounts of water-soluble glucans. Unlike cellulose, these are branched structures linked β1→3 and β1→4 with a relatively low degree of polymerisation. Oats and barley are particularly good sources of this type of polysaccharide.

(d) *Xylans.* Polymers of xylose have to be found in virtually all cell walls. The main xylan chains are frequently branched and also carry short side chains of arabinose (arabinoxylans); 4-O-methylglucuronyl side chains are frequently present. This arabinoxylans are particularly characteristic of the cell-wall matrix of cereals such as wheat, rye and barley.

(e) *Mannans.* Polysaccharides with mannose backbones are found in many cell walls; the chain usually carries galactose side chains (galactomannans) or galactose and glucose side chains (galactoglucomannans). These polysaccharides are a storage form in many legumes and may be stored within thickened cell-wall structures.

(f) *Xyloglucans.* Glucose polymers with xylose side chains are found in many cell walls and are often closely bound to the cellulose fibrils. Many cellulose preparations give traces of xylose on hydrolysis and this may be due to the intimate association of the xyloglucan polysaccharides with the cellulose.

C.   Non-carbohydrate components

These form a minor proportion of the cell wall but their presence may significantly modify the properties of the cell wall and the polysaccharide components of the wall. Lignin, by usage, has been regarded as part of dietary fibre but we do not consider that the other non-carbohydrate components should be regarded in such a way. Figures for "total" dietary fibre, which include lignin and other components, are of little value in themselves.

1.   Lignin

This is a complex polymer of phenyl propane which is formed in the matrix by the condensation of the phenolic alcohols (coniferyl and cinnamyl). The polymer is formed within the matrix and infiltrates through the matrix. The volume of the wall expands as lignification proceeds and the process is initiated in the outer layers of the wall and progresses inwards. When the cell wall is fully lignified, the cell itself is usually dead.

In less mature conducting tissues, the lignin is confined to regions of the wall giving the characteristic annular or spiral bands of lignification. Lignin has a very complex structure (Freudenberg, 1965) and varies from source to source; therefore it is probably more correct to talk of the "lignins".

Despite the presence of many organic functional groups, the polymeric lignin is very resistant to degradation and requires very vigorous oxidative conditions for its removal.

2. Protein

All cell walls contain protein that appears to be an integral part of the wall and is not due to contamination of the cell-wall material with cytoplasmic proteins. The proteins are often glycoproteins (Selvendran and O'Neill, 1982) and in some walls appear to contain a high proportion of hydroxyproline.

3. Inorganic materials

Plant cell-wall material invariably contains inorganic constituents; calcium, potassium and magnesium deposits are usually present. The calcium appears to play an important role in the integrity of the intercellular adhesion presumably by an interaction with the pectic substances. Silica is often associated with the cell walls of cereals, notably rice and oats (Jones, 1978).

4. Cutin and suberin

The external surfaces of many aerial plant organs are covered with a thin cuticular layer that contains the substance cutin. This is a complex internal ester of polyhydroxymonocarboxylic acids with 16 or 18 carbon atoms in the molecule.

Many plant organs have layers of cells below the external surface, which become suberinised—suberin is structurally analogous to cutin and produces a hydrophobic layer. Suberinised tissues occur in foods such as the potato and the skin of russet apples.

D.   Non-structural polysaccharides

A range of polysaccharides occur in foods that are not strictly part of the plant cell wall. These are the gums and mucilages. They are complex heteroglycans with branched structures.

1. Gums and mucilages

The main features of their structures are given in Table 3.3. The amounts of these polysaccharides in foods are usually quite small and the overall contribution of these non-structural polysaccharides to total dietary fibre intake is not significant except where they are used as food additives (Wirths, 1980).

TABLE 3.3. Major structural features of plant gums

Type	Core	Side chains	Terminal groups	Examples
Galactan	D-galactopyranosyl 1,3, and 1,6	L-arabinofuranosyl, some L-rhamnopyranosyl	D-glucuronic or 4-O-methyl glucuronic	Gum arabic[a] and other *Acacia* spp., Asafoetida, Araucaria Lemon, Golden Apple
Glucuronomannan	4-O-substituted D-glucuronic acid alternating with 2-O-substituted D-mannosyl residues	L-arabinofuranosyl L-arabinopyranosyl D-glucopyranosyl D-galactosyl	Variable	Gum ghattie *Prunus* gums
	D-galacturonic acid L-rhamnosyl	D-xylopyranosyl L-fucopyranosyl D-galactopyranosyl arabinoxylo	Variable	Tragacanthic acid[a] Khaya gums[a] *Stercularia* gums
Galactomannan	D-mannopyranosyl	D-galactopyranosyl		Locust bean gum,[a] Guar gum[a] (more side chains)
Xylan	D-xylopyranosyl	D-galactopyranosyl L-arabinofuranosyl	Variable	Sapote gum *Watsonia* gum
Xyloglucan	1,4,-D-glucopyranosyl	D-xylopyranosyl	Variable	Tamarind

[a] Used as food additives.

TABLE 3.4. Major polysaccharide additives

Major type	Variants used	Structural features	Summary of properties	Usage
Pectins	High methoxy, low methoxy, modified	Galacturonans with few side chains—methoxyl varies according to source; some amidated pectins are used	High methoxy pectins gell in sugar solutions at low pH. Low methoxy forms gel with Ca in dilute solution. Amidated used where slow-set is desired.	Very widely used in jams, jellies, desserts
Galactomannans Gums	Guar Locust bean	D-mannopyranosides with D-galactosyl side chains	Forms viscous solutions	Wide use
Algal polysaccharides	Agar	Agarose-linear alternating 1→4-3,6 anhydro-L galactose and 1→3-D-galactose and agaropectin—agarose components plus ester sulphate and D-glucuronic acid	Gels at low concentration; gel melts at high temp., stable over range of pH and ionic strengths	Widespread use in past—now not particularly important as a food additive
	Alginates	Copolymers of D-mannuronic and L-guluronic acids	Insoluble in cold water, Ca salts rather insoluble, Na, K, NH_4, salts and propylene glycol esters very soluble	Widespread use in many foods: milk, puddings, dairy products, ice cream, beers, confectionery, etc.
	Carrageenans	1→3-D-galactose-4-sulphate and 1→4-3,6 anhydro-D-galactose 1→4-D-galactose 2,6-sulphate, 1→3-D-galactose or 1→3-D-galactose	Gels strongly with K^+ ions to give a brittle gel Non-gelling	Very widely used in a large number of types of foods. They exhibit synergic effects (on physical properties) with proteins
		1→3-D-galactose-4-sulphate and 1→4-3,6 anhydro-D-galactose-2-sulphate	Gels strong with Ca ions to give an elastic gel	
Xanthan		Glucose mannose and glucuronic acid in a linear chain with mannose side chains with pyruvate as a side chain	Non-gelling, soluble in hot and cold giving viscous solutions, often used in combination	Many uses at up to 1%

2. *Polysaccharide food additives*

Several polysaccharides are in common use as food additives where they are primarily used to control the physical properties and texture of processed foods. The more important polysaccharides are listed in Table 3.4.

III.   Physical properties

The physical properties of dietary fibre can conveniently be discussed at three levels. The first relates to properties that are reflected in the diet as a whole. Our understanding here is largely intuitive and at best semi-quantitative and at the same time there is little evidence that directly relates these properties to effects of physiological significance. The second relates to the properties of dietary fibre in the context of the structure of foods. Here the information is more soundly based on observations and there is greater (albeit still limited) understanding of the importance of physical properties in relation to physiological effects. The third level relates to the physical properties of the components of dietary fibre. For many components there is a growing volume of experimental data and the physical properties are only partially understood. Even so, evidence that directly relates the physical properties to physiological effects is limited.

A.   Effects on the diet as a whole

The plant foods that provide dietary fibre are drawn from virtually the complete range of plant organs and, therefore, dietary fibre is drawn from a wide range of tissues and cell types. Just as the chemical composition of the cell-wall material from this diverse range of structures varies considerably, so do the physical structures and properties; therefore, it is difficult to make any across-the-board generalisations, and it is necessary to discuss some examples of the different types of structure and properties that are likely to be present.

It is, however, possible to make a few generalisations about dietary fibre-containing foods that affect some gross properties of the diet. Plant foods fall into three broad compositional classes: cereal grains, grain legumes, fruits and other vegetables. Characteristically, the cereal grains are low in fat, rich in starch and, although they are harvested at a low moisture content, they are frequently cooked and eaten with some added water; for example, bread contains around 40% water. Grain legumes are higher in fat but also rich in starch and other storage polysaccharides; again they are often harvested in the mature dry state but eaten after cooking with added water. The fruits and other vegetables are low in fat and high in water content, both when harvested and when consumed. Thus, a diet rich in these foods tends to be of low-energy density (kilojoules per gram) because of a low-fat, high-water content. The cellular structure of most plant foods also tends to make the food less dense (weight per volume) so that a high-fibre diet is often a bulky diet. The starch associated with the cereal grains also swells when cooked with water and the resulting foods are again bulkier and of a lower energy density than all animal products except milk.

B.   Effects on the structure of foods

It is probable that a major factor in determining the physiological behaviour of dietary fibre is that it is consumed as cell-wall structures. These will vary in composition and properties, depending on the plant organ and the types of tissues within that organ. In this section it is only possible to review briefly the outlines of the vast amount of information relating to the anatomy of plant tissues and to focus attention on features that appear to be relevant to our understanding of the physiological significance of dietary fibre.

1.   Development of cell walls

The cell wall develops on a cell plate that is rich in uronic acid-containing polysaccharides. Initially a network of cellulose micro-fibrils is laid down on this plate in a matrix of non-cellulosic polysaccharides, which is rich in pectic substances and arabinogalactans. The primary wall is generally thin and relatively unspecialised. A secondary wall forms on this primary wall; in this the cellulose fibrils are deposited in an ordered arrangement. Several secondary wall layers are clearly distinguishable both from the orientation of the fibrils and from the types of matrix polysaccharides found. This type of cell wall is found in the parenchymatous tissues of most fruits and vegetables. The rigidity of these structures is due to the turgor pressure of the cells exerted on the non-elastic cell-wall structure. In other tissues, differentiation alters the chemical composition and properties.

2.   Protection of cell contents

The cellular structures surround the cell and the protein and carbohydrates it contains. The carbohydrates may be present in solution in the cell sap or deposited as insoluble storage polysaccharides. The cell wall acts as a physical barrier to free diffusion of contents and the entry of digestive secretions.

   In the preparation of foods for consumption, cooking procedures and ingestion, a variable degree of disruption of the cellular material occurs. This releases cell contents and partially removes any barriers to diffusion. Moreover, cooking of starch-rich materials, for example in cereals and potatoes results in considerable cellular disruption due to the swelling of starch granules. Although in man mastication is relatively inefficient compared with the ruminant, the disruption of cellular matter continues once it is consumed in the mouth and in the stomach, where the action tends to move contents from boluses of food. Faecal residues, however, still contain discrete pieces of plant tissues. The survival of the plant debris that can be identified depends on cell structure. Cutinised and lignified tissues can usually be readily identified and seed structures are apparently little altered. The more delicate internal cell walls of fruits and vegetables are difficult to distinguish, except for the lignified elements.

C. *Physical properties of dietary fibre and its components*

A number of physical properties of dietary fibre and its components have been shown to be of physiological consequence and in this section it is proposed to discuss these particular properties. It may be anticipated that other properties will subsequently be shown to be important; the final part of this section includes a speculative assessment of what these might be.

1. *Particle size*

The cellular components of dietary fibre are consumed as cell-wall material and the size of the cellular fragments depends primarily on the type of food contributing these fragments and the food processing. The material from cereals will thus greatly depend on the degree of fineness of milling. The size of wheat bran particles will depend on the type of mill used; in the roller mill the bran is separated from the endosperm as a flake early in the process (Horder *et al.*, 1954), but in the stone ground flour, this separation is not made and the bran is sieved from the wholemeal to prepare the white flour (Broadribb and Groves, 1978). The sizes of the cellular fragments from fruits and vegetables will depend on the preparation of the food. Cooking brings about a loss of cell turgor. The collapse of this tissue and boiling in water disrupts the intercellular adhesion; in the potato, for example, fragments of one or two cells can be seen.

Mastication brings about further cellular fragmentation, but the human dentition is not adapted for grinding vegetable matter to the extent seen in ruminants. The particle size of the cellular dietary fibre will determine the surface area of cell walls directly accessible to digestive secretions and bacteria, and in very fine particles the cellular structure can be completely disrupted. Vigorous treatments such as [prolonged (ie. many hours)] dry ball-milling may depolymerise and partially solubilise cell-wall polysaccharides. Reduction in particle size also removes the cellular envelopes from cell contents.

2. *Water-holding capacity: viscosity and gelling*

The polysaccharides in the cell wall and particularly some of the isolated polysaccharides used as food additives are hydrophilic. The hydrophilic character varies considerably depending on the polysaccharide; cellulose, for example—although swelling in aqueous solutions—has a limited capacity to absorb water; typical values are around 10 to 15%. The matrix polysaccharides such as the arabinoxylans have a much greater water-binding capacity and some preparations will bind several times their own weight of water. Eastwood and his colleagues have measured the capacity of cell-wall preparations to bind and hold water (McConnell *et al.*, 1974; Robertson and Eastwood, 1981a). There are considerable technical difficulties in measuring this capacity, but it is clear that cereal preparations such as bran bind rather poorly, whereas vegetable materials are quite effective. The integrity of the cell-wall material is an important factor and quite mild treatments can alter this binding capacity (Robertson and Eastwood, 1981b).

The expression of this property in foods will depend on particle size and the rate of hydration of the cell-wall material consumed. Vegetables that have been boiled in water are probably consumed with their cell-wall material fully hydrated. The water-holding capacity of isolated polysaccharides (which have been used extensively as models for dietary fibre components) must be assessed in a different way (Stephen and Cummings, 1979). It seems probable that the most important property of these materials, mainly used as food additives, is their capacity to form gels and viscous solutions.

This property is very dependent on the type of polysaccharide and on interactions with other food components. The behaviour of pectin and alginates is very dependent on the proteins and ions. While there have been extensive studies *in vitro* of these gelling polysaccharides (Rees, 1972), the quantitative expression of these properties *in vivo* has not been studied to any degree. Blackburn and Johnson (1981) have shown the effects *in vivo* of guar feeding on the intestinal contents of rats, and related these effects to the viscosity on glucose transport *in vitro* and in vivo.

3. *Ion binding*

The uronic acid-containing polysaccharides and the lignin components of dietary fibre possess acidic functional groups that react with ions—*in vitro* binding of divalent ions has been shown for calcium (James *et al.*, 1978). Binding of other divalent ions such as iron and zinc has been demonstrated (Rheinhold *et al.*, 1982) but it is not clear which components of the cell wall are involved. Fairweather-Tait (1982) has shown that in wheat preparations dietary fibre has little effect on iron availability to the rat compared with phytate, although some effects on zinc appear to be present (Caprez and Fairweather-Tait, 1982).

Binding of other substances such as bile salts (Selvendran, 1978) has been demonstrated with many cell-wall preparations, but it is not clear which components are involved (Topping *et al.*, 1980).

TABLE 3.5. Some methods used for the measurement of fibre[a]

Method	Reference	Type of procedure	Fractions measured[b]
Crude fibre	AOAC (1980)	G	Ce + Li
Neutral detergent fibre (NDF)	Van Soest and Wine (1967)	G	Ce + L + H (St)
Modified NDF	AACC (1981)	G	Ce + L + H
Biochemical fibre	Williams and Olmsted (1935)	R, G	Ce, H, L
Indigestible residue	Hellendoorn et al. (1975)	G	Ce + H + L (St + P)
	Asp (1978)	G, C	Ce, NCP, L
	Asp et al. (1983)	GLC, G	Ce, NCP, L
Unavailable carbohydrate	McCance et al. (1936)	D	Ce + H + P + L
	Southgate (1969)	C, G	Ce, NCP_s, NCP_i, L
Cell-wall polysaccharides	Sloneker (1971)	GLC	Ce, H
Dietary fibre	Englyst (1981)	GLC, G	Ce, NCP_s, NCP_i, L
	Theander and Amen (1982)	GLC	Ce, NCP_s, NCP_i, L
	Selvendran and Du Pont (1980)	GLC, C	Ce, NCP, L
Non-starch polysaccharides	Englyst et al. (1982)	GLC, C	Ce, NCP_s, NCP_i (RS)

[a] Abbreviations: G = gravimetric; R = reductionmetric; C = colorimetric; GLC = gas–liquid chromatography; D = by difference; Ce = cellulose; L = lignin; H = hemicelluloses; NCP = non-cellulosic polysaccharides; NCP_s = soluble NCP; NCP_i = insoluble NCP; St = starch; P = protein; RS = resistant starch.

[b] + = fractions combined; , = fraction separately; ( ) = contaminating material.

IV. Analysis and the amounts of dietary fibre in foods

A. Different methods of analysis

It is both difficult and undesirable to present a discussion on the amounts of dietary fibre in foods without reference to analytical methods. Much confusion has resulted from comparisons of data for specified foods because few of the published methods seem to give comparable values. This is due, first, to problems of definition in that many methods do not claim or attempt to measure the same fractions of plant materials; second, the fractions may be defined in different ways; and third, the techniques used for the measurements have different levels of specificity and, therefore, accuracy and reproducibility.

Table 3.5 lists a number of methods that have been used together with an indication of the fractions they measure.

McCance et al. (1936) used a "by difference" procedure to measure total unavailable carbohydrate plus lignin; like all "by difference" procedures it includes the errors from the other direct measurements. These can be quite important for foods with a high starch content.

The crude fibre method gives only an approximate estimate of cellulose plus lignin; the neutral detergent fibre (NDF) method of Van Soest and

Wine (1967) did not include soluble components in its published data, although attempts are being made to include these components. The modified NDF procedure [American Association of Cereal Chemists (AACC), 1981] was developed specifically for cereals to eliminate starch contamination. The procedure of Williams and Olmsted (1935) was designed to eliminate the worst aspects of the crude fibre procedure by using enzymatic methods to remove starch and protein; these same principles were revived by Hellendoorn et al., (1975) who, however, chose a gravimetric end assay compared with the more specific carbohydrate methods used by Williams and Olmsted (1935). The residue in the Hellendoorn procedure is grossly contaminated with starch and protein. Asp (1978) and Asp et al. (1983) extensively modified this procedure to measure the carbohydrates more specifically and to correct for interferences.

Most of the methods just mentioned gave a single value and consequently offered no information about the composition of the fraction measured. Southgate's (1969) procedure was an attempt to measure unavailable carbohydrate directly as its components. This involved an enzymatic hydrolysis of starch and sequential hydrolysis of the NCP and cellulosic fractions. The method gave the most satisfactory dietary fibre values for most foods but, compared with the more specific gas–liquid chromatography (GLC) methods developed later, the colorimetric measurement of sugars was less accurate, primarily because these procedures are relatively non-specific and suffer from cross-interferences (Southgate, 1969, 1976; Hudson and Bailey, 1980). Sloneker (1971) measured the component sugars released by the two-stage Saeman hydrolyis by GLC; this approach was a major advance although limited in terms of dietary fibre analysis because neither uronic acids nor lignin were measured and all the non-cellulosic glucose was considered to be derived from starch. Englyst (1978) combined the GLC measurements with the enzymatic removal of starch and colorimetric measurements of uronic acids in the "available carbohydrate" procedure (Southgate, 1969). Theander and Amen (1982) followed Sloneker's (1971) procedure for Saeman hydrolysis but measured starch separately after enzymatic hydrolysis. These approaches have formed the basis of the most recent methods designed to measure the carbohydrate components separately (Selvendran and Du Pont, 1980; Theander and Amen, 1982; Englyst et al., 1982). The latter also developed procedures for measuring resistant starch, i.e., starch resistant to enzymatic hydrolysis under the conditions used in the analytical procedure.

Resistant starch is produced when starch, especially high amylose starch, dispersed in cooking, retrogrades and becomes resistant both to redispersion in water and to hydrolysis with α-amylase. Such resistant starch is often produced during treatment of the sample before analysis. This resistant material is only partially hydrolysed with MH_2SO_4 unless previously solubilized with 12 MH_2SO_4 as in the Saeman hydrolysis. In the sequential hydrolysis by dilute acid followed by strong acid (Southgate, 1969), some resistant starch appears in the cellulosic fraction. Resistant starch is clearly not part of the non-cellulosic or the cellulosic fractions, but it may be argued that it should be included in the "total dietary fibre" because it is not hydrolysable by enzymes. If this argument is accepted, it means that the total dietary fibre in white bread would be higher by some 50% than that of the white flour from which it is made, and that of cornflakes would be five times higher than that of the original corn material. The amount of resistant starch in a food depends on the precise conditions of processing or cooking and length and conditions of storage and is, therefore, highly variable and unpredictable. The inclusion of resistant starch in values for total dietary fibre would make calculations from food composition tables very unreliable and these total values may be unrelated to the amounts of cell-wall material in the foodstuffs.

B.   The preferred method of analysis

A satisfactory analytical method for dietary fibre must measure all the NSP (cellulose, NCP, soluble and insoluble). For this reason, values obtained by the crude fibre method, the original and the modified NDF methods, and the Hellendoorn method, are not satisfactory.

Furthermore, it is clear that both physiological and physical properties of dietary fibre are related to specific components so that a method that gives information about the composition of dietary fibre is highly desirable. Characterising the individual NCP is not, at least at the present time, realistic for a routine method. However, separation of the cellulosic, and the soluble and insoluble NCP, with characterisation in terms of the monosaccharide and uronic acid components, can give valuable information about the composition of dietary fibre (Southgate et al., 1978; Selvendran, 1983). The measurement of the non-carbohydrate components of the plant cell wall, lignin, cutin, etc. may be of interest and importance for some foods, but they should be measured separately and not included with the complex carbohydrates.

A method such as that described by Englyst et al., (1982) meets these criteria and has the advantage that, unlike most other procedures, it provides a measure of resistant starch.

The method is summarised in Fig. 3.1. Three replicate samples are analysed in parallel.

1.   Procedure A

The sample is treated with enzymes to remove starch and the residual polysaccharides are precipitated with ethanol. These are then subjected to a Saeman type hydrolysis. The component monosaccharides are measured as their alditol acetates and the uronic acids colorimetrically (Scott, 1979). These values give total NSP plus resistant starch (RS).

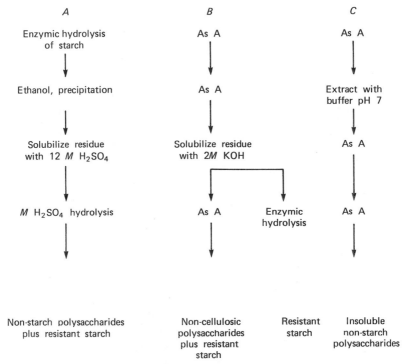

FIG. 3.1. Schematic outline of method for measurement of non-starch polysaccharides. Redrawn from Englyst, *et al.* (1982)

2. *Procedure B*

The initial stages are identical but $2\,M$ KOH is used to solubilise RS which is measured separately in an aliquot. The remainder is hydrolysed with H_2SO_4.

Thus, values for NCP + RS and RS are obtained directly and for NCP by subtraction. Furthermore, subtraction of NCP + RS from values in procedure A give glucose values for cellulose.

3. *Procedure C*

This provides values of NSP insoluble at pH 7 and for soluble NSP by difference.

A simple modification of this method has been developed for the direct measurement of RS and free values for NSP.

C. *Preferred values for dietary fibre in foods*

A detailed systematic study of all foods using these procedures has not been undertaken, but values for some foods are given in Tables 3.6–3.8. Englyst *et al.*, (1983) give values for a range of cereal foods.

TABLE 3.6. Non-starch polysaccharides (NSP) in some foods
[g/100 g dry matter (proportion of total NSP)]

| | Non-cellulosic polysaccharides | | | | Total | Resistant |
	Soluble	Insoluble	Total	Cellulose	NSP	starch
White bread	1.92 (0.71)	0.60 (0.22)	2.52 (0.93)	0.17 (0.08)	2.69	1.24
Wholewheat bread	2.75 (0.26)	5.93 (0.57)	8.68 (0.83)	1.79 (0.17)	10.47	1.14
Wheat bran	3.22 (0.08)	30.07 (0.73)	33.59 (0.81)	7.98 (0.19)	41.57	—
Porridge oats	3.98 (0.55)	2.96 (0.41)	6.94 (0.96)	0.28 (0.04)	7.22	—
Whole rye flour	4.61 (0.34)	7.68 (0.56)	12.29 (0.90)	1.40 (0.10)	13.69	0.21
Cornflakes	0.18 (0.26)	0.24 (0.35)	0.42 (0.61)	0.26 (0.38)	0.68	3.11
White rice	0.16 (0.26)	0.35 (0.52)	0.51 (0.76)	0.16 (0.24)	0.67	Trace
Brown rice	0.14 (0.07)	1.18 (0.58)	1.32 (0.65)	0.70 (0.35)	2.02	—
Butter beans	6.31 (0.39)	5.71 (0.35)	12.02 (0.74)	4.32 (0.26)	16.34	0.54
Chick peas	2.47 (0.24)	5.50 (0.54)	7.97 (0.78)	2.22 (0.22)	10.19	0.33
Potatoes, boiled	2.64 (0.54)	0.57 (0.12)	3.21 (0.66)	1.63 (0.34)	4.84	2.08
Cabbage, raw	13.5 (0.48)	4.21 (0.15)	17.74 (0.63)	9.86 (0.36)	27.60	—
Banana	2.10 (0.55)	0.76 (0.20)	2.86 (0.75)	0.97 (0.25)	3.83	—
Tomato	9.86 (0.42)	4.83 (0.21)	14.69 (0.63)	8.78 (0.37)	23.47	0.21
Hardnuts	2.43 (0.39)	1.86 (0.30)	4.29 (0.69)	1.94 (0.31)	6.23	—

These illustrate the type of information this analytical approach gives about the dietary fibre in foods. Table 3.6 gives the amounts of soluble and insoluble NCP, cellulose, total NSP, and RS in a selection of foods. The proportion of the total NSP present in the fractions is also given.

The soluble NCP vary considerably, both absolutely and as a proportion of the total. In white bread it is the major component of the NCP, while in wholemeal bread it represents about one-third of the total NCP and in bran about one-tenth. One would, therefore, expect the NCP from white bread to be more extensively degraded in the colon than that from wholemeal bread.

The soluble NCP represent about one-quarter to one-third of the total NSP in all the foods except bran. This demonstrates the extent to which values, obtained by use of methods that only measure insoluble material, underestimate the total amount.

The NCP are the major components of the NSP in most foods, providing 60–90% of the total. In white flour and porridge oats, cellulose is a very minor component. The values for NSP do not include lignin and are therefore slightly lower than values obtained that include this component. RS is significant in cooked cereal products, for example, in cornflakes it is five times the NSP value; analogously it is also high in cooked potato. Raw cereals and vegetables contain only minor amounts of RS.

This method also characterises the NCP; this is illustrated in Table 3.7 for cereals and Table 3.8 for the other foods.

The wheat NCP are characterised by their high proportion of arabinose

TABLE 3.7. Non-cellulosic polysaccharides (NCP) in cereals [g/100 g dry matter (proportion of NCP)][a]

		NCP	Rha	Ara	Xyl	Man	Gal	Glu	U
White bread	s	1.92	—	0.63 (0.33)	0.89 (0.46)	Trace	0.15 (0.08)	0.25 (0.13)	—
	i	0.60	—	0.20 (0.33)	0.26 (0.43)	0.06	Trace	0.08 (0.13)	—
Wholemeal bread	s	2.75	—	0.81 (0.29)	1.31 (0.48)	0.01 (tr)	0.15 (0.05)	0.41 (0.14)	0.06 (0.02)
	i	5.93	—	1.86 (0.31)	3.08 (0.52)	0.07 (0.01)	0.10 (0.02)	0.65 (0.11)	0.17 (0.03)
Wheat bran	s	3.22	Trace	1.0 (0.31)	1.58 (0.49)	0.01 (tr)	0.14 (0.04)	0.22 (0.07)	0.27 (0.08)
	i	30.37	Trace	8.79 (0.29)	17.18 (0.57)	0.12 (tr)	0.57 (0.02)	2.81 (0.09)	0.90 (0.03)
Porridge oats	s	3.98	—	0.23 (0.06)	0.18 (0.05)	0.01 (tr)	0.11 (0.03)	3.37 (0.85)	0.08 (0.02)
	i	2.96	—	0.74 (0.25)	1.06 (0.35)	0.09 (0.03)	0.08 (0.03)	0.84 (0.28)	0.15 (0.05)
Whole rye flour	s	4.61	—	1.41 (0.31)	2.14 (0.46)	0.15 (0.03)	0.10 (0.02)	0.73 (0.16)	0.08 (0.02)
	i	7.68	—	2.22 (0.29)	3.62 (0.47)	0.18 (0.02)	0.21 (0.03)	1.33 (0.17)	0.12 (0.02)
Cornflakes	s	0.18	—	0.03 (0.17)	0.06 (0.33)	—	—	0.06 (0.33)	0.03 (0.17)
	i	0.24	—	0.09 (0.38)	0.12 (0.50)	—	—	—	0.03 (0.12)
White rice	s	0.16	—	0.03 (0.19)	0.03 (0.19)	0.02 (0.12)	0.01 (0.06)	0.03 (0.19)	0.04 (0.25)
	i	0.35	—	0.06 (0.17)	0.09 (0.25)	0.03 (0.08)	—	0.16 (0.46)	0.01 (0.03)
Brown rice	s	0.14	—	0.02 (0.14)	0.01 (0.07)	—	0.03 (0.21)	0.04 (0.28)	0.04 (0.28)
	i	1.18	—	0.41 (0.35)	0.48 (0.41)	—	0.08 (0.07)	0.11 (0.09)	0.10 (0.08)

[a] Abbreviations: s = soluble; i = insoluble; Rha = rhamnose; Ara = arabinose; Xyl = xylose; Man = mannose; Gal = galactose; Glu = glucose; U = uronic acids.

50

TABLE 3.8. Non-cellulosic polysaccharides in vegetables, fruits and a nut [g/100 g (proportion of NCP)][a]

		NCP	Rha	Ara	Xyl	Man	Gal	Glu	U
Butter beans	s	6.31	0.14 (0.02)	2.56 (0.41)	0.64 (0.10)	0.44 (0.07)	0.27 (0.04)	0.33 (0.05)	1.93 (0.31)
	i	5.71	0.04 (Tr)	2.64 (0.46)	1.38 (0.24)	0.76 (0.13)	0.26 (0.05)	—	0.63 (0.11)
Chick peas	s	2.47	0.18 (0.07)	0.44 (0.18)	0.09 (0.04)	0.03 (0.01)	0.18 (0.07)	0.15 (0.06)	1.40 (0.57)
	i	5.50	0.06 (0.01)	3.75 (0.68)	0.42 (0.07)	0.07 (0.01)	0.33 (0.06)	—	0.87 (0.16)
Potatoes, boiled	s	2.64	0.12 (0.04)	0.23 (0.09)	0.01 (Tr)	0.03 (0.01)	1.19 (0.45)	0.19 (0.07)	0.87 (0.33)
	i	0.57	Trace	0.08 (0.14)	0.08 (0.14)	0.06 (0.11)	0.32 (0.56)	—	0.03 (0.05)
Cabbage, raw	s	13.53	0.85 (0.06)	3.14 (0.23)	0.19 (0.01)	0.05 (Tr)	1.26 (0.09)	0.38 (0.03)	7.56 (0.55)[b]
	i	4.21	0.05 (0.01)	0.84 (0.20)	1.33 (0.32)	0.64 (0.15)	0.76 (0.18)	—	0.52 (0.12)[c]
Banana	s	2.10	—	0.08 (0.03)	0.04 (0.02)	0.44 (0.21)	0.09 (0.04)	0.21 (0.10)	1.24 (0.59)
	i	0.76	—	0.19 (0.25)	0.19 (0.25)	0.13 (0.17)	0.10 (0.13)	—	0.15 (0.20)
Tomato	s	9.86	0.38 (0.04)	0.64 (0.06)	0.05 (Tr)	0.06 (0.01)	1.01 (0.10)	—	7.72 (0.78)
	i	4.83	0.02 (Tr)	0.40 (0.08)	1.09 (0.03)	1.12 (0.03)	0.79 (0.16)	0.84 (0.17)	0.57 (0.12)
Hazelnuts	s	2.43	0.20 (0.08)	0.65 (0.27)	0.15 (0.06)	0.04 (0.02)	0.24 (0.10)	0.18 (0.07)	0.97 (0.40)
	i	1.86	0.10 (0.05)	0.54 (0.29)	0.32 (0.17)	0.12 (0.06)	0.28 (0.15)	—	0.50 (0.26)

[a] Abbreviations: s = soluble; i = insoluble; Rha = rhamnose; Ara = arabinose; Xyl = xylose; Man = mannose; Gal = galactose; Glu = glucose; U = uronic acids.
[b] Contains 0.10 fucose.
[c] Contains 0.07 fucose.

and xylose, with the soluble and insoluble fractions having similar composition, as does rye where arabinose and xylose contribute over 70% of the total. In porridge oats, the soluble component is rich in glucose whereas the insoluble component is rich in arabinose and xylose. The fractions from the cornflakes show a similar pattern.

The rice fractions are not rich in arabinose and xylose except for the insoluble material in brown rice; the latter has a comparable composition to wheat, wholemeal and whole rye. All the other cereal products, except for porridge oats, are poor in mannose and galactose, and contain small amounts of glucose. Whole cereal products such as wheat wholemeal, whole rye flour and brown rice are richer in all NCP than the more refined products, white flour and white rice. Without exception uronic acids are low.

Table 3.8 gives the amounts of NCP in some vegetables, fruits and a nut. The NCP from these foods, especially the soluble fraction, are rich in uronic acid, galactose and arabinose, which is characteristic of pectic substances.

The insoluble fractions are often richer in xylose. The two legumes given show that even within a family the NCP may differ; it is interesting to note the low galactose and mannose, which shows that seed legumes as a class are not necessarily rich in galactomannan.

In general, the soluble and insoluble fractions show marked differences in composition, once again emphasising that even total NCP values will hide difference of potential physiological importance.

Such details as can be drawn from this one type of procedure illustrate the difficulty of making predictions from total NSP or dietary fibre values.

V.   Use of food composition tables for estimating intakes of dietary fibre

The general guidance given by Paul and Southgate (1978) on the limitations of food composition tables is especially relevant in relation to dietary fibre. It is essential to be familiar with the sources of the data in the composition tables and the modes of expression that have been used in the tables.

In the case of dietary fibre, the sources of the data have a special significance because the analytical method used to obtain the data has a profound influence on the values obtained; this was described in the previous section.

It is therefore essential to establish the analytical origins of the data. Many tables give values for crude fibre (Southgate, 1976) under the heading "fibre". These values are not numerically related to values for dietary fibre as used in the present context. They provide a guide for ranking foods in an approximate order of dietary fibre content but cannot be used to derive values for dietary fibre. Crude fibre values grossly underestimate dietary fibre content.

Some sources quote values obtained by one of the Van Soest (1963) detergent fibre methods. NDF has been used by many authors (AACC, 1981) to signify "insoluble", dietary fibre. This method gives values for some cereals, especially wheat products, that are numerically of the same order as total dietary fibre values obtained by the summation of cellulose, NCP and lignin. However, carbohydrate analysis of the residue shows that this agreement is fortuitous (Selvendran and Du Pont, 1984). In fruits and vegetables and cereals containing water-soluble NCP, the NDF method underestimates dietary fibre content very significantly (Southgate, 1976; Englyst, 1981).

Where an attempt has been made to measure all the components (Southgate et al., 1976; Paul and Southgate, 1978; Englyst, 1981; Theander and Amen, 1982; Asp et al., 1983), it is primarily necessary to be sure whether the values include lignin or only the NSP (Englyst et al., 1982), and second, whether the values are expressed as monosaccharides (Paul and Southgate, 1978) or as the anhydro-components (Englyst et al., 1982); the latter will be approximately 10% lower than the former.

Finally, when making comparisons between different authors' values it should be remembered that foods are biological materials (Paul and Southgate, 1978), and as such show biological variation; many of the differences between values cited by different authors are due, in part, to differences in the samples analysed. In using food composition tables to estimate intakes, these natural variations reduce the predictive accuracy of all calculations. The calculations should become more reliable when used to estimate intakes over a considerable period of time or with large groups of individuals. At the present time information on the natural variation is insufficient for any real guidance to be given on the predictive accuracy of such calculations.

References

American Association of Cereal Chemists (AACC), (1981). *Cereal Foods World* **26**, 295–297.

ALBERSHEIM, P. (1965). *In* "Plant Biochemistry" (J. Bonner and J. E. Varner, eds), pp. 298–321 Academic Press, New York and London.

ALBERSHEIM, P. (1977). *In* "Plant Biochemistry" (J. Bonner and J. E. Varner, eds), 2nd edition, pp. 226–277. Academic Press, New York and London.

ASP, N.-G. (1978). *In* "Dietary Fibre" (K. W. Heaton, ed), pp. 21–25. Newman Publishing, London.

ASP, N.-G., JOHANSSON, C. G. HALLMER, H. and SILJESTROM, M. (1983) *J. Agric. Food. Chem.* **31**, 476–482.

Association of Official Analytic Chemists (AOAC) (1980). "Official Methods of Analysis" (W. Horwitz, ed), AOAC, Washington, D.C.

BLACKBURN, N.A., and JOHNSON, I. T. (1981). *Br. J. Nutr.* **46**, 239–246.

BROADRIBB, A. J. M. and GROVES C. (1978), *Gut* **19**, 60–63.

BURKITT, D. P. and TROWELL, H. C. (eds) (1975). "Refined Carbohydrate Foods and Disease. Some Implications of Dietary Fibre". Academic Press, New York and London.

CAPREZ, A. and FAIRWEATHER-TAIT, S. J. (1982). *Br. J. Nutr.* **48**, 467–475.

CUMMINGS, J. H., SOUTHGATE, D. A. T., BRANCH, W., WIGGINS, H. S., HOUSTON, H., JENKINS, D. J. A., JIBRAJ, T. and HILL, M. W. (1979). *Br. J. Nutr.* **41,** 477–485.

ENGLYST, H. (1978). *Ugeskr. Agron. Hort. Forst. Lic.* **27,** 626–627.

ENGLYST, H. (1981). *In "Analysis of Dietary Fibre in Foods"* (W. P. T. James and O. Theander, eds). pp. 71–93. Dekker, New York.

ENGLYST, H., WIGGINS, H. S. and CUMMINGS, J. H. (1982). *Analyst* **107,** 307–318.

ENGLYST, H., ANDERSON, V. and CUMMINGS, J. H. (1983). *J. Sci. Food Agric.* **34,** 1434–1440.

FAIRWEATHER-TAIT, S. J. (1982). *Br. J. Nutr.* **47,** 243–249.

FREUDENBERG, K. (1965). *Science* **148,** 595–600.

HELLENDOORN, E. W. NORDHOFF, M. G. and SLAGMAN, J. (1975). *J. Sci. Food Agric.* **26,** 1461–1468.

HIPSLEY, E. H. (1953). *Br. Med. J.* **2,** 420–422.

HORDER, LORD, DODDS, E. C. and MORAŃ, T. (1954). "Bread." Constable, London.

HUDSON, G. J. and BAILEY, B. S. (1980). *Food Chem.* **5,** 210–216

JAMES, W. P. T., BRANCH, W. J. and SOUTHGATE, D. A. T. (1978). *Lancet* **1,** 638–639.

JONES, L. H. P. (1978). *Am. J. Clin. Nutr.* **31,** S94–S98.

MCCANCE, R. A. and LAWRENCE, R. D. (1929), *Med. Res. Counc. (G. B.), Spec. Rep. Ser.* **SRS-135.**

MCCANCE, R. A., WIDDOWSON, E. M. and SHACKLETON, L. R. B. (1936). *Med. Res. Counc. (G. B.), Spec. Rep. Ser.* **SRS–213.**

MCCONNELL, A. A., EASTWOOD, M. A. and MITCHELL, W. D. (1974). *J. Sci. Food Agric.* **25,** 1457–1464.

PAUL, A. A. and SOUTHGATE, D. A. T. (1978). *In "McCance and Widdowson's The Composition of Foods",* 4th edition. HM Stationery office, London.

PRYNNE, C. J. and SOUTHGATE, D. A. T. (1979). *Br. J. Nutr.* **41,** 495–503.

REES, D. A. (1972). *Biochem. J.* **126,** 257–273.

RHEINHOLD, J. G., GARCIA P. M., ANAS ARNADO, L. and GARZON, P. (1982). *In "Dietary Fibre in Health and Disease"* (G. V. Vahouny and D. Kritchevsky, eds), pp. 117–132. Plenum, New York.

ROBERTSON, J. A. and EASTWOOD, M. A. (1981a). *Br. J. Nutr.* **46,** 247–255.

ROBERTSON, J. A. and EASTWOOD, M. A. (1981b). *J. Sci. Food Agric.* **32,** 819–825.

SCOTT, R. W. (1979). *Anal. Chem.* **51,** 936–941.

SELVENDRAN, R. R. (1978). *Chem. Ind. (London),* pp. 428–430.

SELVENDRAN, R. R. (1983). *In "Dietary Fibre"* (G. G. Birch and K. J. Parker, eds), pp. 95–147. Applied Science Publishers, London.

SELVENDRAN, R. R. and DU PONT, M. S. (1980). *J. Sci. Food Agric.* 31, 1173–1182.

SELVENDRAN, R. R. and DU PONT, M. S. (1984). *In "Food Analysis Techniques"* (R. D. King, ed.), Vol. 3, pp. 1–68. Applied Science Publishers, London.

SELVENDRAN, R. R. and O'NEILL, M. A. (1982). *In "Plant Carbohydrates"* (F. A. Loewus and W. Tanner, eds), pp. 515–583. Springer-Verlag, Berlin and New York.

SIEGEL, S. M. (1968). *In "Comprehensive Biochemistry"* (M. Florkin and E. H. Stotz, eds), Vol. 26A, pp. 1–51. Elsevier, Amsterdam.

SLONEKER, J. H. (1971). *Anal. Biochem.* **43,** 539–546.

SOUTHGATE, D. A. T. (1969). *J. Sci. Food Agric.* **20,** 3331–335.

SOUTHGATE, D. A. T. (1976). "Determination of Food Carbohydrates". Applied Science Publishers, London.

SOUTHGATE, D. A. T. (1982). *In "Dietary Fibre in Health and Disease"* (G. V. Vahouny and D. Kritchevsky, eds), pp. 1–7. Plenum, New York.

SOUTHGATE, D. A. T., BAILEY, B., COLLINSON, E. and WALKER, A. F. (1976). *J. Hum. Nutr.* **30,** 303–313.

SOUTHGATE, D. A. T., HUDSON, G. J. and ENGLYST, H. (1978). *J. Sci. Food Agric.* **29,** 979–988.

STEPHEN, A. M. and CUMMINGS, J. H. (1979). *Gut.* **20,** 722–729.

THEANDER, O. and AMEN, P. (1982). *J. Sci. Food Agric.* **33,** 340–344.

TOPPING, D. L., STORER, G. B., CALVERT, D. G., ILLMAN, R. J., OAKENFULL, D. G. and WELLER, R. A. (1980). *Am. J. Clin. Nutr.* **33,** 783–786.

TROWELL, H. (1972). *Am. J. Clin Nutr.* **25,** 926–932.

TROWELL, H. C., SOUTHGATE, D. A. T., WOLEVER, T. M. S., LEEDS, A. R., GASSULL, M. A. and JENKINS, D. J. A. (1976). *Lancet* **1,** 967.

VAN SOEST, P. T. (1963). *J. Assoc. Off. Agric. Chem.* **46,** 825–829.

VAN SOEST, P. J. and WINE R. H. (1967). *J. Assoc. Off. Agric. Chem.* **50,** 50–55.

WILLIAMS, R. D. and OLMSTED, W. H. J. (1935). *J. Biol. Chem.* **108,** 653–666.

WIRTHS, W. (1980). *In* "Pflanzenfasern-Ballaststaffe in menschen Ernahrung" (H. Rottka. ed.), pp. 76–82. Thieme, Stuttgart.

Chapter 4

Dietary fibre methodology

LEON PROSKY and BARBARA HARLAND

I. Introduction

The development of methodology for the determination of dietary fibre has evolved over a long period of time and has been hampered by lack of a definition of "fibre". Part of the complication has arisen because fibre is not a single entity but in fact is a mixture of many complex organic substances. Although there was a need for a definition and method for dietary fibre for many years, this need was further stimulated by the publication of a paper by Burkitt *et al.* (1972) who represented dietary fibre as a food ingredient that would cure a number of chronic degenerative diseases. By the time a U.S. Government publication (U.S. Department of Agriculture, 1980) made the recommendation that Americans should "eat foods with adequate starch and fiber", the Food and Drug Administration (FDA), through the Association of Official Analytical Chemists (AOAC), had begun work toward arriving at an acceptable definition and method for dietary fibre.

Dietary Fibre, Fibre-Depleted Foods
and Disease

ISBN 0-12-701160-9

The measurement of dietary fibre was to be the first step in identifying the quantity of fibre in the diet and subsequently an assessment would be made of the physical and physiological effects of dietary fibre, including its interactions with other essential nutrients. This chapter tells the story of the development of the definition and method for its determination. Dietary fibre was first defined by Hipsley (1953) to include lignin, cellulose and hemicellulose, and has been broadened by some to include soluble substances, such as oligosaccharides, pectins, gums, mucilages and modified celluloses (Trowell et al., 1976).

This broader definition has been suggested because additional non-digestible carbohydrate components have been discovered to have physiological actions. Components such as pectins, gums and mucilages may speed gastric emptying time and may bind bile acids. Other components such as cellulose and alginic acid increase the liver cholesterol content in cholesterol-fed rats while lignin, which increases steroid excretion, may bind trace elements. Pectin, on the other hand, has been shown to have a cholesterol lowering effect. The measurement of crude fibre, "the residue of plant food left after extraction with solvent, dilute acid and dilute alkali" (Van Soest and Mc-Queen, 1973), does not differentiate the fibre components and therefore is of little value to the clinician.

In 1975, the AOAC published as official first action a method for acid detergent fibre (ADF), which measures cellulose and lignin (Van Soest, 1963), while a neutral detergent fibre (NDF) method was adopted as an official method by the American Association of Cereal Chemists (AACC) as an alternative to the crude fibre method (Van Soest and Wine, 1967). The NDF method is a rapid chemical method that gives higher estimations of fibre than the crude fibre method because of improved recoveries for cellulose, hemicellulose and lignin. Since complete removal of starch by conventional methods is difficult in some food samples, the method was modified by adding an α-amylase treatment to remove residual starch (AACC, 1978). Neither the ADF nor NDF methods include the newer components that have been encompassed by the term "dietary fibre" nor have these methods been subjected to collaborative analyses in diverse foods and feeds. It is only recently that dietary fibre has achieved recognition as an important component of food: at the "Marabou Food and Fibre" Symposium (1976) held in Sweden; the Symposium (Roth and Mehlman, 1978) on "Role of Dietary Fiber in Health" held in Bethesda, Maryland, March, 1977; the European Economic Community Working Group (Theander and James, 1979); the George Washington University Fiber Symposium (Vahouny and Kritchevsky, 1982); the International Symposium on Dietary Fibre held at the University of Reading in March (1982b); and the International Symposium on Fibre in Human and Animal Nutrition at Massey University, New Zealand, in May (1982a).

In 1978 at the dietary fibre workshop of the XI International Congress of

Nutrition, in Rio de Janeiro, Brazil (Spiller and Kay, 1979), several scientists met to discuss the current state-of-the-art with respect to the definition and methodology of dietary fibre. The following recommendations were made:

1. Both the water-insoluble and the water-soluble carbohydrate polymers that are not hydrolyzed by human digestion enzymes should be included in the overall definition of fibre.

2. Crude fibre bears no consistent quantitative relationship to dietary fibre in a food and the use of this procedure should be abandoned.

3. The NDF method is acceptable for the routine determination of insoluble fibre. In foods containing starch, hydrolysis of the amylose fraction must precede the neutral detergent steps.

4. Determination of water-soluble components (gums, mucilages, pectic substances) must be included in routine methods for dietary fibre.

5. Enzymatic methods may have widespread applicability in fractionation procedures.

6. Although rapid quantitative methodologies are acceptable for routine use such as industry quality control, more tedious methods are essential for defining the chemical characteristics of specific fibres with known physiological effects.

7. Food and feed standards should be made available for quality control and for further characterization of their physicochemical properties. Standards should include defined fibre isolates (cellulose, lignins, pectins) as well as chemically characterized native food sources.

At the AOAC 93rd Annual Meeting in Washington, D.C. Prosky and Harland (1979) announced their intention of seeking a definition and a method for the analysis of total dietary fibre (TDF) which would then be subjected to collaborative study. In the spring of 1981 at an AOAC Workshop in Ottawa, Canada (Prosky, 1981), Asp, Baker, Heckman, Southgate, and Van Soest reported on their fibre research. It was the conclusion of the scientists present that from these reports, two methods for the determination of total dietary fibre should be developed: (1) a rapid gravimetric method (an enzyme modification of the methods developed by Asp, Schweizer, and Furda); and (2) a more comprehensive method, such as a modification of Southgate's procedure (Southgate, 1969) to determine the individual dietary fibre components. In the initial method, the sum of the soluble and insoluble polysaccharides and lignin would be defined and measured as a unit, while in the second method, each of the specific components of TDF would be identified and measured separately (Prosky and Harland, 1981). There was recognition that the needs of cereal chemists were different from those of physiologists who were primarily interested in identifying the fibre fractions that most consistently elicited physiologic responses.

By 1981, at the 95th AOAC Annual Meeting in Washington, D.C., more than 100 responses had been received expressing an interest in the area of dietary fibre and suggesting definitions of dietary fibre and a preferred method for analysis. Most respondents preferred the definition of Trowell (1974): "Dietary fibre consists of remnants of the plant cells resistant to hydrolysis by the alimentary enzymes of man". This definition was later modified by Trowell, Southgate and others (Trowell *et al.*, 1976; Van Soest and McQueen, 1973) to include hemicelluloses, celluloses, lignins, oligosaccharides, pectins, gums and waxes. The preferred methods for the analysis of dietary fibre at that time were modifications of Southgate's procedures (Southgate, 1969). Because of the complexities and time involved with this procedure (even though the method gave the most complete answers), there was a desire for an intermediate method, one that would include analysis of the insoluble fractions and the soluble fractions that had been lost in previous methods (ADF, NDF) and yet a simpler method than the Southgate method, i.e. one that could be carried out in most general chemical laboratories. Thus the collaborative study for the enzymatic–gravimetric method developed by Asp, Furda, De Vries and Schweizer was submitted for collaboration in February, 1982. At the AOAC Annual Meeting in October, 1982, Prosky and Harland (1982) reported on the progress of the Collaborative Study for Total Dietary Fibre. Samples of 13 foods or food mixtures as well as the three enzymes necessary to the method had been sent to 42 laboratories representing 14 countries. A computer program was developed to accommodate the data as they arrived. A preliminary examination of the data showed good agreement for the fibre values in the categories of high-fibre, medium-fibre and low-fibre foods, with greater variation in the determination of low fibre.

II. History of dietary fibre methodology development

Einhof, in 1806, obtained fibre values by simply macerating the feeds with subsequent hot water extraction. Crude fibre determinations obtained by the sequential extractions of plant foods by ether, acid and alkali had been developed in the early nineteenth century and in 1887 the method for crude fibre was adopted by the Association of Official Agricultural Chemists (AOAC) (Browne, 1940). The analysis for crude fibre was favored at this time because it involved three easily obtained reagents and was reasonably reproducible. However, major fractions of the plant fibre such as hemicellulose (ca. 85% lost), lignin (ca. 90% lost), and even some of the cellulose, were all lost due to their solubility in acid or in alkali. This crude fibre method was continuously applied for the analysis of foods and feeds for approximately 40 years, and a large data base of values was developed. When it became clear that the ingestion of particular components of the fibre fraction or food containing particular components of the fraction were indeed successful in aiding the management of certain diseases, i.e. diverticular disease and diabetes (Anderson, 1982), the measurement of those components became a need for clinicians. First one had to measure fibre more accurately to discover how much was in the diet. Then one would have to see how our diets had changed over the years with regard to fibre intake, and finally to define fibre's action in metabolic processes. The term dietary fibre was generally applied to this fraction with physiological response, as opposed to the older term crude fibre.

Early in 1974, Kellogg sponsored its first fibre symposium when dietary fibre was beginning to attract the attention of the scientific community and followed with another symposium in 1977 which brought together the leading chemists, food scientists, epidemiologists and practicing physicians to discuss their experimental findings. In 1979, a symposium held at the Royal College of Physicians of London was concerned mainly with the relationships of fibre and metabolic disease although there was some discussion of methodology and the measurement of dietary fibre (Baird and Ornstein, 1981). In December 1977, the European Economic Community and the International Agency for Research on Cancer (WHO) held a workshop in Lyon, France. Some of the recommendations pertaining to the analysis of dietary fibre made by the representatives of 10 European countries and the United States were: (1) crude fibre analyses should be replaced; (2) dietary fibre analyses should be based on a thorough understanding of the molecular structure of the complex carbohydrates, (3) all properties of dietary fibre such as solubility, density, hydration, ion-exchange capacities, particle size and susceptibility to microbial fermentation should be researched; and (4) fat extraction should be a prerequisite to dietary fibre analyses. Guidelines for analyses of nine different food samples were set, with plans to assemble again in Cambridge, England, in December, 1978 to discuss progress to date.

These early conferences represented a commitment to the tremendous effort that would be required to change concepts, approaches and above all the food and feed fibre data bases. There had been acceptance of the fibre values determined by the crude fibre method, but it was time to discard them in favor of some new values, i.e. TDF, fractions of which had been shown to have a role in the management of diabetes and diverticular disease.

One approach was to name the fibre fraction based on its method of preparation, i.e., ADF or NDF. If one were to reflux foods or feeds for 1 h in a water solution of 1 N sulphuric acid and 2% cetyltrimethylammonium bromide (Van Soest, 1973), the residue, consisting mainly of cellulose and lignin, plus the Maillard products of heating and cooking, was then called ADF. In this procedure, hemicelluloses were lost as well as the water-soluble portions of the fibre. An advantage of this procedure is that further analysis for cellulose and lignin could be performed on the residue.

The chemical analysis that is used to measure NDF consists of boiling plant materials with neutral sodium lauryl sulphate and EDTA. Lignin, cellulose and hemicellulose and such cell-wall components as cutin, minerals and protein are salvaged, although soluble carbohydrates, lipids and pectins are lost (Van Soest *et al.* 1966).

Very early, the need to eliminate starch and protein interferences was recognized. During methodology development, pectins and gums, although lacking the structural characteristics of true plant fibers, possessed properties that elicited characteristic metabolic effects specific to certain fruits, vegetables and grains. The analyses of foods for cellulose, hemicellulose and lignin could be performed with relative agreement by any of a number of procedures; however, when the matrix that binds these components was altered, for instance, during food processing, then the physiological actions of the fibre fraction could be changed. The properties that must be considered are solubility, density hydration and ion-exchange capacities, particle size and susceptibility to microbial fermentation (Theander, 1976). It is also a mistake to believe that a faecal analysis for fibre will accurately reflect the intake of dietary fibre. A great deal occurs to fibre throughout the digestive tract, and a simple faecal analysis would underestimate the dietary fibre intake (Southgate, 1976a, b).

Because of the complexities involved in the analysis of all fibre components, it was the wish of the analysts to develop a method that would be a compromise between the ideal (all identifiable fractions quantitated individually) and a second method that would be a practical approach (the major components identified as TDF without destruction of residues so that further fractionations could be performed if desired).

Historical use of enzymatic methods was initiated by Williams and Olmsted (1935). Pancreatin was used to remove starch and protein followed by acid hydrolysis and subsequent identification and measurement of sugar fractions. Hellendoorn *et al.* (1975) employed pepsin for the hydrolysis of protein and subsequent starch hydrolysis by pancreatin. Asp (1978) and Schweizer and Würsch (1979) evaluated some of the more widely used methods for the analysis of dietary fibre and proposed enzymic modifications that utilize pepsin, pancreatin and α-amylase, the former employing a gravimetric method and the latter a chemical method for the individual components.

At the 93rd AOAC Meeting in Washington, Furda *et al.* (1979) proposed the use of physiological enzymes such as pancreatin and pepsin (free from hemicellulose and pectinase activity), which more nearly simulated human processes. In addition, they sought a measurement of the soluble fractions of dietary fibre. Heckman and Lane (1981) analyzed several foods by various dietary fibre methods: (1) ADF; (2) NDF by the Schaller modification employing hog pancreatic amylase; (3) Robertson's and Van Soest's enzyme-modified NDF employing *Bacillus subtilis* amylase; (4) Furda's method for soluble and insoluble dietary fibre using physiological enzymes; (5) Hellen-doorn's method for TDF; and (6) Southgate's method for TDF. Results showed that enzyme-modified NDF (3) were lower than NDF (2), depending principally upon the starch content of the foods examined. The Furda method (4), with its capability of measuring soluble dietary fibre, and its additional features of simplicity and rapidity, was thought to be the most promising.

Englyst *et al.* (1982) measured the non-starch polysaccharides (the major components of "dietary fibre") from plant foods. They removed starch from samples by use of hog pancreatic α-amylase together with pullulanase and amyloglucosidase and then analyzed the starch-free material by gas–liquid chromatography.

Finally, Theander and Åman (1982) also proposed a chemical method for dietary fibre. They measured the uronic acids and lignin after removal of starch by Termamyl (heat stable α-amylase) and amyloglucosidase.

In the end it was apparent that an enzyme-modified gravimetric method was the most practical and simplest way to meet the second challenge, i.e. the practical approach with the major components identified as fibre.

III. Additional dietary fibre methods in collaboration

There are at least two other major collaborative efforts under way at this time for the determination of fibre in foods and feeds. A study is being conducted by D. O. Holst, University of Missouri, Columbia, Missouri, U.S.A., to test the use of a ceramic fibre in place of asbestos (determined to be carcinogenic) as a filtering aid in the analysis for crude fibre.

R. Wood, of the Ministry of Agriculture, London, England, is conducting a comprehensive Fibre Collaborative Trail to obtain fibre methods which may be used to enforce labelling/claims regulations made in the U.K. Wood enclosed a copy of the AOAC Collaborative Method for TDF with his proposed methods when he sent the information to his collaborators in England. Wood alludes to the advantages of a common AOAC/U.K. procedure for the determination of TDF. Wood's study seeks collaboration in several methods including: (1) an assay for insoluble dietary fibre in cereals; (2) "a simple method for TDF based on obtaining the alcohol insoluble residue followed by starch, total nitrogen, ash and water determinations on that residue", proposed by D. A. T. Southgate; (3) a procedure for TDF based on starch gelatinization and removal by enzyme digestion, adapted by H. Englyst, similar to the one proposed by the AOAC except the AOAC method is gravimetric and Englyst's is a chemical method; (4) a method for the deter-mination of crude fibre; and (5) lignin determination by the Morrison method.

IV.   Development of the total dietary fibre method of Asp, De Vries, Furda and Schweizer for the AOAC collaborative study

The final version of the method under collaborative study was based on several methods (Asp, Englyst, Furda, Schweizer, Southgate, Theander, Van Soest) and was developed at General Mills, Inc., Minneapolis, Minnesota, U.S.A. by De Vries and Furda, at Kemicentrum, University of Lund, Sweden, by Asp and at Nestlé Research Department, La Tour-de-Peilz, Switzerland by Schweizer. It is quite possible that this method will lend itself to further modification (for example, chemical analysis of dietary fibre components) which would warrent another collaborative study in the future.

Since the method requires enzymes, first for the gelatinization and initial starch breakdown, then for protein and further starch digestion, the activity of enzymes was critical to the success of the method.

Termamyl [120 L, KNU/g (Kilo NOVO α-amylase unit)] employed for gelatinizatin and starch breakdown was graciously supplied by NOVO Laboratories, Inc., Wilton, Connecticut, U.S.A. Protease (P-5380 Subtilisin Carlsberg; Subtilopeptidase A, Type VIII, Bacterial, from a strain of *B. subtilis,* crystallized and lyophilized) was used for the hydrolysis of protein and possesses the following activity: one unit will hydrolyze casein to produce color equivalent to $1.0~\mu M$ of tryosine $(181~\mu g)$ per minute at pH 7.5 at 37°. Amyloglucosidase (A-9268, E.C.3.2.1.3), with the activity that one unit will liberate 1.0 mg of glucose from starch in 3 min at pH 4.5 and 55°C, was employed for starch digestion. Both the protease and the amyloglucosidase were purchased from Sigma Chemical Co., St. Louis, Missouri, U.S.A.

A sufficient quantity of the three enzymes necessary to the collaborative method had been pre-tested before shipment to the collaborators.

A.   Collaborators

The number of collaborators who expressed an interest in becoming a part of the study (42 collaborators from 14 countries) far exceeded the number required by the AOAC for a valid study (from 6 to 10). The countries represented were Canada, Denmark, Finland, France, Germany, Israel, Italy, The Netherlands, New Zealand, Norway, Sweden, Switzerland, United Kingdom, and the United States. Approximately one-half of the laboratories were in the United States.

The method was tested by chemists in the food industry, private institutes, universities, pharmaceutical houses, government and in clinical settings, attesting to the widespread interest in and desire for a standardized method to meet a variety of research and practical needs.

B.   Preparation of samples

The foods chosen for analysis and their preparation steps are described below. Unless otherwise stated, all foods were purchased in the metropolitan Washington area and sample preparation was conducted in the laboratories of the FDA.

1. Corn bran, A.E. Staley Manufacturing Co., Decatur, Illinois, U.S.A., Lot CFJ 3101 A-G Regular, was donated by the company and used as provided.

2. Iceburg lettuce. For every 350 g lettuce, 50 ml deionized water was added and the mixture was blended in a Waring blender for 2 min until homogeneous. The slurry was freeze-dried for 48 h and stored in tightly sealed plastic bags at room temperature until ready for shipment.

3. Oats, quick cooking, donated by The Quaker Oats Co., Barrington, Illinois, U.S.A., were blended in a Waring blender for 3 min and stored in plastic bags at room temperature until used.

4. Potatoes, instant, Giant Foods, Inc., Washington, D.C., U.S.A., were used directly.

5. Raisins, seedless, Giant Foods, Inc., Washington, D.C., U.S.A., were blended with enough water to make a thick paste, freeze-dried for 48 h, removed from the pan with a spatula and placed into the sample vials.

6. Rice, enriched, long grain, Giant Foods, Inc., Washington, D.C., U.S.A., was ground for 5 min in an electric Straub mixer (Philadelphia, Pennsylvania, Model number 4E) to a uniform powder. There was visible separation of the outer coating, leading to lack of uniformity of particles.

7. Rye bread (Deli-Rye) from Giant Foods, Inc., Washington, D.C., U.S.A., was broken into pieces about 1 × 3 cm in diameter, placed in an aluminum loaf pan and dried for 4 h at 80°C. The bread pieces were blended in a Waring blender for 2 min.

8. Soy isolate, donated by Ralston-Purina Co., St. Louis, Missouri, U.S.A., was used as received.

9. Wheat bran, American Association of Cereal Chemists Certified Food Grade, was purchased from the AACC in St. Paul, Minnesota, U.S.A.

10. Whole wheat flour,* high extraction, was donated by General Mills, Inc., Minneapolis, Minnesota, and used as received.

11. White wheat flour, low extraction, donated by General Mills, Inc., Minneapolis, Minnesota, was used as received.

12 and 13. These samples consisted of a non-vegetarian mixed diet and a lacto–ovo vegetarian mixed diet. The foods comprising the diet were taken from Oberleas and Harland (1981). Casseroles and baked goods were either purchased ready-to-eat, or prepared in the FDA laboratory. The 17 foods in

* Called wheat wholemeal in Britain.

TABLE 4.1. Daily diet for an adult non-vegetarian

Description of food[a]	Weight (g)
Wheat flakes (Grape Nut Flakes, Post's)	30.0
Sugar, granulated	5.0
Milk, 2% fat	350.9
Egg, medium, raw	51.0
White bread, sliced	75.0
Margarine	15.0
Orange juice	240.0
Coffee, brewed, Maxwell House, Electra-Perk	360.0
Roast beef	90.0
Tomato soup, Campbell Soup Co.	120.0
Carrots, raw	119.5
Banana	110.8
Green bean casserole with cheddar cheese	236.0
Corn, whole kernel, cooked	100.0
Iceberg lettuce wedge	155.0
Rolls, hard, French	50.0
Peach pie	131.0
	2239.2

[a] All foods were from Giant Foods, Inc., Washington D.C.

the non-vegetarian and 20 foods in the vegetarian diet are presented in Tables 4.1 and 4.2, with the amounts of each food expressed as grams per approximately 2200 grams of diet. After purchase or preparation of all foods listed in the diets, homogenates were prepared by adding foods one at a time and blending without the addition of water until a uniform homogenate was formed. The total time necessary to homogenize an entire diet was 1 h. The homogenates were freeze-dried for 48 h, and the powder was again blended in a Waring blender for 2 min before placing into sample vials.

Because the collaborative method recommended fat extraction if samples contained greater than 5% fat, we calculated the fat content of each diet (U.S. Department of Agriculture, 1963, 1976). Calculations showed both diets to contain greater than 5% fat, so fat extraction was recommended for samples 12 and 13.

All samples were placed in 25-ml scintillation vials with screw caps and the sample number was taped to each vial. Because lettuce had such a low density, two vials of lettuce were shipped to each collaborator.

C. The method, incorporating collaborators' suggestions

The AOAC Collaborative Study was initiated on January 25, 1982. Many valuable suggestions for improving the method were received from the collaborators, from simple hints for a more expeditious assay, to clarification of

TABLE 4.2. Daily diet for an adult lacto–ovo vegetarian

Description of food[a]	Weight of food added to composite (g)
Wheat germ pancakes, 1 Tbl. wheat germ/pancake	90.0
Margarine	25.0
Sugar, granulated	10.0
Apple, fresh	181.6
Granola mix consisting of almonds, coconut, sunflower seeds and raisins in equal proportions	32.6
Cheddar cheese	15.0
Grain and spice beverage, Celestial Seasonings Roast Aroma	180.0
Peanut butter, Peter Pan, Crunchy	30.0
Whole wheat bread,[b] sliced	56.0
Sliced tomatoes	120.0
Five-bean salad: navy, kidney, lima, wax and green beans; sugar and vinegar dressing	277.0
Fresh peach	188.0
Milk, fluid, vitamin D, homogenized	232.0
Spinach greens with lemon butter	219.0
Potato salad with egg	194.1
Corn pudding	62.0
Deli-rye bread, sliced	18.0
White cake, lightly iced	73.0
Peanuts for cake, salted, roasted, crushed	30.8
Coffee, brewed, Maxwell House, Electra-Perk	180.0
	2214.1

[a] All foods were from Giant Foods, Inc., Washington D.C.

[b] Called wheat wholemeal bread in Britain.

the formula to reflect the analytical steps actually performed. The basic method has not changed, but many of the improvements have been incorporated into the methodology. Some suggestions, such as substituting sand for Celite to facilitate filtering (suggested by Hellendoorn), must await further testing. The results of this interlaboratory study are reported in detail in Prosky *et al.* (1984a).

D.   Second collaborative study

A second collaborative study initiated and completed using a modified version of the previously described enzymatic–gravimetric procedure was presented (Prosky *et al.*, 1984b) at the AOAC International Meeting on October 30, 1984. This method was accepted as Official First Action by the AOAC.

1.   Definition

This method determines the amount of total dietary fibre in food ingredients and products.

Method Development: Asp, De Vries, Furda and Schweizer

Sample preparation, dried, pulverized and extracted with 25 ml petroleum ether
to remove lipids.

↓

Extraction repeated two times with 25 ml petroleum ether.
Weighing of duplicate samples, 1 g. Addition of 50 ml phosphate buffer, pH 6.0.
Addition of Termamyl for gelatinization, 100 μl.

↓

Incubation, boiling water bath, 15 min, shaking at 5-min intervals.
Adjustment to pH 7.5 with 0.285 N NaOH.

↓

Addition of protease, 5 mg. Incubation, 60°C, 30 min, continuous agitation.
Adjustment to pH 4.5 with 10 ml 0.329 M phosphoric acid.
Addition of amyloglucosidase, 0.3 ml. Incubation, 60°C, 30 min, continuous agitation.
Addition of 280 ml 95% ethyl alcohol, preheated to 60°C.

↓

Formation of precipitate, 60 min. Filtration through bed containing 0.5 g Celite 545.
Washed with three 20-ml portions of 75% ethyl alcohol, two 10-ml portions of 95% ethyl alcohol
and two 10-ml portions of acetone.

↓

Drying of crucibles, 70°C vacuum oven or 105°C air oven, overnight.
Cooling and weighing of crucibles.

↙   ↘

Protein determination, use entire crucible   Ash determination 525°C, 5 h, cool and
contents. Factor = 6.25   weigh.

Calculation of % TDF: weight of residue, minus weight of protein, minus weight of ash,
minus weight of blank

FIG. 4.1. Steps in the analysis of total dietary fibre.

2. *Scope*

This method is applicable to foods, food products and ingredients.

3. *Principle*

Duplicate samples of dried food extract are gelatinized with Termamyl, then
enzymatically digested with protease and amyloglucosidase to remove the
protein and starch present in the sample. Four volumes of 95% ethyl alcohol
are added to precipitate the soluble dietary fibre. The total residue is filtered
and washed with 75% ethyl alcohol, 95% ethyl alcohol and acetone. After
drying, the residue is weighed. One of the duplicates is analyzed for protein,
and the other is incinerated at 525°C and the ash measured. Total dietary
fibre is the weight of the residue minus the weight of the protein and ash
present. (See Fig. 4.1 for a flow chart of the method).

E. Reagents

1. Distilled water (DW).
2. 95% ethyl alcohol—technical grade.
3. 75% ethyl alcohol—place 250 ml of DW into a 1-litre volumetric flask.

Dilute to volume with 95% ethyl alcohol. Mix and bring to volume again with 95% ethyl alcohol if necessary. Mix.

4. Acetone—reagent grade.

5. Phosphate buffer pH 6.0—dissolve 1.5 g of sodium phosphate dibasic and 10.0 g sodium phosphate monobasic monohydrate in approximately 700 ml of DW. Dilute to 1 litre with DW and adjust pH to 6.0 by dropwise addition of phosphoric acid if necessary.

6. Termamyl (heat stable α-amylase) solution—120 litres (NOVO Laboratories, Inc., Wilton, Connecticut 06897). Store the enzyme solution in refrigerator after each use.

7. Protease-P-5380 (Sigma Chemical Co., St. Louis, Missouri 63178). Refrigerate the dry enzyme after each use.

8. Amyloglucosidase A-9268 (Sigma Chemical Co., St. Louis, Missouri 63178). Keep refrigerated when not in use.

9. Sodium hydroxide solution (0.285 N)—dissolve 11.4 g of sodium hydroxide AR in approximately 700 ml DW in a 1-litre volumetric flask. Dilute to volume with DW.

10. Phosphoric acid solution (0.329 M)—dissolve 37.9 g of phosphoric acid AR (85%) in DW in a 1-litre volumetric flask. Dilute to volume with DW.

Collaborators' Comments

Sodium hydroxide and phosphoric acid solutions prepared as instructed may not produce pH's within the ranges specified in either the blanks or the samples analyzed. To maintain correct pH, reagents of greater ionic strength may be used (0.333M NaOH, 0.376 M phosphoric acid). After testing the pH of all samples, minor dropwise additions of reagent may be necessary.

11. Celite 545 (Fisher Scientific Co., Fair Lawn, New Jersey, U.S.A.).

F. Apparatus

1. Balance, analytical, capable of weighing to 0.1 mg.

2. Fritted crucible (porosity No. 2, see note 1, p. 73). Clean thoroughly, ash at 525°C, soak in distilled water and rinse in same. Dry at 130°C for 1 h, cool, and store in desiccator until used in step 15.

Collaborators' Comments

Crucibles indicated in the procedure may not be available in Europe. Porosity No. 2 in Europe signifies pores of 40 to 90 μ whereas it means 40 to 60 μ in the United States. One-half gram of Celite is adequate for crucibles with a diameter of 3 cm. Greater diameters need more Celite, but then problems may arise during the analyses for residual protein. In Kjeldahl determinations, Celite presented "bumping" problems during the digestion stage, necessitating careful watching of flasks and the addition of more digestion acid.

3. Vacuum source—a vacuum pump or aspirator equipped with an in-line double vacuum flask should be used to prevent contamination in case of water backup.

4. Vacuum oven—70°C and desiccator (see note 2, p. 73).

5. Boiling water bath.

6. Constant temperature water bath adjustable to 60°C, and equipped to provide constant agitation of the digestion flasks during enzymatic hydrolysis. This can be accomplished with either a multistation shaker or multistation magnetic stirrer.

7. Vortex mixer.

8. Beaker—tall form, 400 ml.

G. Enzyme purity

To assure that undesirable enzymatic activity is not present in the enzymes used in this procedure, the materials listed in the table below should be run through the entire procedure each time the lot of enzymes is changed, or at a maximum interval of 6 months.

Test sample	Activity tested for	Sample weight (g)	Expected recovery (%)
Citrus pectin	Pectinase	0.1	95–100
Stractan (larch gum)	Hemicellulase	0.1	95–100
Wheat starch	Amylase	1.0	0–1
Corn starch	Amylase	1.0	0–2
Casein	Protease	0.3	0–2
β-glucan (oat gum)	β-glucanase	0.1	95–100 (see note 3)

H. Sample preparation

For this study, no sample preparation was required other than drying overnight at 70°C in a vacuum oven and cooling in a desiccator before weighing out the samples. If the fat content is higher than 5%, defat with petroleum ether (three times with 25-ml portions per gram of sample) before milling. Record the loss of weight due to fat removal and make the appropriate correction to the final percentage TDF. Store dry, milled sample in a capped jar in desiccator until analysis is carried out. When sample preparation is necessary, homogenize sample and dry overnight as described above and then dry mill a portion to 0.3 to 0.5 mm mesh. If sample cannot be heated, freeze dry before milling.

Collaborators' Comments:

When dealing with unknown samples it is best to fat-extract all samples. For fat extraction, place approximately 10 g of sample in a 250-ml beaker. Add 25 ml of petroleum ether. Stir with a magnetic stirrer for 15 min. Let beaker stand for 1 min. Decant the petroleum ether. Repeat two times, using 25 ml of petroleum ether each time. Place beaker into an oven (70°C) and dry overnight. If apparatus is unavailable for milling samples to pass a 0.3- or 0.4-mm mesh screen, grinding in a mortar may be sufficient.

I. Procedure

1. Run a blank through the entire procedure along with the samples to measure any contribution to the residue from the reagents. Measure the pH of the blank solutions in steps 5 and 8 to assure that desired pH is being obtained. (Make adjustments to reagents 9 and 10 if necessary.)

2. Weigh, in duplicate, 1 g of sample accurate to 0.1 mg into 400 ml tall form beakers. Add 50 ml of pH 6.0 phosphate buffer to each beaker.

3. Add 100 µl Termamyl solution.

4. Cover beaker with aluminum foil and place in boiling water bath for 15 min. Shake gently at 5-min intervals. Increase the length of incubation time when the number of beakers added to the boiling water bath makes it difficult for the beaker contents to reach an internal temperature of 100°C. Thirty minutes should be sufficient.

5. Cool. Adjust to pH 7.5 ± 0.1 by adding 10 ml of 0.285 N NaOH solution.

6. Add 5 mg of protease.

Collaborators' Comments

Since protease sticks to the spatula, it may be preferable to make an enzyme solution just prior to use with PO_4 buffer, pH 7.5, and pipette the required amount.

7. Cover with aluminum foil. Incubate at 60°C for 30 min with continuous agitation.

8. Cool. Add 10 ml of 0.329 M phosphoric acid solution to adjust pH to 4.5 ± 0.2.

9. Add 0.3 ml of amyloglucosidase solution.

10. Cover with aluminum foil. Incubate at 60°C for 30 min with continuous agitation.

11. Add 280 ml of 95% ethyl alcohol preheated to 60°C.

12. Allow precipitate to form at room temperature for 60 min.

13. Add approximately 0.5 g of Celite 545 to a dried crucible (porosity No. 2).

Collaborators' Comments

Add Celite to the crucibles before drying to obtain constant weight of crucibles and Celite.

Under step No. 14 of the procedure, after taring the crucible containing the Celite, re-distribute the bed of Celite in the crucible, using a stream of 75% ethyl alcohol from a wash bottle. Suction is then applied to the crucible to draw the Celite onto the fritted glass as an even mat. When the fibre is filtered, i.e. step 15, Celite effectively separates the fibre from the fritted glass of the crucible, allowing for easy removal of the crucible contents.

14. Tare crucible weight containing Celite to nearest 0.1 mg.

15. Filter enzyme digest from step 12 through crucible.

16. Wash residue successively with three 20-ml portions of 75% ethyl alcohol, two 10-ml portions of 95% ethyl alcohol, and two 10-ml portions of acetone.

Collaborators' Comments

With some samples, a gum is formed, trapping the liquid. If the surface film that develops after the addition of the sample to the Celite is broken with a spatula, filtration is improved. The time for filtration and washing varied from 1 to 6 h, averaging 1/2 h per sample.

17. Dry crucible containing residue overnight in a 70°C vacuum oven or a 105°C air oven.

18. Cool in desiccator and weigh crucible, Celite and residue to nearest 0.1 mg.

19. Analyze the residue from one sample of the set of duplicates for protein. (Factor = 6.25.)

Collaborators' Comments

Protein is probably most easily analyzed by carefully scraping the Celite and the fiber mat onto a suitable piece of filter paper which can then be folded shut and analyzed for protein. A piece of filter paper should be analyzed to ensure that it will not affect the protein value obtained or that it can be corrected for in the calculation of protein value. Various collaborators used an automated micro-Kjeldahl setup or proceeded according to the Kjeldahl analysis as specified in the Association of Official Analytical Chemists (1980). Use 6.25 for the protein factor in all cases for which the nature of the protein is unknown. The appropriate protein factor for the particular protein (if known) should be used. For example, for plant protein the factor may be 5.7.

20. Incinerate second sample of the duplicate for 5 h at 525°C.

21. Cool in desiccator. Weigh crucible containing Celite and ash to nearest 0.1 mg.

Collaborators' Comments

Runs should be made in quadruplicate so that duplicate protein and ash values would then be available to increase confidence in the results. Formula for calculating total dietary fibre

$$\% \text{ TDF} = \left[\frac{R(1 - P) - (A - C)}{W} - B\right] \times 100$$

where R = average weight, in milligrams, of residues obtained from duplicate samples, i.e. $R = (R_1 + R_2)/2$; P = fraction of protein present in residue expressed as a decimal, i.e. for a sample containing 5% protein, $P = 0.05$; A = weight of crucible, Celite, and ash, in milligrams; C = weight of crucible and Celite, in milligrams; B = blank correction factor, i.e. $B = R' (1 - P') - (A' - C')$. R', P', A' and C' are values, in milligrams, obtained from duplicates run on blank; W = average weight of duplicate samples, in milligrams.

Notes

1. The fritted crucible is a Pyrex 32940, Coarse ASTM 40–60μ, and may be purchased from: (a) Scientific Products Co., C-8525-1; (b) V.W.R. Scientific Co., 23863-040; (c) Fisher Scientific Co., 08237-1A; (d) Sargent Welch Co., F-243-90-B or -C depending on size needed.

2. Alternatively, an air oven capable of operating at 105°c may be used.

3. The enzyme system used here should be tested for β-glucanase activity when this method is used for analysis of glucan-containing materials. Methods for the preparation of β-glucan can be found in reference 3 below. The β-glucan source may be oat gum or barley gum.*

J.   Results

As results came in, they were verified by a computer program developed for this purpose. From time to time, tests were run to determine the within-and between-laboratory variation. Further tests were made using the Dixon outlier and Youden rank sum tests (Youden and Steiner, 1975). Table 4.3 shows a summary of the data from 29 laboratories that had sent in their results as this chapter went to press. Results are given as the average together with the standard error of the mean and the coefficient of variation. It is apparent from the data that the analysis of several foods does present a large coefficient of variation; however, when one considers the components that are being determined, the variations become understandable. The rice and soy isolate presented us with the major problems but also gave us insight into their solutions. Rice was highest in starch; therefore the enzymatic methodology

* High-purity barley gum is commercially available from Biocon U.S., Inc., 2348 Palumbo Drive, Lexington, Kentucky 40509.

TABLE 4.3. Association of Official Analytical Chemists
Collaborative Study (% total dietary fiber[a])

Food	Mean	Standard error	Coefficient of variation (%)
Corn bran	88.76	0.51	2.96
Lettuce	23.75	0.48	0.59
Oats	12.93	0.59	24.60
Potatoes	7.04	0.27	20.60
Raisins	4.63	0.23	26.56
Rice	4.14	0.47	58.45
Rye bread	6.02	0.29	25.08
Soy isolate	7.98	1.42	95.99
Wheat bran	42.43	0.35	4.36
Whole wheat flour[b]	12.76	0.25	9.72
White flour	3.28	0.22	34.76
Mixed diet (non-veg.)	7.59	0.34	24.11
Mixed diet (veg.)	8.93	0.47	28.00

[a] Values represent duplicate determinations performed in
29 laboratories.
[b] Called wheat wholemeal in Britain.

TABLE 4.4. A comparison of values obtained in the AOAC Collaborative
Study with values obtained using four other analytical procedures[a]
(% total dietary fibre)

Food	AOAC	(A)	(B)	(C)	(D)
Corn bran[b]	88.76	78.23	76.50	82.40	85.62
Lettuce	23.75	18.69	25.40	20.31	21.85
Oats	12.93	7.59	10.00	7.00	10.25
Potatoes	7.04	6.07	9.50	7.03	7.26
Raisins	4.63	1.89	4.90	4.03	2.83
Rice	4.14	0.62	2.60	1.49	1.95
Rye bread	6.02	3.89	7.90	2.90	4.59
Soy isolate	7.98	0.97	5.70	—	2.33
Wheat bran	42.43	32.29	37.20	34.80	39.84
Whole wheat flour[c]	12.76	9.98	10.30	11.30	11.41
White flour	3.28	1.83	3.10	3.90	2.22
Mixed diet (non-veg.)	7.59	4.65	6.80	6.16	5.50
Mixed diet (veg.)	8.93	5.51	6.20	6.90	6.70

[a] References: (A) Englyst (1982); (B) Theander and Åman (1982); (C)
Schweizer and Würsch (1979); (D) N-G., Asp (modified Hellendoorn)
(personal communication).
[b] Called maize bran in Britain.
[c] Called wheat wholemeal in Britain.

for its removal was critical from the point of view of the activity of the enzyme and the temperature and time of incubation. The soy isolate was probably complicated by a high protein value, which has led us to call for a standardization in the protein determination (Kjeldahl). Both of these errors in our methods writeup have been corrected and/or clarified.

Table 4.4 lists the values of dietary fibre obtained in the AOAC Collaborative Study along with those values obtained in four laboratories where the investigators used their own method for determining dietary fibre. The greatest disparity of results occurred in the two previously mentioned foods, rice and soy isolate. What is remarkable is the similarity of values from the various laboratories using different methods. The greatest disagreement was between the method of Englyst et al. (1982) and the four other methods. Values by this method were always lower, probably because of the incomplete starch removal in the other methods. However, the results of all four methods fell within the coefficient of variation of the AOAC method, and this coefficient of variation will surely be reduced by the modifications that have been introduced. A more complete working of the data will be presented to the AOAC when all the data have been received and evaluated by the personnel involved in the development of the method.

Acknowledgements

We would like to acknowledge the invaluable contributions of Dr. Richard Albert, statistician, Ms. Clarisse Jones, technician, and Ms. Donna Waldrop, typist, in the preparation of this chapter.

References

American Association of Cereal Chemists. (AACC) (1978). "Approved Methods of the AACC", Revisions: Method 32-20. AACC, St. Paul, Minnesota.

ANDERSON, J. W. (1982). In "Dietary Fiber in Health and Disease" (G. V. Vahouny and D. Kritchevsky, eds), pp. 151–167. Plenum, New York.

ASP, N.-G. (1978). In "Dietary Fibre" (K. W. Heaton, ed), pp. 21–26. Newman Publishing, London. Association of Official Analytical Chemists (AOAC) (1980). "Official Methods of Analysis" (W. Horwitz, ed). 13th edition, Sects. 47.021, 47.033, 47.022, p. 858. Washington, D.C.

BAIRD, I. M. and ORNSTEIN, M. H. (eds). (1981). "Dietary Fibre: Progress Toward the Future." Kellogg Company of Great Britain, Manchester.

BROWNE, C. A. (1940). J. Assoc. Off. Agric. Chem. 23, 102–108.

BURKITT, D. P., WALKER, A. R. P. and PAINTER, N. S. (1972). Lancet 2, 1408–1412.

EINHOF, H. (1806). Ann Ackerb. 4, 627.

ENGLYST, H. N. and CUMMINGS, J. H. (1984). Analyst 109, 937–942.

ENGLYST, H., WIGGINS, H. S. and CUMMINGS, J. H. (1982). Analyst 107, 307–318.

FURDA, I., GENGLER, S. C., JOHNSON, R. R., MAGNUSON, J. S. and SMITH, D. E. (1979). AOAC 93rd Ann. Meet. Abstract, p. 87.

HECKMAN, M. M. and LANE, S. (1981). J. Assoc. Off. Anal. Chem. 64, 1339–1343.

HELLENDOORN, E. W., NOORDHOFF, M. G., and SLAGMAN, J. (1975). *J. Sci. Food Agric.* **26**, 1461–1468.

HIPSLEY, E. H. (1953). *Br. Med. J.* **2**, 420–422.

International Symposium (1982a). "Fibre in Human and Animal Nutrition." Massey University, Palmerston North, New Zealand.

International Symposium (1982b). "Dietary Fibre." National College of Food Technology, University of Reading, Weybridge, Surrey.

"Marabou Food and Fibre" Symposium (1976). Marabou, Sundbyberg, Sweden, reprinted in *Nutr. Rev.* **35**, 4–72. (1977).

OBERLEAS, D. and HARLAND, B. F. (1981). *J. Am. Diet. Assoc.* **79**, 433–436.

PROSKY, L. (1981). AOAC Spring Workshop, Ottawa, Canada.

PROSKY, L. and HARLAND, B. F. (1979). *AOAC 93rd Ann. Meet.*

PROSKY, L. and HARLAND, B. F. (1981). *AOAC 95th Annu. Meet.* Abstract 63.

PROSKY, L. and HARLAND, B. F. (1982). *AOAC 96th Annu. Meet.* Abstract 103.

PROSKY, L., ASP, N.-G., FURDA, I., DE VRIES, J. W., SCHWEIZER, T. F., and HARLAND, B. F. (1984a). *J. Assoc. Off. Anal. Chem.* **67**, 1044–1052.

PROSKY, L., ASP, N.-G., FURDA, I., DE VRIES, J. W., SCHWEIZER, T. F., and HARLAND, B. F. (1984b). AOAC 98th Annu. Meet. Abstract 270.

ROTH, H. P. and MEHLMAN, M. A. (1978). *Am. J. Clin. Nutr. Suppl.* **31**, S1–S291.

SAUNDERS, R. M. and BETSCHART, A. A. (1980). *Am. J. Clin. Nutr.* **33**, 960–961.

SCHWEIZER, T. E. and WURSCH, P. (1979). *J. Sci. Food Agric.* **30**, 613–619.

SOUTHGATE, D. A. T. (1969). *J. Sci. Food Agric.* **20**, 331–335.

SOUTHGATE, D. A. T. (1976a). *J. Hum. Nutr.* **30**, 303–313.

SOUTHGATE, D. A. T. (1976b). *In* "Marabou Food and Fibre Symposium", Vol. 20, Suppl. 14, pp. 31–37. Reprinted in *Nutr. Rev.* **35**, 31–37. (1977).

SPILLER, G. A. and KAY, R. M. (1979). *Am. J. Clin. Nutr.* **32**, 2102–2103.

THEANDER, O. (1976). *In* "Marabou Food and Fibre Symposium", Suppl. 14, pp. 23–30. reprinted in *Nutr. Rev.* **35**, 23–30. (1977).

THEANDER, O. and ÅMAN, P. (1982). *J. Sci. Food Agric.* **33**, 340–344.

THEANDER, O. and JAMES, P. (1979). *In* "Dietary Fibres: Chemistry and Nutrition" (G. E. Inglett and S. Falkehag, eds), pp. 245–249. Academic Press, New York and London.

TROWELL, H. (1974). *Lancet* **1**, 503.

TROWELL, H., SOUTHGATE, D. A. T., WOLEVER, T. M. S., LEEDS, A. R., GASSULL, M. A. and JENKINS, D. J. A. (1976). *Lancet* **1**, 967.

U.S. Department of Agriculture (1963). "Composition of Foods, Raw, Processed and Prepared", Handbook No. 8. Agric. Res. Serv., USDA, Washington, D.C.

U.S. Department of Agriculture (1976). "Composition of Foods, Raw, Processed and Prepared", Handbook No. 8-1. Agric. Res. Serv., USDA, Washington, D.C.

U.S. Department of Agriculture and U.S. Department of Health and Human Services (1980). "Nutrition and Your Health. Dietary Guidelines for Americans." USDA, HHS, Washington, D.C.

VAHOUNY, G. and KRITCHEVSKY, D. (eds). (1982). "Dietary Fiber in Health and Disease." Plenum, New York.

VAN SOEST, P. J. (1963). *J. Assoc. Off. Agric. Chem.* **46**, 825–829.

VAN SOEST, P. J. (1973). *J. Assoc. Off. Anal. Chem.* **56**, 781–784.

VAN SOEST, P. J. and McQUEEN, R. W. (1973). *Proc. Nutr. Soc.* **32**, 123–130.

VAN SOEST, P. J. and WINE, R. H. (1967). *J. Assoc. Off. Anal. Chem.* **50**, 50–55.

VAN SOEST, P. J., WINE, R. H. and MOORE, L. A. (1966). *Proc. Int. Grassl. Congr. 10th, 1966*, p. 438.

WILLIAMS, R. D. and OLMSTED, W. D. (1935). *J. Biol. Chem.* **108**, 653–666.

YOUDON, W. J. and STEINER, E. H. (1975). "Statistical Manual of the Association of Official Analytical Chemists." AOAC, Arlington, Virginia.

Chapter 5

Dietary fibre intakes: intake studies, problems, methods and results

SHEILA BINGHAM

I. Introduction

The present time is one of radical change in medical opinion concerning the quality of the "Western" diet and its relation to health. A major impetus to this change is the dietary fibre hypothesis which states that low intakes of fibre in Western industrialised countries, when compared with rural Africa, are responsible for a number of common diseases such as heart disease, diabetes, obesity and bowel disorders (Burkitt, 1969; Burkitt and Trowell, 1975).

However, the dietary fibre content of most of the world's foods is unknown, and existing methods for the measurement of fibre give widely differing values for the same food (Englyst and Cummings, 1983). Furthermore, there are many different ways to assess the amount of food people eat and

Dietary Fibre, Fibre-Depleted Foods
and Disease

each method is associated with some error. Apparent differences in dietary fibre consumption between populations may thus be blurred due to differences in methodology.

Because of these problems in fibre analysis and in the measurement of food consumption, there have been few good epidemiological studies in the past 15 years of dietary fibre research. There is little useful information available on the consumption of dietary fibre in most of the world's populations, and for some areas, such as South America, parts of Asia, the middle East, Russia and China, there are no data at all. Some information for Europe, Africa, Australasia, Japan and North America does exist, and is summarised in the later sections of this chapter.

Future progress in dietary fibre epidemiology lies in the establishment of a clear relationship in individuals between dietary fibre intake and eventual outcome of disease. Since there are many other differences in diet, lifestyle, and individual response that will tend to obscure any relationship at the individual level within a population, if it exists, it is of great importance that the errors in assessing dietary fibre intake are minimised. These errors are discussed in the first part of this chapter.

II.   Assessment of dietary fibre intake in individuals

A pre-requisite for the estimation of dietary fibre intake is accurate information about the amount of food eaten. The most widely available data, which have been used in many correlation studies, are based on the "per capita" method whereby food available at a national or household level is divided by the number of people for which it is intended. The limitations of this method are easily recognised; for example, no information can be obtained about distribution of intake amongst men and women of different ages. In the United Kingdom, per capita intakes calculated from national statistics overestimate actual food consumption by about 25% (Ministry of Agriculture, Fisheries and Food, 1953–1979, see 1971). With a stable population base, however, these data can be used to give an idea of secular trends, seasonal variation and geographical differences within a country.

A.   Methods for assessing food consumption of individuals

For specific groups or individuals within a population, there are a variety of ways in which average food intake can be estimated (Marr, 1971; Pekkarinen, 1970; James *et al.*, 1981; Bazarre and Myers, 1980). Subjects may be sent a questionnaire through the post asking for information about usual diet, or they may be interviewed by a person trained in the technique of obtaining a history of food consumption during the past weeks or months, or of a single report of the preceding day (the 24-h recall). These methods depend on the ability of the subject to remember not only how often but also the type of food eaten and the amount. There are obvious potential sources of error which, until recently, have been assumed to be random and therefore unimportant. If the number of subjects included in a study is sufficiently large, random errors cancel eliminating bias in the overall mean.

Recent comparative studies of one method with another on the same individuals suggest the contrary. Reports of food intake assessed from a single 24-h recall tend to give overall mean estimates of consumption which are up to 30% less than those assessed by more objective measures (Isaksson, 1980; Acheson et al., 1980; James et al., 1981). Food intake measured by diet history of usual food consumption gives values up to 30% greater compared with detailed records of food intake (Jain et al., 1980; Huenemann and Turner, 1942). Different methods of assessing food consumption thus create difficulties of interpretation if the fibre consumption of different populations is to be compared.

Furthermore, results using different methods in the same individual rarely agree, particularly at the extremes of intake (Bazarre and Myers, 1980; Linussen et al., 1974). These inaccuracies will attenuate relationships at the individual level between diet and disease (Liu et al., 1978; Beaton et al., 1979). Gross misclassification of individuals will, of course, invalidate any attempt to group people into classes of disease incidence according to dietary intake.

The most objective method currently available for measuring food consumption relies on careful weighing and recording of all food eaten. Such scrutiny itself may disturb a person's normal eating pattern and so it is preferable to validate this (or any other method) using an independent indicator of food intake. The 24-h urine nitrogen excretion (Isaksson, 1980; Bingham et al., 1982) has been used to validate dietary methods, although the urine collections must be shown to be complete (Bingham and Cummings, 1983). However, the usual 1 week of weighing may not be enough to assess a person's average intake due to both seasonal variation and the magnitude of daily fluctuations in dietary fibre intake.

B. Seasonal variation

There is little information on seasonal variation in fibre intake of individuals, but published data from two household surveys show that seasonal changes occur. As a consequence, dietary surveys to assess fibre intake must take into account the time of the year.

Between 1963 and 1965, a dietary survey was carried out for Euratom in 11 rural areas of the European Economic Community (EEC) to determine radioactive contamination of foodstuffs (Cresta et al., 1969). The areas were chosen on the basis of their dietary patterns and likely cooperation rates and

TABLE 5.1. Monthly coefficients of variation
in dietary fibre intake in 11 regions
of the European Economic Community[a]

Area[b]	Vegetables[c]	Cereal	Total
Friesland (H)	8.1	13.1	7.3
Gent (B)	8.2	14.3	7.4
Liege (B)	7.2	6.4	4.7
Luxembourg	17.1	6.9	13.7
Hessen (G)	13.6	5.3	5.2
Normandy (F)	10.9	8.9	7.4
Bretagne (F)	17.2	13.1	11.8
Vendee (F)	25.0	6.8	14.8
Fruili (I)	20.8	16.6	12.0
Campania (I)	23.0	13.4	12.3
Basilicata (I)	18.6	5.9	6.4
Between regions	30.0	26.1	9.1

[a] Values given as percentages.

[b] H, Holland; B, Belgium; G, Germany; F, France; I, Italy.

[c] Includes potatoes.

over a period of 3 years about 30 families per month were studied. Each family weighed all their food after preparing it, thus eliminating the need to correct for inedible wastage, and the total food intake was then divided by the number of persons in the household. Monthly food consumption figures have been used to calculate dietary fibre intakes, using the British food tables (Paul and Southgate, 1978).

Table 5.1 shows the coefficients of variation from month to month in each of the 11 regions for total, cereal and vegetable dietary fibre intake. In some areas (Luxembourg, Bretagne, Vendee, Fruili and Campania), the variation between months was greater than the variation between areas—for example, over the whole year Normandy and Fruili had identical intakes of 25 g of dietary fibre per head per day. If, however, dietary fibre intakes had been assessed in April, in Fruili they would have been 19 g, and in Normandy 27 g—a difference of 8 g/day.

The second survey for which data on food consumption by season is available is the British National Food Survey (Ministry of Agriculture, Fisheries and Food, 1953–1979). In the National Food Survey, housewives are asked to keep a record of their food purchases for 1 week, together with details of food grown by the family. The amount of food coming into the household is calculated from these records and divided equally by the number of people living there. About 6500 households randomly selected from the electoral registers of England, Scotland and Wales take part throughout the year, and the survey has been conducted annually since 1950. Fibre intakes for the four

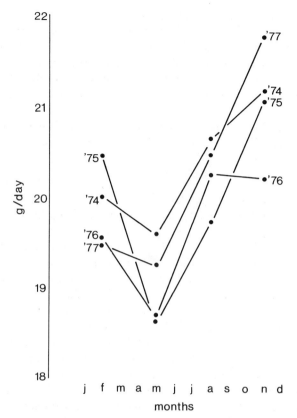

FIG. 5.1. Total dietary fibre intakes for each quarter of the year (January–March; April–June; July–September; October–December) calculated from the U.K. National Food Survey for 1974, 1975, 1976 and 1977 (g/person/day).

quarters of the year from 1974 to 1977 have been calculated using the British Food Tables, taking account of inedible wastage. Figure 5.1 shows the value for total dietary fibre, and Fig. 5.2 for vegetable fibre (excluding potatoes). In contrast to the EEC study, seasonal variation in total dietary fibre intake is much less, although fibre intakes are significantly lower in the second quarter (April–June) and highest in the fourth (October–December). Vegetable fibre intakes are highest in the winter months because the type of vegetables eaten in winter (root vegetables, brussel sprouts, etc.) contain more fibre than the traditional summer salad vegetables (tomatoes, lettuce, cucumber, etc.).

C. Daily variation

In the past, food intake in individuals has been estimated on the basis of traditional patterns in food habits over 1 week. Recently, using statistical techniques, the extent to which an individual can be expected to vary from

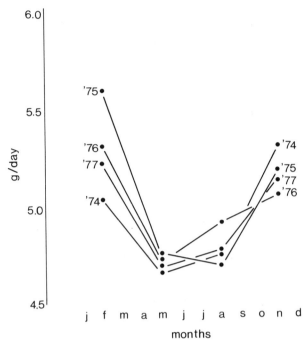

FIG. 5.2. Dietary fibre intake from vegetables (excluding potatoes) for each quarter of the year calculated from the U.K. National Food Survey (g/person/day). See Fig. 5.1 for details.

day to day in dietary intake has been calculated. This is an important development because this variation is in fact very large and the precision, and therefore the significance of findings in a dietary study, is to a large extent dependent on the number of days over which an individual is studied (Liu *et al.*, 1978; Beaton *et al.*, 1979; Marr, 1981; James *et al.*, 1981). Not infrequently the coefficient of variation in nutrient intake from day to day in individuals is 50% and the resulting large standard error associated with individual mean intakes assessed for only a short period of time can give highly misleading results.

The extent of daily variation, and the distribution of intakes amongst individuals, is characteristic of a population. Two recent surveys specifically designed to assess fibre intake in randomly selected population samples show that individual daily variation is greater than that from season to season. From these surveys, an idea of the number of days of recording necessary to classify an individual to a given level of precision can be shown.

In the first survey, in 1977, 31 men aged 20–80 years were randomly selected from the electoral register of a Cambridgeshire village and asked to weigh all food and drink eaten for 7 days (Bingham *et al.*, 1979a). In the second survey, in 1978, groups of 30 men aged 50–59 were randomly selected

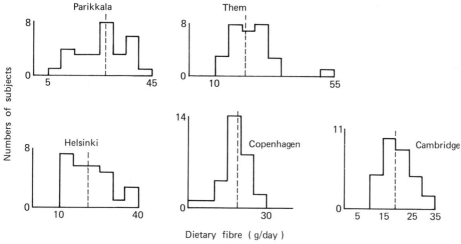

FIG. 5.3. The distribution of average individual daily dietary fibre (expressed as monosac-charides plus lignin) intakes calculated from 4- and 7-day records in Scandinavia and Cambridge.

from population registers in four areas of Scandinavia: Them in rural Den-mark; Parikkala in rural Finland; Helsinki; Copenhagen; and Cambridge. A standard protocol, consisting of a 4-day weighed food record, was used in each of these four areas, and dietary intake data validated using 24-h urine and faecal nitrogen excretion (Bingham *et al.*, 1982). The food records were then processed using a computer programme based on the British Food Tables and values for rye flour (Englyst, 1981).

In Fig. 5.3, the distribution of individual daily dietary fibre intakes are shown. The large range suggests that it might be easy to distinguish the intake of one individual from another within a population, as is necessary for example in a prospective study. However, the ability to do this depends on the ratio of the between subject and the within (daily) variation in fibre intake (Gardner and Heady, 1973; Marr, 1981). The within person variation can be calculated using analysis of variance of the dietary records. For these five populations, the standard deviations for daily dietary fibre intake for indi-viduals are shown in Table 5.2 together with the standard deviations between subjects in each area. It can be seen that the extent of daily variation was such that the pooled daily (within) person variation was almost as great as the between person variation in all five areas. As an illustration of the way in which people vary from day to day, the course of one individual's intake of dietary fibre over the 4 days in which he weighed his food was 37, 29, 10 and 14 g/day. This individual spanned virtually the whole range of fibre intakes, and if he had been assessed solely on the first day of the survey he would have been classified as eating 37 g of dietary fibre; however, if he had been assessed

TABLE 5.2. Standard deviations (g/day) for total non-starch polysaccharides[a] and lignin[b]

	Parikkala	Them	Helsinki	Copenhagen	Cambridge
Between individuals	8.7	7.1	6.5	4.2	4.7
Within individuals	7.3	5.0	6.4	5.1	6.9

[a] As monosaccharides.
[b] NSP and lignin are alternative terms for dietary fibre.

on the third day, he would have been thought to have been consuming under a third of this.

If the variance between and within individuals is known, it is then possible to work out the number of days necessary to record dietary intake before individuals can be classified into groups within the population (Gardner and Heady, 1973). The number of days will vary depending on the level of precision one wishes to attain (Marr, 1981) but simply to have classified 80% of the men in these populations into their correct third of intake of dietary fibre would have taken up to 10 days of weighing and recording food (Table 5.3). Table 5.3 shows that vegetable fibre intakes are particularly difficult to assess.

These calculations are based on pooled variances and assume that every individual varies to the same extent from day to day. However, there is a distribution in the extent of daily variation with some individuals varying little, whereas others vary markedly. This has to be taken into account if one wishes to classify each individual to within a stated level of accuracy. Table 5.4 for example, shows the number of records necessary to classify 50, 70 and 90% of individuals within the Cambridge population to within $\pm 10\%$ (SE) of each individual's mean intake of fibre, fat, protein and energy.

Prolonged periods of observation may be necessary, taking into account seasonal variation, to establish an individual's dietary fibre intake. It is unlikely that diet histories, designed to assess several months' intake in one interview, can short-circuit this problem since individual results from interviews do not agree with records kept over a comparable period of time (Huenemann and Turner, 1942; Jain et al., 1980). The problem of in-

TABLE 5.3. Number of days required to classify 80% of men into their correct third of dietary fibre intake at $p < .05$

Item	Parikkala	Them	Helsinki	Copenhagen	Cambridge
Total dietary fibre	4	3	5	7	10
Pentose	6	2	4	12	12
Cereal fibre	4	2	3	8	10
Vegetable fibre	25	8	27	49	18

TABLE 5.4. Number of days required to determine
the mean nutrient intake[a] of individual subjects[b]
with a standard error of ± 10%

	Number of days for:		
Nutrient	50% of population	70% of population	90% of population
Energy	5	7	13
Protein	5	7	14
Fat	9	13	23
NSP	12	13	28

[a] Fibre, fat, protein and energy.
[b] Randomly selected Cambridgeshire men aged 20–80
years ($n = 32$).

terpretation is increased by the varied individual responses to a given dietary
intake (Cummings and Stephen, 1980; Ahrens, 1979) and interrelations with
other dietary components that will attenuate relationships in even the most
carefully conducted epidemiological studies.

D. Definition and analysis of dietary fibre

A further difficulty in establishing dietary fibre intake is the lack of an agreed
method for its analysis in food. Even if accurate information on food consumption is available, this has then to be converted into fibre intake using
tables or direct analysis. With only two exceptions, food tables throughout
the world contain values for fibre measured as crude fibre. This measurement
of fibre was developed originally for animal foodstuffs and is irrelevant to
human nutrition since the majority of cellulose and hemicellulose is not
measured in the analytical procedure. Its deficiencies have been reviewed by
Van Soest and McQueen (1973). Reports of fibre intake using crude fibre
data are not included in this chapter.

The various chemical methods that exist for dietary fibre differ markedly
in their approach. They are discussed in detail elsewhere in this volume
(Southgate and Englyst, Chapter 3). Briefly, one approach is the gravimetric
one whereby other constituents of food are removed and the residue designated dietary fibre. A well researched example of this is the neutral detergent
method (Goering and Van Soest, 1970). Other gravimetric methods include
a digestion stage using starch- and protein-removing enzymes to simulate
what is happening in the human small intestine (Hellendoorn et al., 1975;
Asp, 1978). With these techniques there is uncertainty as to exactly what is
being measured, although collaborative studies have shown that incomplete
starch removal, loss of water-soluble polysaccharides and contamination with

other cell-wall constituents account for some of the variation between them (James and Theander, 1981).

The method for measuring dietary fibre described by Southgate first in 1969, with its subsequent modifications (Southgate, 1976; Southgate *et al.*, 1978b) has been the most suitable available for human nutrition in recent years. It is based on removal of starch using α-amylase and hydrolysis of the remaining cellulose and non-cellulosic polysaccharides. The resulting sugars are measured colorimetrically. Most of the data in this chapter are based on food analyses using this method (Southgate *et al.*, 1976; Southgate, 1978; Paul and Southgate, 1978) supplemented with data from McCance *et al.* (1936) and for a few foods, the method of Englyst (Englyst *et al.*, 1982b). The efficacy of starch removal, however, is of great importance. Food processing, cooking and even the way in which samples are prepared may affect the structure of starch so that it becomes resistant to the action of α-amylase (Englyst *et al.*, 1982b). The Southgate method thus has been criticised (Selvendran *et al.*, 1979).

Dietary fibre, in chemical terms, is mainly polysaccharide (Cummings, 1980) and in terms of food composition is best seen as such. Lignin is difficult to measure and in fact is present in only small amounts in the human diet. The isolation of dietary polysaccharides and their separation into starch and non-starch polysaccharides (NSP) (or dietary fibre) has been the objective of more recent methods for measuring dietary fibre in food (Englyst *et al.*, 1982b; Theander and Aman, 1979). Until tables of food composition are available using these more precise methods, the data in this chapter are open to revision.

III.   Dietary fibre intakes worldwide

Few papers of food intake record dietary fibre values, and those that do are usually based on the British Food Tables (Paul and Southgate, 1978). It is possible, however, to add fibre calculations to studies where details of food consumption are available. Some data on African diets were obtained as long ago as the 1920s, but the wealth of detail in these studies makes retrospective analysis of them possible. Bearing in mind the methodological problems in assessing dietary fibre intake, it may be some time before the final values are known.

A.   Europe

1.   United Kingdom

(a) *Present day intakes.* In an attempt to measure dietary fibre intakes in the United Kingdom, the food intake of 63 men and women, aged 20–80 years and randomly selected from the electoral register in part of Cambridgeshire, was determined by asking them to weigh all items of food over 1 week (Bingham *et al.*, 1979a). Dietary fibre intake was 19.9 ± 5.3 g/day, with no differences in total fibre intake between the sexes. Vegetables contributed 41.3% (8.2 g) to the total intake, cereals 30.5% (5.8 g) and fruit 11.7% (2.3 g). Dietary fibre intake was also calculated from the National Food Survey for 1976 and found to be 19.7 g/day. The close agreement between the average data from the National Food Survey and the individual survey was notable, because the two methods of assessing food consumption were quite different. From a completely different data base, that of food supplies for the whole population, Southgate *et al.* (1978a) calculated that dietary fibre intakes in 1970 were 22.7 g/day. These independently derived data taken together reinforce the view that fibre intakes are around 20 g/day at present in the United Kingdom.

(*b*) *Geographical variation.* Data from the National Food Survey also show that there are differences amongst the various geographical regions in Britain in food consumption. For example, more fruit, vegetables and brown bread are consumed in the Southeast, more beef and less vegetables in Scotland, and more butter in Wales. Using these data, the intake of dietary fibre for each of the nine standard regions from 1969 to 1973 was calculated and intakes of fibre–pentose were shown to be lowest in Scotland (Bingham *et al.*, 1979b).

Scotland. Two surveys of randomly selected population samples, in Edinburgh and the Orkney Islands, have shown fibre intakes to be lower than those in Cambridge, in line with the National Food Survey data. In Edinburgh, 40-year-old men were randomly selected from population registers in 1976 as part of a study to identify factors which might explain the threefold difference in mortality from ischaemic heart disease between Edinburgh and Stockholm, Sweden (Thomson *et al.*, 1982). The 97 men who took part were asked to weigh their food for 1 week and dietary fibre and other nutrients were calculated using the British Food Tables. Average energy intakes (±SE) were 12.1 ± 0.2 MJ of which 38% was supplied by fat and 9% by alcohol. The P:S ratio of 0.23 was similar to that of 0.20 assessed from the National Food Survey. Average dietary fibre intake was 17.5 ± 0.6 g in these men, significantly lower than the Cambridge average of 19.9 g, although more dietary fibre came from cereals (7.6 g). There was a sixfold range in total intake, from 6 to 36 g, in the individual values. Even lower intakes of dietary fibre were found by Eastwood *et al.* (1982), also in Edinburgh, but this time in a group of volunteers. Average fibre intakes were 15.9 ± 6.1 g in men, and only 12.7 ± 4.6 in women.

The second survey was in one of the most northerly islands of Scotland, Westray, which is part of the Orkney Islands. The island was chosen because of its stable local population, and because no previous quantitative survey had been carried out in this region (Bull *et al.*, 1982). Sixteen men and 27 women, aged 21–69, randomly selected from the population, took part and kept a food diary over a month in August, 1979. Energy intakes in the men were high (11.3 MJ/day) because most were engaged in moderately active occupations, such as fishing. Apart from fish and some vegetables most of the food eaten was imported. Dietary fibre intakes were again low in comparison with the National average, 16.5 g for the men, and 15.0 g for the women.

(*c*) *Vegetarians.* Another group whose fibre intakes differ from the average in England are vegetarians, who in two studies have been shown to eat from 33 to 41 g/day. In the first, dietary intakes were measured, by use of a dietary questionnaire, in 189 subjects selected from the patient lists of family doctors in Oxford, and in 55 members of the United Kingdom Vegetarian Society (Gear *et al.*, 1979). All the subjects were 45 years of age or older. Total dietary fibre intake in the general practice population was similar to the national average, 21.4 ± 8.2 g/day, and a similar amount was derived from cereals (37%), vegetables (45%) and fruit (12%). The vegetarians, however, had a fibre intake which was almost double that of the general practice group, 41.5 ± 12.6 g/day and contained more fibre from cereals (40%), less from vegetables (35%) and much more from fruit (23%).

In the second study, 25 vegetarians living in Cardiff, Bristol and Brighton weighed and recorded their food intake for 1 week and dietary fibre intakes were also calculated from the British Food Tables (Burr *et al.*, 1981). The vegetarians ate 33.0 ± 10.5 g dietary fibre per day which was significantly more than 46 non-vegetarians who were recruited through publications of the health food movement. Their dietary fibre intake was close to the national average at 21.3 ± 6.8 g/day.

(*d*) *Long-term trends.* It has been suggested that there was a fall in dietary fibre consumption in Britain in the nineteenth century due to the introduction of roller milling, which allowed cheap white flour to be available to the population as a whole, rather than to only the higher income groups. However, little adequate data on food consumption for this period exist, and while it is clear that all types of bread were eaten throughout the nineteenth century, exactly how much and by whom is difficult to determine. Table 5.5 shows that a range of possible dietary fibre values has to be given to these years. Furthermore, there are no figures for the consumption of fruit, vegetables other than potatoes, or cereals other than wheat in 1860 and 1880. If, however, the consumption of these items during the period 1909–1913 is assumed to be similar to that in 1860 and 1880, it can then be added to the earlier data. Dietary fibre intake for these years then becomes 37–47 g in 1860, and 29 g in 1880. Hughes and Jones (1979) estimated that Welsh farm labourers' diets contained 65 g of dietary fibre in 1870. Overall, the trend has been for a

TABLE 5.5. Long-term trends in dietary fibre available for consumption: United Kingdom[a,b]

Year(s)	Total	Cereal	Potato	Other
1860	37–47	22–32[c]	10	(5.1)
1880	28.6	(13.9)	9.6	(5.1)
1909–1913	23.9	10.9	7.9	5.1
1938	22.3	9.2	6.1	7.0
1942–1944	32–39.6	18.7–24.6	7.3–8.9	6.0–6.2
1957	23.3	8.7	7.3	7.3
1970	22.7	8.1	7.3	7.3

[a] From Southgate et al., 1978a.

[b] Values are given in grams per person per day.

[c] Calculated assuming white bread made from stoneground flour contained 2.7–4.0 g dietary fibre per 100 g.

decrease in dietary fibre consumption from cereals which has been offset by an increase in vegetable consumption. A most striking change was the doubling of fibre intakes in Britain during the period 1940–1953. From Table 5.5, it can be seen that this was due mainly to an increase in cereal fibre and was a result of the raising of flour extraction rates, thus more than doubling the fibre content of bread, during and after World War II. At the same time, bread and vegetable consumption was encouraged whilst other foods, such as milk and cheese, were in short supply, so that more bread was eaten.

2. The Netherlands

(a) Individual intakes. Information on intakes of dietary fibre were obtained from adults randomly selected from population registers in the town of Rhenen, Netherlands (Van Staveren et al., 1982). Forty-four men and 56 women aged 25–65 kept a record of all food eaten over 7 days, and dietary fibre intakes were calculated from the data of Southgate et al. (1976), Hellendoorn et al. (1975), and Katan and Van de Bovenkamp (1981). Average dietary fibre intakes were 24.0 ± 6.9 g/day, with men consuming 27.5 ± 7.8 g/day, and women 21.3 ± 4.7 g/day; 32% of the dietary fibre was supplied by cereals and 41% by potatoes and vegetables. Fruit contributed 15%. Intakes were significantly lower on the weekend than on weekdays.

In another study (Van Dokkum et al., 1982), dietary fibre intakes in the Netherlands were found to be lower, 17.7 g; 41% of this came from cereals and 46% from vegetables. The data refer to 16- to 18-year-olds and, although it is possible that adolescents were eating rather less dietary fibre than 25- to 65-year-olds, perhaps more importantly, the methods used in these two studies were very different. In the latter study, composites of diets were analysed directly by the method of Hellendoorn (Hellendoorn et al., 1975) rather than

TABLE 5.6. Dietary fibre consumption in the Netherlands
per capita per day as determined from Dutch
food balance sheets, 1951–1976

	Dietary fibre intake (g/day)		
Foods	1951	1961	1976
Bread and cereals	13.6	9.9	8.0
Potatoes	6.4	5.5	5.2
Other vegetables	4.6	5.1	6.3
Fruit	1.7	2.3	3.5
Other (nuts, raisins, chocolate, etc.)	0.7	1.2	1.6
Total	27.0	24.0	24.6

using food tables. The composite diets were made up from data obtained at interviews in several schools in Amsterdam.

(b) *Long-term trends.* Some indications of long-term trends in dietary fibre intake are available for the Netherlands, where dietary fibre intake has been calculated from Dutch food balance sheet data, 1951–1976 (Van Staveren *et al.*, 1982). Dietary fibre values of foods were obtained from the same sources as above. From Table 5.6 it can be seen that dietary fibre intakes decreased from 27 to 24 g/day between 1951 and 1961, mainly because of a decline in the consumption of bread, other cereals and potatoes. Although the consumption of these foods continued to decrease in the following years, total dietary fibre consumption did not decrease because of greater consumption of other vegetables and of fruit. The decline in cereal dietary fibre has been even more marked than in Britain, from 50% of total intake in 1951 to 32.5% in 1976.

3.   *Scandinavia*

(a) *Denmark and Finland.* Denmark and Finland are of particular interest because there is a well established three- to fourfold range in large bowel cancer incidence between rural Finland and Copenhagen (Jensen *et al.*, 1982). Consequently, there have been a number of surveys of dietary intake and faecal output in these areas, and data from the latest (Englyst *et al.*, 1982a) is probably the best for dietary fibre intake at the present time. The study has already been outlined in detail (p. 82). Four randomly selected groups of men aged 50–59 living in Parikkala, rural Finland, Them in rural Denmark, Copenhagen and Helsinki were asked to weigh their food for 4 days. Dietary fibre intakes were calculated from 4-day records, using the British Food Tables supplemented with values for rye flour (Englyst, 1980). In addition, each of the 120 men collected a complete duplicate of all food

TABLE 5.7. Analysed intakes of non-starch polysaccharides[a] in Scandinavia

Study area (No. of diets)	Intake of NSP (g/day)				
	Total	Pentose	Hexose	Uronic acid	Cellulose
Them (25)	18.0 ± 6.4[b]	6.6 ± 3.0	5.5 ± 1.9	2.2 ± 1.3	3.7 ± 1.8
Copenhagen (29)	13.2 ± 4.8	4.5 ± 2.1	3.6 ± 1.3	1.9 ± 1.1	3.2 ± 1.4
Parikkala (30)	18.4 ± 7.8	7.4 ± 4.0	5.3 ± 1.9	1.9 ± 1.1	4.2 ± 1.8
Helsinki (28)	14.5 ± 5.4	5.5 ± 2.7	3.7 ± 1.1	2.0 ± 1.2	3.4 ± 1.3

[a] Alternative term for dietary fibre.
[b] All NSP intake values are given as the mean ± SD.

eaten on the last day of the survey. These samples were frozen and transported to Cambridge, England where their completeness was established
(Bingham *et al.*, 1982), and their dietary fibre content analysed by the method of Englyst *et al.*, (1982b). In this method, no attempt is made to analyze
for lignin content, and, following a recommendation of an EEC working
party (James and Theander, 1981), the values for NSP are expressed as such,
rather than as monosaccharides as is customary in food tables. This conversion causes a 10% reduction in apparent NSP content. For these reasons, and
because of an overestimation in the calculated values, which were based on
the British Food Tables, the analytical values are less than those shown in
Fig. 5.3.

Table 5.7 shows the analysed intakes of NSP in each of these four areas.
Intake was significantly higher in both of the rural areas compared with their
respective urban capitals, but not significantly different between the two rural
areas (Them, 18.3 ± 6.4 g, Parikkala, 18.4 ± 7.8 g) nor between the two urban
areas (Copenhagen, 13.2 ± 4.8 g, Helsinki, 14.5 ± 5.4 g). Despite these small
differences in intake, there was a significant inverse relationship with large
bowel cancer incidence (Jensen *et al.*, 1982). These fibre values are substantially lower than those previously found in rural Finland and Copenhagen
(IARC, Intestinal Microecology Group, 1977). This is largely due to problems in the analysis of rye flour. Table 5.8 shows that 30–50% of NSP intake in
these populations was from rye products and any errors in their chemical
analysis will make a large difference to the final value.

(b) *Long-term trends in Denmark.* Since 1927, surveys of the food eaten in
farming households in the Jutland peninsular of rural Denmark have been
carried out, and the intake of dietary fibre has been calculated from these data
using the early analyses of Englyst (Englyst, 1978; Helms and Englyst,
1978). Table 5.9 shows that there has been a 25% reduction in dietary fibre
intake over this period (Helms *et al.*, 1982), coupled with a marked increase
in fat and decrease in carbohydrate consumption.

TABLE 5.8. Contribution of different sources of food to total dietary fibre intake in Scandinavia

NSP source	Contribution to total intake of NSP (%)			
	Them	Copenhagen	Parikkala	Helsinki
Fruit	11 ± 13[a]	10 ± 9	6 ± 6	7 ± 9
Vegetables	28 ± 15	26 ± 17	17 ± 11	29 ± 18
Cereals[b]	58	59	73	60
Rye	41 ± 20	41 ± 19	52 ± 22	34 ± 22
White wheat products	16 ± 11	15 ± 10	8 ± 11	8 ± 10
Brown, bran, and wholemeal wheat products	1 ± 3	3 ± 9	13 ± 19	18 ± 22
Other	3	5	4	4

[a] Values represent means ± SD.
[b] Standard deviation not available.

4. Yugoslavia

In the early 1960s, the food intake of heads of 24 families in villages in Dalmatia and 25 in Slavonia was carefully measured by weighing and collecting duplicate foods (Buzina *et al.*, 1964). This was part of an international collaborative study using standardised dietary methods to investigate the effect of diet on the incidence of ischaemic heart disease (The Seven Countries Heart Study; Keys, 1970). Records of the average quantities of foods eaten by the 49 men have been made available to us (R. Buzina, personal communication) and dietary fibre intakes have been calculated from these records. Total fibre intake was 25.5 ± 7.5 g/day, 13 g (50%) of which was from cereal, mainly white bread. The 9 g of vegetable dietary fibre was from potatoes, root vegetables, legumes and green vegetables. The contribution of fruit to the total was small (4 g).

5. Germany

In 1973, a dietary survey of 135,000 people was undertaken throughout all the states in Germany. Details of food intake were obtained by a food diary,

TABLE 5.9. Dietary fibre and contribution of fat, protein and carbohydrate to energy in rural areas in Denmark, 1927–1977

Items	Calculated from farmers' organizations food surveys						
	1927	1933	1944	1950	1960	1971	1977
Total dietary fibre (g)	34.1	31.8	37.0	30.8	24.9	23.4	25.3
Energy percentages (excluding alcohol)							
Fat	29	34	32	34	38	39	43
Protein	11	12	12	13	12	13	12
Carbohydrate	60	54	56	53	50	48	44

and fibre intakes were calculated as crude fibre. Dietary fibre has now been calculated and average intakes for men were 25.1 g/day and for women 22.3 g/day (Rottka, 1980). Cereal intakes of dietary fibre were higher than in Britain, 12 g or 51% of the total, largely because of the consumption of rye bread. Vegetables supplied 8 g and fruit 4 g/day.

6. Sweden

Two surveys in Sweden have quantitated dietary and neutral detergent fibre intakes at 14 g/day. The first (Lindegarde et al., 1979) was obtained by asking 55 middle-aged men in Malmo to recall all food eaten over the previous 7 days. The men were randomly selected out of a group of 1121 attending a medical health-screening clinic. Dietary fibre intakes, calculated using Southgate's data, were 14.2 ± 4.6 g/day with that from cereals being 5.5 ± 3.4 g/day. In this study, the individuals with above-average cereal fibre intakes had "better" glucose tolerance.

In the second study, 35 men and women pensioners were asked to collect replicate portions of a day's food intake, which were then analysed for neutral detergent fibre (Asp et al., 1979). Daily intakes were 17.8 ± 6.9 g/day for men and 11.1 ± 3.5 g/day for women; analysis as undigestible residues gave higher values (women, 21.1 ± 4.8 g/day; men, 27.5 ± 5.9 g/day).

7. Ireland

In a group of 16 women and 9 men in Dublin, dietary fibre intakes were 22.7 ± 4.3 g/day and 22.6 ± 4.1 g/day (Fielding and Melvin, 1979). These intakes were obtained with a retrospective diet history over 1 week, in which data on the portions of food and the frequency with which they were eaten were obtained. Fibre intakes were calculated from the British Food Tables. No details of the sources of fibre were given.

8. Other areas of Europe

Table 5.10 summarises the average intakes of dietary fibre and its sources calculated from the Euratom study (Cresta et al., 1969) of 11 rural areas of the EEC, as described on p. 79. White bread was the staple food in most of the areas, although in the southern regions it was supplemented with pasta and maize flour, and in the north more brown and rye bread and potatoes were eaten. A greater proportion (on average 45%) of dietary fibre came from cereals and less from vegetables and potatoes (44%) than in the United Kingdom. The Italian regions derived the greatest proportions of their fibre from cereals (51–63%) largely as a result of their consumption of pasta. Fibre intake from vegetables was highest in the Vendee (45%) where large quantities of beans and peas were eaten in the winter months.

TABLE 5.10. Sources of dietary fibre in 11 regions
of the European Economic Community[a]

Area[b]	Cereal	Vegetable	Fruit, nuts	Potato	Total
Friesland (H)	8.2	5.6	2.6	6.3	22.6
Gent (B)	10.9	4.1	1.7	12.3	28.9
Liege (B)	8.0	6.0	2.3	10.5	26.8
Luxembourg	7.3	6.5	2.1	13.2	29.1
Hessen (G)	11.6	4.9	2.6	8.2	27.3
Normandy (F)	9.1	5.7	2.2	7.8	24.8
Bretagne (F)	10.2	4.9	1.8	6.9	23.8
Vendee (F)	10.1	12.7	2.8	4.0	29.6
Fruili (I)	14.7	5.1	1.3	3.8	24.9
Campania (I)	13.4	7.7	4.3	1.6	26.9
Basilicata (I)	13.5	5.7	3.9	0.7	23.8

[a] Values are given in grams per person per day.
[b] H, Holland; B, Belgium; G, Germany; F, France; I, Italy.

B. Africa

While much has been written about dietary fibre intakes in Africa, in fact, very little is known about it. No dietary surveys have been done specifically to measure fibre intake and nothing is therefore known of its main sources and composition. Dietary surveys to quantitate intakes of other nutrients have been done and these have been used as a basis for obtaining some preliminary figures for fibre intakes. These are summarised in Table 5.11. The main

TABLE 5.11. Dietary fibre intakes in Africa[a]

Source of data	Total	Cereal	Vegetable	Fruit, nuts
Orr and Gilkes (1931)				
Kenya	130	79[b]	54	NA[c]
Masai				
Warriors	0	0	0	0
Women	25	25	NA	NA
Platt (unpublished)				
Malawi (foothill village)	55	40	10	4
Jones (undated)				
Swaziland (middle veld)	60	40	19	1
Ruitsihauser (unpublished)				
Uganda (Buganda)	150	0	147	3

[a] Values are given in grams per person per day.
[b] Calculated assuming maize meal contained 10% dietary fibre.
[c] Not available.

problem in using these food intake data for dietary fibre calculations is that very few of the staple African foods have been analysed for fibre. Therefore, the closest approximate figure has to be taken from existing food tables. Notwithstanding these compromises, it is clear from Table 5.11 that large differences in fibre intakes exist between populations in the African continent and those in the West.

1. *Kikuyu and Masai*

In 1931 the Medical Research Council of Great Britain published a report on the diet and health of two African tribes, the Kikuyu and the Masai in Kenya (Orr and Gilkes, 1931). A research team had visited the areas and observed the preparation and eating of food. They were able to weigh some foods, but this was limited because of local superstitions, particularly amongst the Kikuyu. Furthermore, food consumed while the tribesmen were at work in the field could not be recorded. The Masai diet was apparently easier to quantitate. Samples of food from both regions were sent back to England for analysis although not for fibre analysis. There were big differences in food intake between men and women, and between warriors and non-warriors.

The diets of the two tribes were very different, the Masai being a pastoral tribe living mainly on meat, milk and blood. The Masai warriors live almost entirely on these items, but the rest of the tribe also consume bananas, beans, millet, arrowroot, maize, sugar and honey. Fibre intakes amongst the warriors would usually have been zero and for the rest of the tribe about 25 g/day, mostly from maize.

The Kikuyu, however, have a very different diet, largely vegetarian. It consists of cereals, tubers, plantains, legumes and green leaves. Meat is rarely eaten. The vegetables are made into a thick porridge or into a gruel, and an average male was observed to eat between 3 and 6 lb of the porridge per day and 2 and 3 pints of gruel. We have calculated this to contain 130 g of dietary fibre.

2. *Malawi*

From 1938 to 1939, Dr. B. S. Platt studied the food intakes of two villages and one urban area in what was then Nyasaland. The survey was not published, although the records have been kept by the School of Hygiene and Tropical Medicine in London. The staple diet of villagers living on the shores of Lake Nyasa included cassava, fresh fish, green leaves and mango, and villagers living in the foothill region ate mainly maize, potato, green leaves, beans and a little meat. Their intake of dietary fibre was about 55 g/day (Table 5.11). Interestingly, the diet eaten in urban areas was similar to that of the foothill villages at that time, except that slightly more milk, oil and sugar were eaten.

3. *Swaziland*

In a report prepared for the government of Swaziland in the 1950s (Jones, undated), the food intakes of rural and urban Swazis were recorded, having been studied in detail using the weighing technique. Great diversity exists in climate and land form throughout Swaziland and hence in the diets eaten in rural areas. There was also an abundance of food in spring but shortage and semi-starvation in winter. The winter diet of Swazis living in the middle velt was mostly maize, beans, potatoes and green vegetables and contained about 60 g of dietary fibre (Table 5.11).

4. *Uganda*

The staple food of villagers living in the central (Buganda) region of Uganda is the plantain, of which at least 1 kg will be eaten by men at each main meal (I. H. E. Ruitishauser, personal communication, 1976). This is steamed or boiled and eaten with vegetable and groundnut relishes or very occasionally with meat. The dietary fibre content of plantain is 6 g/100 g (Paul and Southgate, 1978), and total dietary fibre intakes in this region are consequently probably the highest known at 150 g/day (Table XI).

5. *South Africa*

A classic paper in 1971 (Lubbe, 1971) described marked differences in diet between rural and urban Venda males. In the rural areas, maize meal porridge was eaten in large amounts (up to 3.8 kg/person/day). The amount of maize used in the porridge was not reported and its dietary fibre content has not been measured. Nevertheless, an average intake of 1.7 kg/day together with large quantities of vegetable relishes (average intake 586 g/day) suggests dietary fibre intakes of at least 100 g/person/day.

C. *Australasia*

1. *New Zealand*

Two reports from New Zealand suggest that dietary fibre intakes are similar to those in Britain, at least so far as women are concerned. In the first study (Stace *et al.*, 1981), 5-day weighed records were obtained from four groups of women: 25 Europeans, 18 Maoris, 24 Tongans living in New Zealand, and 25 Tongans living in Tonga (see the following section). All were healthy women, matched for age (29–67 years) and dietary fibre intakes were calculated using the British Food Tables. In the three groups living in New Zealand, dietary fibre intakes were all low: Europeans, 18 ± 5; Maori, 16 ± 6; and New Zealand Tongans 19 ± 6 g. Typically, vegetables supplied most dietary fibre, 45–54%, followed by cereals, 25–37%, and fruit and nuts, 16–23% (Pomare *et al.*, 1983).

In the second report (Hillman *et al.*, 1982), 25 normal women aged 26–58 from Wellington were used as controls in a study to investigate fibre intake in patients with the irritable bowel syndrome. Total dietary fibre intakes, also calculated from the British Food Tables, were the same as in the study of Stace *et al.* (1981) at 18.1 ± 4.7 g. Again, vegetables were the major source (8.2 g), followed by cereals (5.7 g), and fruit (4.2 g).

2. *Polynesia*

Stace *et al.* (1981) also measured dietary fibre intakes of 25 women living in the South Pacific island of Tonga. The main food sources in this area were taro, cassava, and breadfruit and, as a result, the diets were different in many aspects from the typical "western" type diets eaten in New Zealand. Energy intakes were higher (11.2 ± 3.6 MJ) than that of the women living in New Zealand (8.5 ± 7.6 MJ) and protein intakes lower (51 vs. 64–74 g) as were fat intakes (46 vs. 87–95 g). The Tongans ate three times more dietary fibre, 72 ± 29 g, of which 65% was from taro, cassava and breadfruit, and only 4% from greens and cereals. Fruit and nuts supplied 31% of dietary fibre (Pomare *et al.*, 1983).

Intakes of dietary fibre on another Polynesian island, Tokelau, are, however, very different. In Tokelau, 63% of energy is supplied by coconut which is taken with every meal in some form. Some taro and breadfruit also are eaten. The main emphasis in this study was on fat intakes, and average intakes in 26 men were 156 g/day and in 51 women 131 g/day—much higher than in New Zealand (Prior *et al.*, 1981). Using Southgate's analyses, supplemented with analyses of Holloway (Holloway *et al.*, 1977) for taro, breadfruit and coconut, extra information was obtained in 1976 for 95 men and 161 women to calculate dietary fibre intake. Surprisingly reported intakes were only 16.5 g for men and 14.9 g for women.

3. *Australia*

Using a questionnaire and British Food Tables, dietary fibre intakes of 800 randomly selected men and women in Adelaide were calculated and compared with those of patients with large bowel cancer (Potter *et al.*, 1983). Fibre intakes were similar in men and women to that found in Britain, around 20 g/day, with men aged 50 or less eating slightly more (22 g). The dietary fibre intake of 27 elderly men and women living in Victoria estimated from a 3-day weighed record of all food consumed and an interview (diet history) was also about 20 g/day (20.5 ± 1.7 g, SEM) (Flint *et al.*, 1982).

D. *Japan*

With its highly urbanised society, yet disease pattern which contrasts with Western countries, Japan is of special interest to the epidemiologist, particularly since these patterns of disease change within one or two generations in Japanese who migrate (Haenzel and Kurihara, 1968). Traditional Japanese diets are known to be low in fat and high in carbohydrate on which basis dietary fibre intakes might be expected to be high. However, rice contains only little dietary fibre (Paul and Southgate, 1978) and so it might be predicted that the fibre intake of populations where white rice is the staple cereal would be low when compared with diets eaten in rural Africa where lightly processed carbohydrate intake was high. A recent report confirms this, with the present Japanese diet reported to contain only 19.4 g/day in 1979 (Minowa *et al.*, 1983). Mori, using his own technique for analyses of Japanese foods, reported the dietary fibre content of two student meals to be 14.8 and 19.5 g/day (Mori, 1982).

1. *Long-term trends*

In Japan, yearly nationwide household surveys are carried out, and these data have been used by Minowa *et al.* (1983) to calculate dietary fibre intakes using the British Food Tables together with neutral detergent fibre plus pectin values for some seaweed-based foods (Nakamura *et al.*, 1981). Total dietary fibre from rice has fallen from 7.7 g/day in 1965 to 5.1 g/day in 1979, and overall total dietary fibre intake has fallen from 21.2 g in 1965 to 19.4 g in 1979 (Table 5.12). These changes are small compared with a 70-g decline in carbohydrate intake since 1965, a threefold increase in fat intake and a 25% increase in the amount of protein derived from animal products since 1950.

There are no household statistics available prior to 1950, but a dietary record of an artist's family (all adults) in 1925 shows that on a typical day, rice was eaten three times a day, together with pickles, salted fish, soybean curd, radishes, spring onions and soy sauce. Only 12 g/day of fat was eaten

TABLE 5.12. Secular changes in major nutrient intakes, 1950–1979
(per capita per day) in Japan[a]

	Fat	Carbohydrate	Dietary fibre		Protein from animal food
			Total	From rice	
1950	18	418	NA[b]	NA	25.0
1955	20.3	411	NA	NA	32.0
1960	24.7	399	NA	NA	35.4
1965	36.0	384	21.2[c]	7.7[a]	40.0
1970	46.5	368	20.2	7.0	44.1
1975	52.0	337	20.2	5.7	48.6
1979	54.8	315	19.4	5.1	50.3

[a] Values are given in grams.
[b] Not available.
[c] 1966 data.

but the dietary fibre content was the same as today, 18.2 g/day, although at that time rice supplied 11.3 g/day (Minowa *et al.*, 1983).

2. *Present day intakes*

Geographical comparisons within Japan show that these changes in diet have been most marked in the urban areas (Minowa *et al.*, 1983). In the 10 largest cities in 1979, 57.5 g/day of fat were eaten, and 52% of protein derived from animal foods. Carbohydrate and dietary fibre intakes were also lower, 296 and 17.7 g, in these areas. This compares with less fat, 50.6 g, less protein from animal sources, 48.2%, more carbohydrate, 332 g, and more dietary fibre, 20.2 g, in towns and villages. There is a clear trend between these extremes, depending on the size of the city.

E. India

Up to 1980 only one report was available on dietary fibre intakes in India, that of the Hos tribe, who from 1940 to 1941 used no fat and derived 93% of their energy from rice (Mitra, 1942). Fibre intake, calculated from details of food consumption and the British Food Tables, was 38 g/day (Bingham and Cummings, 1980). Since that time, dietary fibre intakes have been calculated using data from a number of dietary surveys carried out by the National Nutritional Monitoring Bureau in 1980 in India (Shetty, 1981). These show a twofold range in fibre intake from 22 g/day in predominantly rice-eating states such as Kerala to 42 g in Karnataka where other cereals are eaten in addition. In Kerala, 9.8 g of dietary fibre came from cereals, compared with 35.9 g in Karnataka.

F. North America

1. *Canada*

National statistics have not yet been used to calculate dietary fibre intakes in Canada, but there are two reports from Toronto and the University of Guelph. In the first, 200 men aged 35–59 from the staff and faculty of the University were asked to recall one previous day's food intake. Dietary fibre intakes were calculated from the British Food Tables for comparison with blood lipids. Average dietary fibre intakes were 17.8 ± 9.4 g, of which 8.9 ± 6.1 was from cereals (Kay *et al.*, 1980).

In the second, 100 women aged 30 ± 6 years were recruited from the University and asked to keep 3-day records of all food eaten, and a duplicate collection of food on the final day for analysis of trace elements (Gibson and Scythes, 1982). Dietary fibre intakes, also calculated from British Food Tables, were slightly higher (19.4 ± 6.6 g) in this group of women than in the men studied above, possibly because the 24-h recall method underestimates food intake (p. 79).

A comparable study, also from the University of Guelph, supports the observations of Gear *et al.*, (1979) and of Burr *et al.*, (1981) of a higher dietary fibre intake in vegetarians compared with omnivores. At the University of Guelph, 56 Seventh-Day Adventist Canadian women aged 53 ± 15 years kept dietary records of their food intake for 3 days. The purpose of the study was to assess iron and zinc status but dietary fibre intakes were also calculated using the British Food Tables (Anderson *et al.*, 1981). Total dietary fibre intake in these women was 30.9 ± 11.0 g/day, with a range from 11 to 68 g/day, and 39% from vegetables, 28% from cereals and 30% from fruit.

2. *United States*

(*a*) *Present day intakes.* From 1965 to 1966 there was a Nationwide Household Food Consumption Survey of the American population from which the average consumption of food items was calculated. A representative sample of these foods was taken and homogenised (Ahrens and Boucher, 1978), and was analysed by Dr. D. A. T. Southgate. Total dietary fibre was 19.1 g in this composite diet.

Similar findings have also been reported by Marlett and Bokram (1981), who asked 57 men and 143 women students at the University of Wisconsin-Madison to record food intake for 2 days using household measures to establish the weights of food eaten in order to investigate the relationship between crude and dietary fibre intake. Dietary fibre intakes, calculated using the British Food Tables were 19.91 ± 9.97 g in the men, and 13.41 ± 6.02 g in the women. Typical of Western diets, the main source of fibre was vegetables (41%), followed by cereals and legumes (32%) and fruits (22%).

(*b*) *Long-term trends.* Based on the published data of Heller and Hackler (1978), long-term trends in dietary fibre intake for the American population were calculated. These showed a 55% decrease in cereal fibre available for consumption from 1909 to 1975 (Bingham and Cummings, 1980).

IV.   Conclusions

Current evidence indicates that average dietary fibre intakes of groups of adults in industrialised affluent communities are in the range of 15 to 30 g/day. Examples are many countries in Europe, also Canada, the United States, Australia, New Zealand and Japan. Within the overall average, there are, however, considerable individual variations, both in average habitual intake and from day to day. Seasonal variations in dietary fibre intake may be marked, particularly in rural communities, and vegetarians often have somewhat higher intakes, up to 40 g/day on average.

Long-term trends in Britain suggest that the adult average dietary fibre intake from cereals may have fallen from about 30 g/day in 1860, to the present day level of 8 g/day. This has been only partially offset by an increase of about 2 g/day from a rising consumption of fruit and vegetables. Similar long-term trends have occurred in Holland, Denmark, the United States and, most strikingly, in Japan where there are marked recent changes towards a more Western diet, containing more animal protein, fat, and less starch, from rice. White rice has a fibre content even lower than that of white wheat flour.

There are almost no data concerning the dietary fibre content of many common tropical foodstuffs and vegetables. There is, therefore, little information concerning dietary fibre intakes in many improverished Third World countries apart from sub-Saharan Africa. The scanty data from these African rural communities indicate dietary fibre intakes to be in the range of 70 to over 100 g/day. This is due to the very high intakes of lightly processed staple foodstuffs, such as plantain, maize and millet, pulses and vegetables. Scanty data from Polynesia reported a comparable high figure in one island, but a much lower figure in another island wherein much coconut oil but less starch was consumed. In areas where white rice is the staple cereal, however, such as in parts of South America, the Far East, and China, data from India and Japan suggest that fibre intakes are likely to be low, around 20 g/day and similar to those found in westernized urban communities.

Relatively little accurate data are available, however, and comparisons between countries are difficult because of bias inherent in the methods used to assess food consumption and continuing difficulties in the definition and analysis of dietary fibre. Relationships on the individual level between diet and disease will be lessened to a marked extent by these factors, also by other dietary factors, the variable individual response, and both seasonal and daily variations in dietary fibre and nutrient intakes.

References

ACHESON, K. J., CAMPBELL, I. T., EDHOLM, O. G., MILLER, D. S. and STOCK, M. J. (1980). *Am. J. Clin. Nutr.* **33**, 1147–1154.

AHRENS, E. H. (1979). *Lancet* **2**, 1345–1348.

AHRENS, E. H. and BOUCHER, C. A. (1978). *J. Am. Diet. Assoc.* **73**, 613–620.

ANDERSON, B. M., GIBSON, R. S. and SABRY, J. H. (1981). *Am. J. Clin. Nutr.* **34**, 1042–1048.

ASP, N.-G. (1978). *J. Plant Foods* **3**, 21–26.

ASP, N.-G. CARLSTEDT, L., DAHLQVIST, A., JOHANSSON, C. G. and PAULSSON, M. (1979). *Scand. J. Gastroenterol.* **14**, 128–137.

BAZARRE, T. L. and MYERS, M. P. (1980). *Nutr. Cancer* **1**, 22–45.

BEATON, G. H., MILNER, J., COREY, P., McGUIRE, V., COUSINS, M., STEWART, E., RAMOS, M., HEWITT, D., GRANBISCH, P. V., KAJSIM, N. and LITTLE, J. A. (1979). *Am. J. Clin. Nutr.* **32**, 2546–2559.

BINGHAM, S. and CUMMINGS, J. H. (1980). *In* "Medical Aspects of Dietary Fiber" G. A. Spiller and R. M. Kay, eds) pp. 261–284. Plenum, New York.

BINGHAM, S. and CUMMINGS, J. H. (1983). *Clin. Sci.* **64**, 629–635.

BINGHAM, S., CUMMINGS, J. H. and MCNEIL, N. I. (1979a). *Am. J. Clin. Nutr.* **32**, 1313–1319.

BINGHAM, S., WILLIAMS, D. R. R., COLE, T. J. and JAMES, W. P. T. (1979b). *Br. J. Cancer* **40**, 456–463.

BINGHAM, S., WIGGINS, H. S., ENGLYST, H., SEPPANEN, R., HELMS, P., STRAND, R., BURTON, R., JORGENSEN, I. M., POULSEN, L., PAERREGAARD, A., BJERRUM, L. and JAMES, W. P. T. (1982). *Nutr. Cancer* **4**, 23–33.

BULL, N. L., SMART, G. A. and JUDSON, H. (1982). *Ecol. Food. Nutr.* **12**, 97–101.

BURKITT, D. P. (1969). *Lancet* **2**, 1229–1231.

BURKITT, D. P. and TROWELL, H. C. (eds) (1975) "Refined Carbohydrate Foods and Disease." Academic Press, London.

BURR, M. L., BATES, C. J., FEHILY, A. M. and ST. LEGER, A. S. (1981). *J. Hum. Nutr.* **35**, 437–441.

BUZINA, R., FERBER, E., KEYS, A., BORADAREC, A., AGNELETTO, B. and HORVAT, A. (1964). *Voeding,* **25**, 629–639.

CRESTA, M., LEDERMANN, S., GARDINER, A., LOMBARDO, E. and LACOURLY, G. (1969). "A Dietary Survey of 11 Areas of the EEC in Order to Determine Levels of Radioactive Contamination", EUR.4218f. Euratom, Leiden.

CUMMINGS, J. H. (1980). *In* "Food and Health—Science and Technology" (G. G. Birch, ed), pp. 441–458. Applied Science Publishers, London.

CUMMINGS, J. H. and STEPHEN, A. M. (1980). *Can. Med. Assoc. J.* **123**, 1109–1114.

EASTWOOD, M. A., BRYDON, W. G., SMITH, D. M. and SMITH, J. H. (1982). *Am. J. Clin. Nutr.* **36**, 290–293.

ENGLYST, H. (1978). *Ugeskr. Agron. Hort. Forst. Lic.* **7**, 626–627.

ENGLYST, H. (1980). *In* "Analysis of Dietary Fibre" (W. P. T. James and O. Theander, eds), pp. 217–239. Dekker, New York.

ENGLYST, H. N., BINGHAM, S., WIGGINS, H. S., SOUTHGATE, D. A. T., SEPPAREN, R., HELMS, P., ANDERSON, V., DAY, K. C., CHOOLUN, R., COLLINSON, E. and CUMMINGS, J. H. (1982a). *Nutr. Cancer* **4**, 50–60.

ENGLYST, H., WIGGINS, H. S. and CUMMINGS, J. R. (1982b). *Analyst* **107**, 307–318.

ENGLYST, H. N., ANDERSON, V. and CUMMINGS, J. H. (1983). *J. Sci. Food. Agric.* **34**, 1434–1440.

FIELDING, J. F. and MELVIN, K. (1979). *J. Hum. Nutr.* **33**, 243.

FLINT, D. M., WAHLQVIST, M. L., PARISH, A. E. and SMITH, T. J. (1982). *Int. Symp. Diet. Fibre, 1983* Abstract No. 200, New Zealand.

GARDNER, M. H. and HEADY, J. A. (1973). *J. Chronic. Dis.* **26**, 781–795.

GEAR, J. S. S., WARE, A., FURSDON, P., MANN, J. I., NOLAN, D. J., BRODRIBB, A. J. M. and VESSEY, M. P. (1979). *Lancet* **1**, 511–514.

GIBSON, R. S. and SCYTHES, C. A. (1982). *Br. J. Nutr.* **48**, 241–248.

GOERING, H. K. and VAN SOEST, P. J. (1970). *U.S., Dep. Agric., Agric. Handb.* **379**.

HAENZEL, W. and KURIHARA, M. (1968). *J. Natl. Cancer Inst. (U.S.)* **40**, 43–68.

HELLENDOORN, E. W., NOORDHOFF, M. G. and SLAGMAN, J. (1975). *J. Sci. Food Agric.* **26**, 1461–1468.

HELLER, S. M. and HACKLER, L. R. (1978). *Am. J. Clin. Nutr.* **31**, 1510–1514.

HELMS, P. and ENGLYST, H. (1978). *Tek. Medd.* **3**, 14–16.

HELMS, P., JORGENSEN, I. M., PAERREGAARD, A., BJERRUM, L., POULSEN, L. and MORSBECH, J. (1982). *Nutr. Cancer* **4**, 34–40.

HUENEMANN, R. and TURNER, D. (1942). *J. Am. Diet. Assoc.* **18**, 502–508.

HILLMAN, L. C., STACE, N. H., FISHER, A. and POMARE, E. W. (1982). *Am. J. Clin. Nutr.*

36, 626–629.

HOLLOWAY, W. D., TASMAN-JONES, C. and MAHER, K. (1977). *N. Z. Med. J.* **85,** 420–423.

HUGHES, R. E. and JONES, E. (1979). *Br. Med. J.* **1,** 1145.

IARC Intestinal Microecology Group (1977). *Lancet* **2,** 207–211.

ISAKSSON, B. (1980). *Am. J. Clin. Nutr.* **33,** 4–6.

JAIN, M., HOWE, G. R., JOHNSON, K. C. and MILLER, A. B.,(1980). *Am. J. Epidemiol.* **111,** 212–219.

JAMES, W. P. T., and THEANDER, O. (eds), (1981). "Analysis of Dietary Fibre in Foods." Dekker, New York.

JAMES, W. P. T., BINGHAM, S. and COLE, T. J. (1981). *Nutr. Cancer* **2,** 203–212.

JENSEN, O., MACLENNAN, R. and WAHRENDORF, J. (1982). *Nutr. Cancer* **4,** 5–19.

JONES, S. (undated). A Study of Swazi Nutrition. Report for the University of Natal for the Swaziland Government.

KAY, R. M., SABRY, Z. I. and CSIMA, A. (1980). *Am. J. Clin. Nutr.* **33,** 2566–2572.

KATAN, M. B. and VAN DE BOVENKAMP, P. (1981). *In* "Analysis of Dietary Fibre in Foods" (W. P. T. James and O. Theander, eds), pp. 217–239. Dekker, New York.

KEYES, A. (1970). *Circulation* **41,** 42–198.

LINDGARDE, F., RASMUSSON, M. and WENDT, B. (1979). *Var Foda, Suppl.* **3,** 193.

LINUSSEN, E. I., SARJUR, D. and ERIKSON, E. C. (1974). *Arch. Latinoaom. Nutr.* **24,** 277–294.

LIU, K., STAMLER, J., DYER, A., McKEEVER, J. and McKeever, P. (1978). *J. Chronic Dis.* **31,** 399–418.

LUBBE, A. M. (1971). *S. Afr. Med. J.* **45,** 1289–1297.

McCANCE, R. A., WIDDOWSON, E. M. and SHACKLETON R. B. (1936). *Med. Res. Counc. (G.B.), Spec. Rep. Ser.* **213.**

MARLETT, J. A. and BOKRAM, R. L. (1981). *Am. J. Clin. Nutr.* **34,** 335–342.

MARR, J. (1981). *In* "Preventive Nutrition in Society" (M. R. Turner, ed), pp. 77–83. Academic Press, London.

MARR, J. W. (1971). *World Rev. Nutr. Diet.* **13,** 105–164.

Ministry of Agriculture, Fisheries and Food (1953-1979). "Household Food consumption and Expenditure, 1950-1977." HM Stationery Office, London.

MILTRA, K. (1942). *Indian J. Med. Res.* **30,** 91–97.

MINOWA, M., BINGHAM, S. and CUMMINGS, J. H. (1983). *Human Nutr.* **37A,** 113–119.

MORI, B. and ARAGANE, K. (1981). *Nutr. Food* **34,** 97–104.

NAKAMURA, H., TAMURA, A., TANAKA, H., MATSUSHITA, C., YAMAMOTO, F., YOSHI, S. and IZUMI, K. (1981). *Nutr. Food* **34,** 71–75.

ORR, J. B. and GILKES, T. L. (1931). *Med. Res. Counc. (G.B.), Spec. Rep. Ser.* **155.**

PAUL, A. A. and SOUTHGATE, D. A. T. (1978). *In* "McCance and Widdowson's The Composition of Foods," 4th edition. HM Stationery Office, London.

PEKKARINEN, M. (1979). *World Rev. Nutr. Diet,* **12,** 145–171.

POMARE, E. W., STACE, N. H., PETERS, S. G., and FISHER, A. (1983). *Bull.—R. Soc. N.Z.* **20.** (Abstract No. 186).

POTTER, J. D., McMICHAEL, A. J. and BONNETT, A. Z. (1983). *Bull.—R. Soc. N.Z.* **20,** (Abstract No. 114).

PRIOR, I. A., DAVIDSON, F., SALMOND, C. E. and CZOCHANSKA, Z. (1981). *Am. J. Clin. Nutr.* **34,** 1552–1561.

ROTTKA, H. (1980). "Pflanzenfasern - Ballastoffe in der menschlichen ernahrung", pp. 63–72. Thieme, Stuttgart.

SELVENDRAN, R. R., RING, S. G. and DU PONT, M. S. (1979). *Chem. Ind. (London)* **7,** 225.

SHETTY, P. S. (1981). *Proc. Annu. Conf. Ind. Soc. Gastrol. Trivardrum.*

SOUTHGATE, D. A. T. (1969). *J. Sci. Food Agric.* **20,** 331.

SOUTHGATE, D. A. T. (1976). *In* "Fiber in Human Nutrition" (G.A. Spiller and R. J. Amen, eds), pp. 73–107. Plenum, New York.

SOUTHGATE, D. A. T. (1978). *Am. J. Clin. Nutr.* **31,** Suppl., S107–S110.

SOUTHGATE, D. A. T., BAILEY, B., COLLINSON, E. and WALKER, A. F. (1976). *J. Hum. Nutr.* **30,** 303–313.

SOUTHGATE, D. A. T., BINGHAM, S. and ROBERTSON, J. (1978a). *Nature, (London)* **274,** 51–52.

SOUTHGATE, D. A. T., HUDSON, G. J. and ENGLYST, H. (1978b). *J. Sci. Food Agric.* **29,** 979–988.

STACE, N. H., POMARE, E. W., PETERS, S., THOMAS, L., and FISHER, A. (1983). Bull.—R. Soc. N. 2. 20 Abst. 1291.

THEANDER, O. and AMAN, P. (1979). *In* "Dietary Fibres: Chemistry and Nutrition" (G. E. Inglett and S. I. Falkehag, eds), pp. 215–244. Academic Press, London.

THOMSON, M., LOGAN, R. L., SHARMAN, M., LOCKERBIE, L., RIEMERSMA, R. A. and OLIVER, M. R. (1982). *Hum. Nutr. Appl. Nutr.* **36A,** 272–280.

VAN DOKKUM, W., DE VOS, R. H., CLOUGHLEY, F. A., HULSHOF, K. F. A. M., DUKEL, F. and WIJSMAN, J. A. (1982). *Br. J. Nutr.* **48,** 223–231.

VAN SOEST, P. J. and MCQUEEN, R. W. (1973). *Proc. Nutr. Soc.* **32,** 123.

VAN STAVEREN, W. A., HAUTVAST, J. G. A. J., KATAN, M. B., VAN MONTFORT, M. A. J. and VAN OOSTEN-VAN DER GOES, H. G. C. (1982). *J. Am. Diet. Assoc.* **80,** 324–330.

Chapter 6

Physiological effects of dietary fibre on the alimentary tract

MARTIN EASTWOOD and W. GORDON BRYDON

I.   Introduction

Dietary fibre has a considerable effect on function and morphology throughout the gastrointestinal tract. This has been thoroughly reviewed by the Royal College of Physicians (1980), Spiller and Kay (1980), and Vahouny and Kritchevsky (1982). Substantial progress has been made in our under-

Dietary Fibre, Fibre-Depleted Foods
and Disease

standing of dietary fibre. As yet, however, there is no methodology available which enables a prediction to be made of how a particular fibre will behave along the gastrointestinal tract. This limits our ability to prescribe the ideal dietary fibre intake.

The progress that has been made in our knowledge has to be interpreted with caution. This is in part because of the broad range of experiments, fibre sources and animals that have been used.

The anatomical areas of the gastrointestinal tract which are useful for discussion of fibre are (1) foregut; (2) exocrine pancreas; (3) mid-gut; (4) hind-gut; and (5) enterohepatic circulation and biliary system.

The influence of fibre at each stage will be in part a function of the residence time or transit. The effects of fibre will also be a consequence of the type and age of fibre, how it is prepared, and the overall diet and for how long a particular fibre was eaten. Experiments have to be interpreted in the light of the previous dietary intake and whether or not the animals or subjects are omnivores, carnivores or herbivores. The fibre will affect the mucosa, absorptive ability and luminal contents throughout the gastrointestinal tract. The mucosa is coated with mucus and the effect of dietary fibre on this may be considerable. The luminal environment will vary throughout the gastrointestinal tract but will consist of phases. The volume of fluid, pH, osmolality and chemistry of the luminal contents will vary from the foregut through the mid-gut to the hind-gut. In the foregut there is a contrast between the digestion of dietary constituents into absorbable fragments and the intactness of the dietary fibre. Here we have fibre providing a continuous large molecular weight phase. On the other hand, the hind-gut dietary fibre undergoes partial or total degradation according to the type of fibre. All of this will influence the luminal environment and the nature and rate of absorption.

The composition of the plant cell wall is not homogenous. As the plant matures, there are changes in the cell-wall composition, lignification and a change from primary cell wall to a secondary cell wall which varies with increasing development, age and between species (Thornber and Northcote, 1961; Siegel, 1968). Fruit and vegetables, e.g. the potato, have cells that are relatively large and open (Robertson and Eastwood, 1981a, b), whereas in cereal bran the cells are smaller and the fibre appears more coarse. Cereal bran shows evidence of lignification of the outer cell layers whereas lignified tissue is rarely found in potato. Bagasse is very fibrous, highly vascularised and does not show much evidence of cell structure. Gums, mucilages and polysaccharide isolates will have no distinctive structure except that produced by processing into flakes or granules.

Fibres from different plant sources will have varied physical and chemical properties. These in turn will be different from homogeneous fibres such as polysaccharide isolates, gums and mucilages (Robertson and Eastwood, 1981a). These differences in chemistry and physical structure will profoundly affect the manner in which dietary fibres behave along the gastrointestinal tract.

Physical properties that influence function along the gastrointestinal tract are in combination of the colligative properties of the water-soluble fibre components and the surface properties of the water-insoluble fibre components. These properties including water holding, cation exchange, organic adsorption, gel filtration and particle size distribution (Eastwood and Mitchell, 1976). These physical properties are interrelated. It has been suggested that dietary fibre can act as an ion exchange and molecular sieve chromatography system throughout the gastrointestinal tract (Eastwood, 1975). The cell wall provides a water-soluble or insoluble matrix or phase through which the soluble contents of the gut can variably penetrate and partition with.

Along the gastrointestinal tract, fibre will interact with different phases. The systems that will develop will include (1) one-phase miscible mixtures; or (2) binary mixtures (multiphase system). These include (a) two-phase systems with one continuous phase and one dispersed phase; and (b) two-phase systems with two continuous phases. There are equations for defining each of these classes of mixtures (Nielsen, 1978). Along the gastrointestinal tract, fibre and other constituents of the luminal and mural phases may act as single-phase systems in which the components are completely miscible or soluble in each other. The properties that then become important are the density of the liquid mixtures, the dielectric constant of the mixture, viscosity, conductivity, surface tension and thermodynamic properties. Alternatively there can be two-phase or multiphase systems in which the components are insoluble or only partially soluble in each other. For two-phase systems, the shape and physical characteristics of the particles, the rate of diffusion through the mixtures, the viscosity of the suspension and the character and physical properties of the two phases become important. The nature of the interface between the phases is very important.

The simplest rule of mixture equation is

$$P = P_1 O_1 + P_2 O_2$$

The given property of the mixture being studied is P, and P_1 and P_2 are the corresponding properties of the components 1 and 2 of the mixture. The concentration of the components are O_1 and O_2. The property of a mixture is a direct combination of the properties of the components making up the mixture; for example, glucose entrapped in a water-soluble polysaccharide gel, like guar, and slowly being released for absorption in the jejunum.

However, these simple mixture rules are not capable of accurately predicting the properties of the binary mixture. Such predictions have to include intermolecular interaction or the way in which the molecules pack in the mixture. It is also necessary to know about the shape and orientation of the dispersed particles and the nature of the interphase; for example, an interaction between a fat dispersion, lipase and fibre in the jejunum, or bacteria, extracellular enzymes, bile acids, electrolytes, water and fibre in the colon. Our understanding of the behaviour of fibre and other intestinal luminal contents of varying molecular weight and type will be dependent on our understanding and prediction of these properties of mixtures. Such an understanding will be complicated in the jejunum with the digestive processes and in the colon where fermentation by bacteria will affect the fibre preparations.

Many fibre preparations have been shown to have an adsorptive ability (Eastwood and Hamilton, 1968; Birkner and Kern, 1974; Kritchevsky and Story, 1974). This is a surface phenomenon and therefore is affected by particle size. The water-holding capacity of the fibre source is not affected by age or plant variety (Robertson et al., 1980), but the fibre particle size does not affect water-holding capacity (Kirwan et al., 1974). It has been shown that water is associated with fibre in different phases, water bound to the fibre surface, water entrapped within the fibre matrix and free water (Labuza and Lewicki, 1979). Water bound to the fibre surface will be difficult to remove and the release of matrix and free water will vary with the fibre source. Bran is very insoluble and will contain little bound water, whereas vegetable fibre is partially water soluble and will contain a larger proportion of bound water. Very little suction pressure is required to produce a highly concentrated bran solution, but for vegetable fibre a relatively high suction pressure is required (Lewicki et al., 1978).

Such a physical approach to how fibre behaves along the gastrointestinal tract enables us to understand a further complicating factor. This is the influence of processing on how fibre behaves. Drying and cooking fibre will cause the collapse of the matrix structure and hence the ability to hydrate. The evaporation of water from the fibre causes the fibre to collapse to a non-porous solid. The heating of fibre can result in a non-enzymic browning (Maillard reaction) which alters the surface structure of the fibre. There is evidence that the metabolic effects of dietary fibre may also be influenced by interaction with other nutrients. It has been shown, for example (Levine and Silvis, 1980), that the ability of the dietary fibre to adsorb lipid depends on the physical form of the fat in the diet and the degree of refinement. Mac-Leod and Blacklock (1979) have shown that the ability of dietary fibre to bind calcium is reduced by the simultaneous administration of a high-carbohydrate diet. Similarly, the protein content of the diet may also influence the metabolic effects of the dietary fibre (Sanstead et al., 1979; Munoz, 1982). There are differences in the metabolism of gum arabic in the colon, depending on the diet given along with the gum arabic (Ross et al., 1984). The reason for these changes is that the physical properties of the fibre are modified and altered in binary mixtures along the gastrointestinal tract.

II. The effect of dietary fibre on gastric emptying

Digestible solids such as liver, egg and meat are probably delivered from the stomach as a result of two processes, grinding of the swallowed particles by antral contraction and propulsion of the finely suspended particles to the duodenum (Carlson et al., 1966). Fibre strands, however, are probably resistant to mechanical and chemical digestion in the stomach. Thus the shape, mechanical resilience and texture of the solid particles of different sizes are not the same. Also the results obtained for gastric emptying studies are very much dependent on which of the many methods are used (Heading et al., 1976). Carryer et al., (1982), using an I^{131}-labelled fibre that was 1 mm in length, showed that this left the stomach more slowly than the liquid but there was some fibre emptying in most periods, which suggests that solid–liquid separation in the post-prandial state is a continuous rather than a clearcut process. It is almost certain, however, that gastric emptying for a fibre on its own will be quite different when taken along with other dietary constituents. Likewise, it has been shown that the gastric emptying time for different fibre sources is variable (Tadesse, 1982). More viscous meals are probably emptied more slowly from the stomach (Holt et al., 1979).

Bueno et al. (1981) showed that the addition of bran, cellulose or guar gum to a meal increased the duration of the post-prandial disappearance of the migrating myoelectric motility pattern. This indicated that the bulking activity of these fibres prolongs the period of rapid gastric emptying and small intestinal flow. The effect was greatest in the diet that contained guar gum and this may relate to the greater water-holding capacity. Only guar gum significantly increased the frequency of the antral contraction.

These effects of fibre on gastric emptying have consequences for satiety and subsequent absorption from the small intestine.

III. The effect of dietary fibre on pancreatic function

Dietary fibre can have an inhibitory effect on pancreatic enzyme activities of human duodenal juice (Isaksson et al., 1979). It is possible that the fibre preparations that have a high viscosity, e.g. guar and a highly methoxylated pectin, may reduce enzyme substrate contact. It has been shown that there is an electrostatic interaction between trypsin and λ-carageenan, which is in keeping with other findings wherein enzymes and ionic polymers interact and the polymers act as competitive inhibitors (Gatfield and Stute, 1972). The in vitro digestibility of casein has been shown to be reduced in the presence of karaya, ghatti, tragacanth and guar (in descending order). The extent to which the protein digestion is reduced appears to be influenced by the structure of the gum, by the degree of branching, and the extent of ionisation

(Acton *et al.*, 1982). Other fibre constituents, lignin, apple pectin and residues from the predigested wheat bran, also reduce casein digestibility. In the presence of pectin, bran or bean, casein hydrolysis was less effective compared with hydrolysis of the casein alone. The restrictive filtration characteristics of the fibre may affect the availability of variable-sized peptides for further enzyme hydrolysis. Studies have been conducted on the hydrolysis rate of starch in food. Fibre appears to have an inhibitory effect on the rate of hydrolysis by forming a physical barrier to the access of the hydrolytic enzymes to the starch, e.g. whole brown rice. Particle size is an important factor in determining the rate of hydrolysis. Cooking makes starch much more readily available for enzymic hydrolysis as a result of gelatinising the starch. Stone ground wholemeal flour is believed to contain a natural amylase inhibitor that makes the starch hydrolyse slower than white flour. This amylase inhibitory activity is destroyed by passage through the roller mill (Snow and Odea, 1981).

Isaksson *et al.* (1982) further showed that the effect of fibre on pancreatic enzymes can be due to several factors. There is a direct enzyme fibre interaction. There are effects of viscosity and pH and adsorption. They showed in man decreased pancreatic enzyme activity in duodenal aspirates after the addition of fibre to the test meal. However, the complexity of the effect of fibre on pancreatic secretion was further shown by Schneeman (1982) in the rat where there are changes in pancreatic excretion of enzymes in response to the feeding of fibre.

IV.   Dietary fibre in the small intestine

A.   The small intestinal morphology

The small intestinal mucosa responds to many stimuli. Not all of the stimuli are identified but it is known that malnutrition, infection and infestation all can affect mucosal structure. In the adult population of Western countries, the mucosa is little different in shape than that in the infant. However, in most of Asia, Africa and Central and South America, the jejunal mucosa is more likely to be composed of leaf and convoluted shapes (Creamer, 1974). These latter areas, in addition to being malnourished and infected by all manner of bacteria and worms, are also the high-fibre-eating populations. It is possible that some variations in the small intestinal morphology are the result of diet.

Several studies have suggested that some sources of dietary fibre can cause morphological changes of the small intestine. Mucosal protein concentrations are lower in rats fed wheat bran or cellulose and mucosal peptidase activity is lower in rats fed cellulose (Schneeman, 1982). Rats fed dietary fibre supplements of 15 g/100 g diet showed variable responses in the enteric morphology according to the fibre source when the jejunal mucosa was looked at by the scanning electron microscope. Bran- and cellulose-fed rats showed no change in the surface mucosa. Animals fed 2% cholestyramine or 2% DEAE-Sephadex or 15% pectin or alfalfa were associated with significant morphological changes (Cassiday *et al.*, 1982). These changes are characterised by erosive damage to the mucosal epithelial cells.

B. Small intestinal contents

Physical properties of fibre will influence intestinal luminal contents. One of the striking effects of dietary fibre on small intestinal contents is to increase the dry weight (Eastwood and Boyd, 1967). The viscosity of the intestinal contents can be changed by the addition of fibre; high methoxy pectin and guar gum increase the viscosity of human duodenal fluid tenfold or more, and wheat bran increases the viscosity threefold (Schneeman, 1982).

In the small intestine during digestion and adsorption, endogenous and exogenous materials interact. Dietary fibre and bile acids both in solution and micelles interact so that the endogenous bile acids in the small intestine are adsorbed to dietary fibre. This adsorption is influenced by pH, osmolality, structure of the bile acids, the nature of the micelle and the physical and chemical form of the fibre (Eastwood and Hamilton, 1968; Kritchevsky and Story, 1974; Eastwood and Mowbray, 1976; Vahouny, 1982). Fibre can affect the distribution of bile acids between the small intestine and colon (Brydon *et al.*, 1980).

Vahouny (1982) has shown that certain dietary fibres may either interfere with the formation of micelles within the lumen of the small intestine or effectively alter the normal diffusion and accessibility of micellar lipids to the absorptive surface. Sequestration of lipids by fibre results in a reduced availability of fatty acids, monoglycerides and cholesterol for absorption in the upper intestine. This may mean a slowing down of the rate of absorption or even an increase in faecal fat and cholesterol and its bacterial metabolites. The reduced availability of biliary lecithin for absorption may be very important in the ability of the upper small intestine to snythesise and secrete the lipoproteins.

Carbohydrates, fats and proteins in the diet will be affected in a variety of ways in the small intestine. Low molecular weight sugars, glucose, maltose and oligosaccharides will be sequestrated within the water held in the matrix of the fibre. Thus, there will be a slowing of release of solute from the matrix and hence availability for absorption. The more viscous the fibre source the more effective it is in delaying solute release and absorption (Jenkins *et al.*, 1978). Studies with whole apples and apple juice show that the fibre present in fruits reduces the insulin response to the sugar within it and prevents rebound hypoglycaemia (Haber *et al.*, 1977; Bolton *et al.*, 1981). Following experiments with oranges, orange juice, grape and grape juice, satiety was found to be greater after whole food than after juice, and return of appetite was delayed with whole fruit. With oranges there was a significantly smaller insulin response to fruit than to juice and a smaller decrease in plasma glucose thereafter. However, with grapes the insulin response to the whole fruit was more than with the juice, whilst the post-absorptive glucose concentrations were similar.

It is apparent that the sequestration of nutrients and biliary and pancreatic secretions within fibre will influence intestinal absorption.

C. Mouth to caecum transit times

Investigation of the rate of passage from the mouth to the caecum in man requires indirect methods of study, e.g. to measure from the time of ingestion of lactulose to the increase in excretion of hydrogen in the breath caused by anaerobic bacterial metabolism in the caecum. By this means, Jenkins *et al.* (1978) showed that the addition of guar gum delayed the appearance of hydrogen in the breath by 1 to $1\frac{1}{2}$ h. Gum tragacanth and wheat bran have less delaying effects whilst pectin and methyl cellulose have none. Viscosity appears to have an effect on this mouth to caecum transit time. A complicating factor in the interpretation of the result is gastric emptying time. A further complicating factor is the molecular weight of the sugar used in the test. The mouth to caecum transit time for lactulose has been found to be 90 ± 7 min; for raffinose, 168 ± 38 min; and for stachyose, 290 min. Fasting and varying the osmolarity of the same oligosaccharide did not alter the mouth to caecum transit time. Yet, giving the three oligosaccharides directly into the colostomy of the patient did not show any difference in the hydrogen evolution time as measured in the colostomy orifice (Tadesse *et al.*, 1980).

D. The influence of dietary fibre on the release of gastrointestinal hormones

The effect of dietary fibre on the release of gastrin, glucagon, gastric inhibitory polypeptides (GIP) and insulin have been studied by Schrezenmeir and Casper (1981). These authors used wheat bran of fine or coarse particle size, apple pectin and carob seed flour. When wheat bran of small particle size is given as a 10-g addition to the diet, along with a standardised formula diet, the effect was an increase in the serum gastrin and a decrease in the GIP. The opposite effect was obtained by wheat bran of large particle size in that GIP concentration increased but the glucagon concentration decreased. The effect of 5 g of pectin was a decrease in the glucagon concentration. Similarly, carob seed flour decreased the glucagon concentration and the GIP concentration. The only significant effect on gastrin release was obtained by adding fine wheat bran to the diet.

E. The ileum

The ileum absorbs bile acids, vitamin b_{12} and intrinsic factor and chloride ions. The mechanism by which certain gel-forming polysaccharides, e.g. pectin, influence serum cholesterol and the enterohepatic circulation of bile acids is unknown. These polysaccharides increase faecal bile acid excretion. It is possible that the mechanism of such a hypocholesterolaemic effect is mediated through trapping bile acids in a gel which prevents absorption in the ileum and increases faecal loss.

V. The effect of fibre on the colon

The colon should be regarded as two organs. The right side, or caecum, is a fermenter. Here a large mass of bacteria live in anaerobic conditions where they metabolise and ferment materials passing out of the ileum. The left side of the colon, or descending and sigmoid colon, is involved in continence. The whole colon, though primarily the caecum, is involved in the concentration of faeces through the absorption of sodium and water. At the same time some potassium is excreted depending on luminal concentrations. Caecal metabolism also has an influence on the enterohepatic circulation.

A. The effect of dietary fibre on colonic morphology

The studies on colonic structure and mucosal cell growth have all been conducted in the rat. Jacobs and Schneeman (1981) showed that 20% wheat bran-containing diet fed to rats for 2 weeks led to colonic mucosal hyperplasia and muscle hypertrophy. The effect was that the total intestinal wet weight of both the proximal and the distal colon increased in the bran-fed rats compared to the fibre-free controls, whilst the mucosal weight was increased only in the distal colon of the bran-fed group. The increase in mucosal growth in the distal colon of the bran-fed animals was shown by raised amounts of protein, DNA and RNA, whilst in the proximal colon, changes in mucosal growth were less marked. It is known that the proliferative activity of the intestinal mucosa is influenced both in humans and experimental animals by the diet, by the composition of luminal contents, and by a variety of hormones. Both conjugated and unconjugated bile acids of physiological concentration have been reported to affect intestinal ultrastructure and cause disruptive changes (Saunders et al., 1975). It is known that some dietary fibres and pharmaceutical bile acid sequestrants interact with bile acids and hence increase faecal bile acids. Vahouny et al. (1981) looked at the effect of three bile acid sequestrants—cholestyramine, colestipol and DEAE-Sephadex—at 2% or 15% additions of wheat bran, cellulose, pectin or alfalfa. The cholestyramine caused discontinuities of the colonic epithelial barrier, cell destruction and haemorrhage of the tissue surfaces. Similar but less severe changes from the normal morphology were observed in animals fed colestipol or DEAE-Sephadex, pectin or alfalfa. Wheat bran and cellulose had no such effects except for some increased goblet cell numbers. Wheat bran and cellulose were the only feeding situations where there were significantly reduced intestinal transit times. There was a strong correlation between the bile acid-binding capacity of the dietary supplements and the morphological changes observed in the colon.

Bran and citrus pulp affects the microsomal enzyme 3-hydroxy-3-methylglutaryl-CoA reductase (HMG-CoA reductase), the rate-limiting enzyme in cholesterol biosynthesis. This enzyme is present in the colon, small intestine and liver. The small intestine is the second major site of cholesterol synthesis in the body. However, as a result of the administration of wheat bran and citrus pulp, the HMG-CoA reductase activity in the small intestine was 33% lower than the citrus pulp group and 55% lower in the wheat bran group compared with a control group. HMG-CoA reductase activity was significantly lower in the colon in rats that consumed the wheat bran diet than those that consumed the control diet (Smith-Barbaro et al., 1981). Similarly, the cytochrome p-450 was reduced in the colon as a result of increase in the fibre content of the diet with wheat bran and citrus pulp. Elsanhans et al. (1981) showed the long-term effect of the feeding of fibre sources on the small intestine and colon. They studied some polysaccharides, guar, tragacanth, gum arabic, carageenan, karaya and methylcellulose. They used a period of 7 to 8 weeks, which is longer than most experiments where 3 weeks is about normal. They assumed that guar, tragacanth and gum arabic would be degraded by bacteria in the colon, whilse carageenan and gum karaya would not. The results confirmed that this was the case; 85% of the former fibre sources were degraded and less than 10% of the inert polysaccharides. The polysaccharides that were microbiologically degraded caused the caecal contents and muscle to double in weight compared to the responses to the inert polysaccharides. In conventional animals, the caecum enlargement resulted from incompletely digested carbohydrates and bacterial proliferation. In germ-free animals, the enlargement is thought to be due in part to the accumulation of mucous materials. It is not clear why the muscle mass as well as the contents appear to increase. Perhaps it is because increased colonic work is needed to propel the more bulky contents along the colon. On the other hand, as will be discussed later, the evolution of nutrients within the colon may result in increased nutrition to the colon.

B.   Caecal contents

The caecal contents contain (1) matrix, the fibrous material of the dietary fibre; (2) bacteria; and (3) intestinal contents, which include (a) solute of varying type and amount derived from unabsorbed nutrients, bile and intestinal secretions, and (b) water.

1.   *Matrix—dietary fibre*

The matrix or support medium will consist of polysaccharides and lignin with physical properties that will affect the behaviour of the caecal contents. The aqueous phase will function as flowing and fixed zones that interact with phases of water in the fibre in a manner similar to that of liquid chromatography.

Partition behaviour in gel chromatography depends on the relative polarities of the gel, solute and solvents in addition to steric exclusion. The polarity of the interphase is important. Adsorption may well occur and there is an inverse relationship between adsorption and solubility of the solute. In the colon, chemicals will be partitioned in the various phases and bacteria will also be distributed throughout the system in a way which will be based on physical characteristics.

2.   *The caecum as a fermenter*

The microbial system of the rumen is the most clearly understood intestinal fermentation system (Wolin, 1981). Ruminants rely on the digestion of food by micro-organisms. However, whilst the knowledge of fermentation in the rumen gives important clues to the events in the human large intestine, the two do not necessarily function in the same manner. In the ruminant, ingested polysaccharides, e.g. grasses, hay and corn, which have been ground in the mouth and swallowed, are then fermented in the rumen to volatile fatty acids (VFA) (acetate, propionate and butyrate), methane, hydrogen and carbon dioxide. The large mass of bacteria and protozoa derive their energy from the ingested food. The VFA are a major source of carbon energy for metabolic activities. The micro-organisms, however, are the primary digestion systems. The large volume of gases and large number of micro-organisms create a highly anaerobic environment and the pH is controlled by the secretion of bicarbonate and phosphate that enters the rumen from saliva. Factors that influence turnover times include the amount of food intake, the cell-wall content and particle size of the diet. An important effect on microbial activity is the turnover time which determines the balance between rates of microbial processes and the rates of passage of the rumen contents. These micro-organisms not only produce VFA but synthesise vitamins and convert protein to organic acids and ammonia. Ammonia is used by almost all bacteria as a source of nitrogen for the generation of protein. Hydrogen is an important intermediate produce of fermentation and is rapidly used by methanogens. Continual reduction and oxidation of pyridine nucleotides are central to any fermentation. The generation of lactate, ethanol, propionate, succinate and butyrate requires the reoxidation of reduced nicotinamide adenine dinucleotide (NADH) or reduced nicotinamide adenine dinucleotide phosphate (NADPH). In the rumen there is an inverse relationship between the formation of VFA and methane. It is desirable to produce more VFA than methane in the cow or sheep for obvious nutritional purposes.

The fibrous constituents of the human diet which are not digested by endogenous secreted enzymes are available for microbial fermentation in the large intestine. A further source of nutrient in the colon are intestinal epithelial cells and mucins from the small and large intestine (Salyers *et al.,* 1977). The hydrolytic conditions in the large intestine are complex. There is a complicated solute–bacterial–fibre interaction. Whilst the products of the large intestinal fermentation are similar to those in the rumen, there are important differences in how they function (McKay *et al.,* 1981).

3. *Bacteria in the caecum*

There are problems in studying the human large intestinal microbial flora, particularly in the caecum. Bacteria are found in the various phases adherent to the epithelium and in the lumen with a variable proportion bound to and associated with fibre. The bacterial population in each phase is different. The bacterial flora of the intestine has been investigated in detail (Wrong *et al.,* 1981). The large intestine contains approximately 10^{11} bacteria per gram. The proportion of the large bowel contents made up of bacteria vary in estimation between 20 and 55%, depending on the fractionation technique. In man, over 95% of faecal bacteria are obligatory anaerobes, the most numerous being bifidobacilli and bacteroides. Problems of identifying bacteria relate in part to available techniques (Hill, 1982). A complication of describing the effects of dietary fibre on caecal bacteria is in part because of the large variety of species. There are 400–500 bacterial species in the colon, colonic contents and faeces and many bacterial species are present in relatively small number. A further complication in identifying bacteria is caused by their variable alignment on the fibre matrix and hence problems of extraction.

Berg *et al.* (1972) looked at cellulytic bacteria grown on cellulose and showed that growth only occurred when the fibres were cut short. Other bacteria grow within the lumen of the fibre. Cellulytic enzymes may be extracellular and pass into fibre pores.

It has been shown that bacteria, adsorbed to DOWEX-1 chloride columns, grow as well as, if not faster than, cells in free solution. However, the oxygen consumption of these adsorbed cells is lower (Hattori, 1972; Hattori and Hattori, 1973). Savage (1978) has suggested that fibre may act to stabilise the epithelial bacteria communities by affecting bowel peristalsis mixing and hence affect colonic microbial activity. Dietary fibre also can add stability to microbial communities by providing nutrients for such microbes that can digest cellulose or other fibres not digested in the small bowel. Fibre may interact with microbes to lower local oxygen tension and oxidation reduction potential by absorbing oxygen or other oxidising molecules. Wilkins (1981) stresses that the interpretation of results in experiments using animals and man where there are microbial differences must be cautious. The bacterial flora of rodents is so very different from that of the human digestive tract, particularly in the colon. Coprophagy causes even more problems.

There are two types of study on the effect of diet on the faecal bacterial flora. One such study is a comparison of the flora of individuals who have taken one lifelong diet with that of another population. This has been investigated with Ugandans and Londoners, Ugandans eating a diet of matoke (plantains) and the Londoners a normal Western diet. There were slight differences between the bacterial flora in these two groups (Hill, 1982). The faecal flora of various populations in India, Japan, Edinburgh, London and Hawaii are somewhat similar (Hill, 1982). An alternative method has been to study the effect of dietary changes on the faecal bacteria. Such studies have failed to reveal any major change with altering dietary fat, protein, meat, wheat bran and various fractions of dietary fibre (Hill, 1982; Bornside, 1978). The total amount of bacteria per gram of faeces remain constant. Therefore, the total output but not concentration of faecal bacteria is related to dietary fibre and stool mass (Bornside, 1978).

Another approach is the use of an *in vitro* semi-continuous culture system (Miller and Wolin, 1981). Whilst it is possible to produce an impressive artefact by such a system, it is possible that important insights into the human large intestinal microbial activity can be obtained. Clearly the initial faecal innoculum has to be carefully described. For example, the previous dietary habits of the individual from whom the innoculum was obtained are important in order that reproducible work results. Miller and Wolin (1981) found that when the nutrient suspension contained lettuce, celery, carrot and unsweetened apple sauce, the predominent non-sporing anaerobes obtained were bacteroides species. When carrots and apple sauce were omitted, the predominent non-sporing isolates were fusobacterium species. In both diets clostridia were isolated.

However, the overwhelming conclusion for all the studies reported is to indicates the stability of the human faecal flora. It is possible, therefore, that any effects of dietary fibre will be functional rather than changes in overall type of bacteria.

The effects of bacteria on fibre. It has been demonstrated in various ways that polysaccharides can be metabolised by colonic bacteria. Electron microscopic observations on the degradation of cellulose fibres demonstrates that compact fibres are slowly degraded (Berg *et al.,* 1972). Bacteria penetrate into the lumen of the fibre and accumulate in large numbers, which indicates that the fibre matrix may disintegrate under bacterial hydrolytic attack.

However, the methods of looking at fibre metabolism are somewhat limited and there is a temptation to over-interpret the results. Part of the problem is the preoccupation with the effect of fibre on stool weight rather than the possibility that, in part, man is coprophagic albiet by absorption from the colon of short-chain fatty acids. The inaccessibility of the caecum and the difficulty to cannulate the portal vein makes the study of the absorption of caecal metabolites a formidable problem. The methods that investigate faeces represent studies on end products and may be an inaccurate reflection of caecal metabolism. For example, after ingesting gum arabic for 3 weeks, there was no increase in faecal VFA output but other indicators of gum arabic fermentation, e.g. breath hydrogen, increased (Ross et al., 1983).

One way of looking at polysaccharide fermentation in the rat colon has been to use gum arabic (Ross et al., (1984). This gum, as with other gums, gives a white precipitate with ethanolic hydrochloric acid. In this way, it was possible to show that the caecum is essential for polysaccharide fermentation in the rat. A caecectomy resulted in a white precipitate of gum arabic being obtained in the stool.

It has been suggested in man that on control diets only about 20% of ingested fibre is recovered in the stools, which suggests that fibre from a wide range of sources is digested (Cummings et al., 1981). Other studies show that pectin and cabbage fibre are metabolised but bran fibre is only partly digested; 60% is recovered in the stool. In wheat bran all the main components of fibre are poorly digested and recognisable bran particles can be seen in the faeces of subjects taking bran (Williams et al., 1978). The likely reason for this is the tightly compressed structure of the bran in the presence of lignin, which is known to inhibit bacterial activity. Polysaccharides that are water soluble, e.g. gum arabic and pectin, appear to be readily broken down. The water-soluble gel appears to allow ready access to bacteria (Robertson and Eastwood, 1981a).

The factors that affect the fermentation of polysaccharides in the colon include the inherent characteristics of fibre, water solubility (Robertson and Eastwood, 1981a), lignification, particle size and molecular structure. The interplay of water, bacteria and fibre must mean that no single factor stands on its own so that bacteria which get ready access to the interior of a fibre such as pectin by virtue of water solubility will also be influenced by particle size and molecular structure. Similarly, the effect of particle size of wheat bran is in part mediated through chemistry, the availability of bacteria and also water-holding capacity.

The duration of fibre feeding is important. Experiments with gum arabic (Ross et al., 1983), carrot (Robertson et al., 1979) and gum karaya (M. A. Eastwood, personal cummunications, 1982) show that a prolonged period of ingestion is required to get objective evidence of fermentation of these fibres. This is in contrast to acute exposure when there may be no evidence of fermentation (Tadesse and Eastwood, 1978).

Few studies on dietary fibre have included dose–response curves. Part of the problem here is an aftermath effect wherein when one fibre source has been stopped and the control diet restored there are consequences of this change which affect the next phase of the experiment (Eastwood *et al.*, 1973; Kay and Truswell, 1977a; Wyman *et al.*, 1976). it would appear that other components of the diet, e.g. starch, which have not been digested by pancreatic amylase, may pass into the colon and be fermented. This again is idiosyncratic to each fibre source and will depend on the type of fibre, its relationship to the starch and how it was cooked. There is no doubt that there are considerable effects of food processing such that dried and heated fibre sources will not behave in the same way as fibres that are raw or cooked (Robertson and Eastwood, 1981a; Wyman *et al.*, 1976). Cogeeners ingested with the fibre source are important. This has not been thoroughly explored, but Ross *et al.* (1984) showed that gum arabic is metabolised differently in the rat when fed with an elemental diet or with a standard rat pellet diet.

C. Evidence of fermentation of fibre in the caecum

1. Gas production

The three major gases formed in the colon are carbon dioxide, hydrogen and methane. Bond and Levitt (1978) have shown that hydrogen in man is derived from bacterial metabolism and that this takes place almost entirely in the colon. Production in the colon depends on the presence of exogenously supplied fermentable substrate such as carbohydrate (Bond and Levitt, 1978).

2. Carbon dioxide

Carbon dioxide results from bacterial metabolism in the colon. The precise mechanism of its production is not known. It has been shown that the effect of beans on intestinal gas is to increase the production of hydrogen and carbon dioxide (Steggarda and Dimmick, 1966). This indicates that plant polysaccharides are involved in carbon dioxide production.

3. Hydrogen production

Hydrogen is produced in the colon (Bond and Levitt, 1978). In anaerobic bacterial metabolism, hydrogen ions are transferred to a number of suitable carriers. An important disposal mechanism for hydrogen ions is through the formation of molecular hydrogen:

$$2e + 2H^+ \xrightarrow{\text{hydrogenase}} H^2$$

Hydrogen once it is formed in the caecum and colon is either passed as flatus per rectum or absorbed into the portal blood stream and excreted unchanged by the lungs (Calloway, 1968).

The evolution of hydrogen has a regular pattern through the day: comparatively high in the morning, falling until about midday and rising during the early afternoon. The mean hydrogen excretion at any time during the day is less than 0.5 μmol/litre and individual breath samples rarely contain more than 0.9 μmol/litre. The average daily breath excretion by an individual is of the order of 50 to 200 ml/day. Fasting decreases the overall hydrogen production and markedly affects the afternoon rise. The early morning increase is probably due to the previous evening meal and the afternoon rise is related to breakfast.

In acute studies, few of the different components of dietary fibre cellulose, pectin and lignin, ingested on a single occasion, resulted in the increased production of hydrogen (Tadesse and Eastwood, 1978). The single dose administration of unprocessed bran results in a modest increase in breath hydrogen (Bond and Levitt, 1978). However, a complicating and variable problem with bran is the coincidental adminstration of starch. Whilst most of the starch will be digested in the small bowel, a proportion of retrograde starch that has evaded or is inaccessible to amylase digestion is carried down to the colon. If a fibre preparation is taken for 3 weeks, e.g. carrot (Robertson et al. 1979) or gum arabic (Ross et al., 1983), then there is an increase in breath hydrogen. Conditions in the colon are important in the production of hydrogen from carbohydrate. Perman et al. (1981) have shown that hydrogen production in the colon is maximal at neutral pH and is strongly inhibited at acid and alkaline pH. This reduction in activity is not due to the disappearance of bacteria but rather to diminished metabolic activity. An endogenous source of substrate for bacterial metabolism which leads to production of hydrogen is intestinal mucopolysaccharide. The amount of hydrogen generated appears to be related to the proportion of carbohydrate in the mucopolysaccharide (Perman and Modler, 1982).

4. *Methane*

The proportion of the population who produces methane differs somewhat from population to population, varying between 30 and 60%. The reasons for this are not at all apparent. The mechanism by which methane is produced is well understood in the rumen but poorly understood in the human colon. There is no obvious daily pattern of excretion in those individuals who excrete methane. Once one is a methane producer, one is always a methane producer. However, individuals who do not produce methane in the breath almost entirely have methane in the flatus gas.

It has always been assumed that methane production is dependent on a strict anaerobic methanobacterium (Nottingham and Hungate, 1968). McKay et al. (1982) showed that small but significant amounts of methane are produced by three strains, *Clostridium histolyticum, C. perfringens* and *Bacteroides thetaiotaomicron*. Fresh or freeze-dried faeces, on incubation, can result in methane production (McKay et al., 1985).

It has been shown in a population study that the concentration of methane in the expired breath of methane-producing subjects was related to the dietary intake of non-cellulosic polysaccharide pentoses and also to the intake of lignin (McKay *et al.*, 1981). The single dose administration of D (+) xylose and L (+) arabinose led to a significant increase in methane excretion in methane producers in a biphasic manner. The first peak of methane production is probably caused by the rapid fermentation of the unabsorbed fraction of pentose passing into the caecum. The second phase possibly is a delayed metabolism caused by unfavourable conditions, e.g. altered pH or as the result of a second slowly reacting methanogenic bacterial species (McKay *et al.*, 1981). However, if a complex polysaccharide source rich in pentoses was given to fasting subjects, this did not result in an increase in methane production when measured over 5 h. There appears to be a period of adaptation because prolonged administration of gum arabic to rats resulted in a steady increase in methane production (Ross *et al.*, 1984).

In man, colonic methane production appears to be quite separate from hydrogen production and does not have the same inverse relationship as in the rumen (McKay *et al.*, 1981). The factors that influence methane production in man are more complicated than in the rumen.

An effect of gas formation is the introduction of a further phase in the luminal environment. This will mean that there will be gas bubbles and pockets of gas in addition to the liquid and solid phases which will influence the contact between luminal content, colonic mucosa and between bacteria and substrate. Some of the distension of the colon will affect mucosal and muscular activity.

5. *Short-chain fatty acids*

The fermentation of bacteria in the colon of both soluble and insoluble carbohydrate results in the formation of short-chain fatty acids of which acetate, propionate and butyrate are the most important end products. In the ruminants they provide 70–80% of the animal's nutritional requirements. Less is known of short-chain fatty acid metabolism in the colon. The fermentation of carbohydrate to short-chain fatty acids is an anaerobic process. The hexose breakdown is through the Embden-Meyerhoff glycolytic pathway to pyruvate and is converted to acetate, propionate, butyrate, carbon dioxide, hydrogen, methane and water (Cummings, 1981b). Short-chain fatty acids constitute a major anion in colonic contents (Argenzio, 1982) with a concentration of approximately 75 mmol/kg wet weight. It has been suggested that approximately 20 g of cell-wall polysaccharides and other carbohydrates are fermented in the human colon each day so that approximately 200 mmol of short-chain fatty acids are produced (Cummings, 1981b).

The proportion of the major fatty acids varies with the diet and other conditions. Gum arabic results in an increase of production of VFA in the rat colon (Ross *et al.*, 1984). Studies in men who have changed from a conventional diet to one containing only carbohydrate demonstrate an overall fall in total VFA concentration in faecal dialysate from 85 to 46 mmol/litre and modest changes in the molar ratios of acetate, propionate and butyrate. If the same subjects took only methylcellulose, a further fall in concentration was seen (Rubenstein *et al.*, 1969).

Whilst a considerable amount of short-chain fatty acids are produced, only 7–20 mmol/day are excreted in the stool; therefore, there must be substantial absorption and metabolism of short-chain fatty acids in the colon (Cummings, 1981).

The absorption of VFA in the human colon is comparable to that observed in animals of the order of 6 to 12 mmol/cm^2/h. There appears to be a substantial metabolism of short-chain fatty acids in the colonic mucosal cells and this may be an important energy source, especially butyrate. This metabolism in the colon and the uptake by the liver results in a very small circulating concentration of acetate, less than 0.02 mmol/l (Skutches *et al.*, 1979). In the rat, VFA from fermented carbohydrate increase in the caecum over 2 h from the time of the last meal. It has been estimated that acetate propionate and butyrate contribute approximately 5% of the caloric intake (Yang *et al.*, 1970). It is clear that in the rat VFA constitute a steady and important source of nutrition through the portal vein (Buckley and Williamson, 1977; Remesy and Demigne, 1976). It is not known how important such sources of nutrition are in man.

D.   Fibre: the caecum and the enterohepatic circulation

Water-soluble conjugates arriving in the caecum, usually biliary excretion products which are unabsorbed in the small intestine, are modified by bacteria to less water-soluble compounds, e.g. bile acids and bilirubin. Such modified metabolites may adsorb to bacteria or fibre or be reabsorbed into the circulation through the colonic mucosa. This is an important but poorly understood aspect of physiology, pathology and drug metabolism. Changes in pH will affect bacterial activity and chemical metabolic activity (Perman *et al.*, 1981).

The enterohepatic circulation contributes to the conservation of compounds in the body, e.g. bile acids and possibly other compounds of intermediate metabolism. This is of physiological importance. The half-life is influenced by the enterohepatic circulation of such compounds, e.g. iophenoxic acid is $2\frac{1}{2}$ years. Recycling contributes to the persistence of stilboestrol, butylated hydroxy toluene, rifomycin SV, chlorinated hydrocarbon pesticides and carcinogenic hydrocarbons. It is possible that the presence of fibre in the caecum may influence the metabolism of these compounds.

VI.   The effect of dietary fibre on intestinal transit time

The gastrointestinal tract is a long tube punctuated by sphincters, the lower oesophageal sphincter, the pylorus, ileal caecal valve and the rectum. Whilst intestinal transit is usually measured as the total intestinal transit time, there are variable periods of delay in the stomach, ileum, caecum and rectum. Each of these will influence the intestinal transit. Transit time lengthens the further along the gut the chyme passes, so that oesophageal, gastric, and small intestinal passage are faster than that through the colon. Yet from a functional point of view, these areas seem to be much more important. The effect of fibre on transit from the stomach and small intestine has already been discussed at the appropriate points.

The movement of contents along the colon is achieved by mass peristalsis but an important role is played by segmentation. This motor activity is much more likely to aid the slow turnover of contents locally to assist water absorption and the conversion from a viscous liquid to a solid or plasticine-like faeces. Movement along the colon is aided by mass peristalsis. Food increases the segmenting motor activity of the colon by distension either directly in the colon or indirectly in the small intestine through the release of cholecystikinin.

A.   Caecal residence time

Very few studies have been done to establish accurately the influence of fibre on caecal residence time. The recent study of McKay et al. (1983) showed that a straight X-ray of the abdomen could separate old people into one of three groups: those with a caecum full of faeces from those with a caecum full of gas, and a group which was intermediate. In the one, the proportion of methane producers was 65% and in the other the proportion of methane producers was 30%. However, using a multiple marker method no difference in caecal emptying time could be distinguished.

B.   Intestinal transit time

The rate of passage of material from mouth to anus varies from person to person and even from time to time in that individual (Wyman et al., 1976). However, a complicating factor is the shortcomings of the methodology (Hinton et al., 1969; Wiggins and Cummings, 1976; Kirwan and Smith, 1974).

Burkitt and Painter (1975), Connell and Smith (1974), Spiller et al. (1977), and Findlay et al. (1974), have all shown a reciprocal relationship between intestinal transit and faecal weight. Spiller has suggested that the transit time decreased to a faecal output of 150 g/day but beyond this there was no further decrease. He suggested that the colonic activity was more predictable at faecal outputs of 140 to 150 g/day where the transit averaged 2–3 days. Payler *et al.* (1975) suggested that this is the normal or perhaps even ideal transit time. Spiller suggested that in order to examine influences on stool weight, 150 g would be the ideal stool weight to start from in order to get reproducible results. Wheat bran is the most effective in reducing transit time. Raw bran with high water-holding capacity is more effective than fine bran and cooked bran which has less water-holding capacity. This has been shown in normal subjects and in patients with diverticular disease (Kirwan *et al.*, 1974; Wyman *et al.*, 1976; Eastwood *et al.*, 1978; Smith *et al.*, 1981). Other sources of fibre are not so effective on transit time, e.g. citrus pectin (Kay and Truswell, 1977b), sugar cane fibre (Baird *et al.*, 1977), and cabbage and apple fibre (Cummings *et al.*, 1978).

VII.   Normal stool weight

It is not really known what normal stool weight is. Variations in stool weight in various communities is almost certainly due to differences in diet. However, a recent study suggests that the personality of the individual affects stool weight (Tucker *et al.*, 1981) so that the more extrovert person excretes more stool on a given fibre diet than an introverted individual, which suggests that the colon is yet another mode of self expression. Estimates of stool weight for the average Western diet are 100–150 g/day (Eastwood *et al.*, 1982; Burkitt *et al.*, 1974; Wyman *et al.*, 1978). The figures for British vegetarians were 225 g/day (Burkitt and Painter, 1975) and for Dutch students, eating a diet rich in fruit and vegetables and wholemeal bread, 184 g/day (Stasse-Wolthuis *et al.*, 1979).

A.   *The effect of fibre on faecal content*

The effect of fibre on faecal content depends on the fibre source. The effect of cereal bran taken daily results in a dilution of the faecal contents (Eastwood *et al.*, 1973; Cummings *et al.*, 1976). The dilution of colonic contents as a result of cereal bran presumably coincides with the reduction of any unfortunate effects of the concentrated stool. Bile acid excretion has been shown to increase 3–4 weeks following a period of bran administration (Eastwood *et al.*, 1973; Kay and Truswell, 1977a). This suggests that changes in bacterial flora are important. However, if water soluble and fermentable fibre sources are given, such as pectin, psyllium seed and certain legumes then there is an enhancement of faecal bile acid loss (Eastwood *et al.*, 1980). Under these circumstances the faecal weight increase is not significant and hence the faecal constituents are more concentrated.

B. *Fibre and stool weight*

The relationship between dietary fibre and stool weight has been substantially reviewed in the recent past (Eastwood *et al.*, 1980; Royal College of Physicians, 1980).

Faeces are a complex mixture of micro-organisms, undigested food residues, soluble ions and organic compounds and water. However, it is not a uniform phase. Scanning electron microscopy (Williams, *et al.*, 1978) shows that faeces contain a large number of bacteria intermingled with small or amorphous particles of food residue. Some of the bacteria are groups in colonies. Within the faecal mass, fragments of cell residues are embedded and bacteria can be seen aligned on the fibre surface.

The most important and possibly only physiological determinant of stool weight is dietary fibre. This has been shown in repeated studies by supplementing the diet with fibre (Royal College of Physicians, 1980; Eastwood *et al.*, 1980) and also in epidemiological studies (Eastwood *et al.*, 1982). However, the effect of fibre on stool weight varies with the fibre source and from person to person (Cummings *et al.*, 1978). Williams and Olmsted (1936) originally suggested that it was the fermentation of carbohydrates in the caecum with the release of short-chain fatty acids that was responsible for stool bulk. Hellendoorn (1978) continued to uphold the view that it is the VFA, lactic acid and bacterial mass which account for the faecal mass. This suggests that it is the disappearance of fibre rather than the persistence of fibre that is important. McNeil *et al.* (1978), however showed that most of the short-chain fatty acids produced can be absorbed by the human large intestine.

An alternative view that has been developed is that it is the water-holding capacity of the fibre that is important. Bran preparations of different water-holding capacity have effects on colon function which parallel the water-holding capacity of that bran. Fine bran with low water-holding capacity has less effect on colon function than coarse bran which has a high water-holding capacity (Kirwan *et al.*, 1974; Brodribb and Groves, 1978; Smith *et al.*, 1981).

It would appear that it is the effect of fermentation on a dietary source which will influence its final faecal bulking effect. Stephen and Cummings (1980) showed that the bacterial content of the stool is an important factor in dictating stool weight. Fermentation enables bacteria to proliferate and hence to influence stool weight. Fibre passing from the ileum into the caecum will be saturated with water. Stephen and Cummings (1980) showed that there is an inverse relationship between water-holding capacity and faecal output. One reason for this is that in fibre preparations with a high water-holding capacity, e.g. pectin, the water is strongly held, whereas in fibre preparation with a low water-holding capacity, e.g. bran, the water is very loosely held when measured against known suction potential (Robertson and Eastwood, 1981b).

A further estimate of the ability of fibre to retain water can be obtained from the measurement of the rate of flow of water through the fibre when it has been packed into a column. The rate of flow at a given pressure difference depends on the mean pore size of the fibre and the affinity of the fibre for water. Cereal fibre, bagasse and cellulose allow a steady flow of water through the fibre, whereas potato fibre and gum arabic hold the water tightly and the flow rate is very slow (Robertson and Eastwood, 1981b).

In the caecum and the colon, there is the conversion of fibre into stool. The water content of stools is almost always between 70% and 80%. Bacteria consist of about 80% water which suggests that the constancy of faecal water percentage is in part dictated by bacteria (Stephen and Cummings, 1980). The other important constituent of stool, i.e. fibre, would require a water-holding capacity of 3 to maintain this constancy of 75% water. Very little pressure is required to change the water-holding capacity of cereal bran which is usually approximately 3, so that suction pressure of only 0–0.1 atm is required. Bagasse only required 0.05 atm; potato fibre and carrot fibre, 0.5–1.2; and gum arabic and pectin, which have large water-holding capacities, require 6–10 atm to reduce the water-holding capacity to 3. These latter bind water much more strongly than bagasse and cereals.

Once the fibre is in the caecum, bacteria begin to ferment it. Bacteria will attack those fibres which are susceptible to hydrolysis. It is possible that there is change over a period of time and adaptation to a new and regularly administered fibre. Bacteria will proliferate as a result of the available nutrient provided by the fibre. There may be inhibition of bacterial activity by osmotic pressure and solutes such as bile acids. However, there will be a residual fibre which may well have a substantial pentosan content and water-holding capacity (Cummings et al., 1978). Physical factors such as compression, chemistry, water insolubility and cooking may influence penetration of the fibre mass by bacteria. The extent to which fermentation takes place appears to depend on the following.

1.   *The chemistry of fibre*

Water-insoluble fibres such as bran and bagasse appear to be less readily available for fermentation than water soluble fibres such as pectin, gum arabic and vegetable fibres. The degree to which bacteria can penetrate the fibre is important so that those fibres that form gels are water soluble and allow penetration and fermentation more readily than water insoluble. Again the mode of cooking and preparation such as drying, influence such penetration.

2. *Solutes in the caecum*

Bile acids are known to influence bacterial activity (Mitchell *et al.*, 1974). pH may influence fibre degradation. The residence time in the caecum is important. The longer the fibre remains in the caecum, presumably the longer the available time for fermenting the fibre. Residence, however, may well be influenced by the generation of fermentation products, e.g. VFA.

Overall the conversion of ileal contents to faeces is a consequence of a redistribution of water. Some water will be retained by the fibre. The remainder will be held as intracellular water by proliferating bacteria or absorbed by the colon. In this way the litre or so of ileal effluent is converted to 100 to 150 g of faecal mass.

The plasticine-like nature of faeces will be a complex between fibre, bacteria, intracellular interfibril water, lipids, VFA, medium- and long-chain fatty acids, calcium and magnesium ions. The complicated physical nature will be due to ionic charges, fatty layers, hydrophobic and hydrophilic characteristics of the residual fibre and bacteria. All of this in physiological terms results in approximately 25% dry weight and 75% water content.

References

ACTON, J. L., BREYER, L. and SATTURLEE, L. D. (1982). *J. Food Sci.* **47**, 556–560.

ARGENZIO, R. A. (1982). *Dig. Dis. Sci.* **26**, 97–98.

BAIRD, I. M., WALTER, R. L., DAVIES, P. S., HILL, M. J., DRASAR, B. S. and SOUTHGATE, D. A. T. (1977). *Metab., Clin. Exp.* **26**, 117–128.

BERG, B., HOFSTEN, B. V. and PETTERSSON, G. (1972). *J. Appl. Bacteriol.* **35**, 215–219.

BIRKNER, H. J. and KERN, F. JR. (1974). *Gastroenterology* **67**, 237–244.

BOLTON, R. P., HEATON, K. W. and BURROUGHS, L. F. (1981). *Am. J. Clin. Nutr.* **34**, 211–217.

BOND, J. H. and LEVITT, M. D. (1978). *Am. J. Clin. Nutr.* **31**, S169–S174.

BORNSIDE, G. H. (1978). *Am. J. Clin. Nutr.* **31**, S141–S144.

BRODRIBB, A. J. M. and GROVES, C. (1978). *Gut* **19**, 60–63.

BRYDON, W. G., TADESSE, K., EASTWOOD, M. A. and LAWSON, M. E. (1980). *Br. J. Nutr.* **43**, 101–106.

BUCKLEY, B. M. and WILLIAMSON, D. H. (1977). *Biochem. J.* **166**, 539–545.

BUENO, L., PRADDAUDE, F., FIORAMONTI, J. and RUCKEBUSCH, Y. (1981). *Gastroenterology* **80**, 701–707.

BURKITT, D. P. and PAINTER, N. S. (1975). *In* "Refined Carbohydrate, Foods and Disease" D. P. Burkitt and H. C. Trowell, eds), pp. 69–84. Academic Press, London.

BURKITT, D. P., WALKER, A. R. P. and PAINTER, N. S. (1974). *JAMA, J. Am. Med. Assoc.* **229**, 1068–1074.

CALLOWAY, D. H. (1968). *In* "Handbook of Physiology" (C. F. Code, ed.), Sect. VI, Vol. 5 pp. 2839-2859. Am. Physiol. Soc., Washington, D.C.

CARLSON, H. C., CODE, C. F. and NELSON, R. A. (1966). *Am. J. Dig. Dis.* **11**, 155–172.

CARRYER, P. W., BROWN, M. L., MALAGELADA, J. R., CARLSON, G. L. and MCCALL, J. T. (1982). *Gastroenterology,* **82**, 1389–1394.

CASSIDAY, M. M., LIGHTFOOD, F. G. and VAHOUNY, G. V. (1982). *In* "Dietary Fibre in Health and Disease" (G. V. Vahouny and D. Kritchevsky, eds), pp. 239–264. Plenum, New York.

CONNELL, A. M. and SMITH, C. L. (1974). *In* "Proceedings of the Fourth International Symposium on Gastrointestinal Motility" (E. E. Daniel *et al.,* eds)., pp. 365–368. Mitchell Press Ltd., Vancouver, B. C., Canada.

CREAMER, B. (1974). *In* "The Small Intestine" (B. Creamer, ed.), pp. 1–24. Heinemann, London.

CUMMINGS, J. H. (1981). *Gut* **22,** 763–779.

CUMMINGS, J. H., HILL, M. J., JENKINS, D. J. A., PEARSON, J. H. and WIGGINS, H. S. (1976). *Am. J. Clin. Nutr.* **29,** 1468–1473.

CUMMINGS, J. H., SOUTHGATE, D. A. T., BRANCH, W. J., HOUSTON, H., JENKINS, D. J. and JAMES, W. P. T. (1978). *Lancet* **1,** 5–8.

CUMMINGS, J. H., STEPHEN, A. M. and BRANCH, W. J. (1981). *In* "Gastrointestinal Cancer: Endogenous Factors" (W. R. Bruce, P. Correa, M. Lipkin, S. R. Tannenbaum and T. D. Wilkins, eds), Banbury Rep. No. 7, pp. 71–81. Cold Spring Harbor Lab., Cold Spring Harbor, New York.

EASTWOOD, M. A. (1975). *Med. Hypothesis* **1,** 46–53.

EASTWOOD, M. A. and BOYD, G. S. (1967). *Biochim. Biophys. Acta.* **152,** 159–166.

EASTWOOD, M. A. and HAMILTON, D. (1968). *Biochim. Biophys. Acta* **52,** 165–173.

EASTWOOD, M. A. and MITCHELL, W. D. (1976). *In* "Fibre in Human Nutrition (G. A. Spiller and R. J. Amen, eds), pp. 109–130. Plenum, New York.

EASTWOOD, M. A. and MOWBRAY, L. (1976). *Am. J. Clin. Nutr.* **29,** 1461–1467.

EASTWOOD, M. A., KIRKPATRICK, J. R., MITCHELL, W. D., BONE, A. and HAMILTON, T. (1973). *Br. Med. J.* **4,** 392–394.

EASTWOOD, M. A., SMITH, A. N., BRYDON, W. G. and PRITCHARD, J. L. (1978). *Gut* **19,** 1144–1147.

EASTWOOD, M. A., BRYDON, W. G. and TADESSE, K. (1980). *In* "Medical Aspects of Dietary Fiber" (G. A. Spiller and R. M. Kay, eds). pp. 1–26. Plenum, New York.

EASTWOOD, M. A., BAIRD, J. D., BRYDON, W. G., SMITH, J. H., HELLIWELL, S. and PRITCHARD, J. L. (1982). *In* "Dietary Fiber in health and disease" (G. V. Vahouny and D. Kritchevsky, eds), pp. 23–33. Plenum. New York.

ELSENHANS, B., BLUME, R. and CASPARY, W. F. (1981). *Am. J. Clin. Nutr.* **34,** 1837–1848.

FINDLAY, J. M., SMITH, A. N., MITCHELL, W. D., ANDERSON, A. J. B. and EASTWOOD, M. A. (1974). *Lancet* **1,** 146–149.

GATFIELD, I. L. and STUTE, R. (1972). *FEBS Lett.* **28,** 29–31.

HABER, G. B., HEATON, K. W., MURPHY, D. and BURROUGHS, L. F. (1977). *Lancet* **2,** 679–682.

HATTORI, R. (1972). *J. Gen. Appl. Microbiol.* **18,** 319–327

HATTORI, R. and HATTORI, T. (1973). *Ecol. Rev.* **16,** 63–70.

HEADING, R. C., TOTHILL, P. and MCLAUCHLIN, G. P. (1976). *Gastroenterology,* **71,** 45–60.

HELLENDOORN, E. W. (1978). *In* "Topics in Dietary Fiber Research" (G. A. Spiller, ed.), pp. 127–146. Plenum, New York.

HILL, M. J. (1982). *In* "Colon and Nutrition" (H. Kasper and H. Goebell, eds), pp. 37–45. M.T.P. Press Ltd., Lancaster, England.

HINTON, J. M., LENNARD-JONES, J. E. and YOUNG, A. C. (1969). *Gut* **10,** 842–847.

HOLT, S., HEADING, R. C., CARTER, D. C. PRESCOTT, L. F. and TOTHILL, P. (1979). *Lancet* **1,** 636–639.

ISAKSSON, G., IHSE, E. and LUNDQUIST, I. (1979). *Dan. Med. Bull,* **26,** 19.

ISAKSSON, G., LUNDQUIST, I. and ISHE, I. (1982). *Gastroenterology* **82,** 918–924.

JACOBS, L. R. and SCHNEEMAN, B. O. (1981). *J. Nutr.* **11,** 798–803.

JENKINS, D. J. A., WOLEVER, T. M. S., LEEDS, A. R. GASSULL, M. A., HAISMAN, P., DILAWARI, J., GOFF, D. V., METZ, G. L. and ALBERTI, K. G. M. M. (1978). *Br. Med. J.* **1,** 1392–1394.

KAY, R. M. and TRUSWELL, A. S. (1977a). *Br. J. Nutr.* **37,** 227–235.

KAY, R. M. and TRUSWELL, A. S. (1977b). *Am. J. Clin. Nutr.* **30,** 171–175.

KIRWAN, W. O. and SMITH, A. N. (1974). *Scand. J. Gastroenterol.* **9,** 763–768.

KIRWAN, W. O., SMTIH, A. N., McCONNELL, A. A., MITCHELL, W. D. and EASTWOOD, M. A. (1974). *Br. Med. J.* **4,** 187–189.

KRITCHEVSKY, D. and STORY, J. A. (1974). *J. Nutr.* **104,** 458–462.

LABUZA, T. P. and LEWICKI, P. P. (1979). *J. Food Sci.* **43,** 1264–1273.

LEVINE, A. S. and SILVIS, S. E. (1980). *N. Engl. J. Med.* **303,** 917–918.

LEVITT, M. D. and BOND, J. H. (1970). *Gastroenterology* **59,** 921–929.

LEWICKI, P. P., BUSK, G. C. and LABUZA, T. P. (1978). *J. Colloid Interface Sci.* **64,** 501–509.

McKAY, L. F., BRYDON, W. G., EASTWOOD, M. A. and SMITH, J. H. (1981). *Am. J. Clin. Nutr.* **34,** 2728–2733.

McKAY, L. F., HOLBROOK, W. P. and EASTWOOD, M. A. (1982). *Acta Pathol. Microbiol. Immunol. Scand,* **90,** 257–260.

McKAY, L. F., SMITH, R. G., EASTWOOD, M. A., WALSH, S. D. and CRUIKSHANK, J. G. (1983). *Age and Ageing* **12,** 105–110.

McKAY, L. F., EASTWOOD, M. A. and BRYDON, W. G. (1985). *Gut* **26,** 69–74.

McLEOD, M. A. and BLACKLOCK, N. J. (1979). *J. R. Nav. Med. Serv., Winter* **65,** 143–146.

McNEIL, N. I., CUMMINGS, J. H. and JAMES, W. P. T. (1978). *Gut* **19,** 819–822.

MILLER, T. L. and WOLIN, M. J. (1981). *Appl. Environ. Microbiol.* **42,** 400–407.

MITCHELL, W. D., FINDLAY, J. M., MACRAE, R., EASTWOOD, M. A. and ANDERSON, R. (1974). *Digestion* **11,** 135–146.

MUNOZ, J. M. (1982). *In* "Dietary Fibre in Health and Disease" (G. V. Vahouny and D. Kritchevsky, eds), pp. 85–89. Plenum, New York.

NIELSEN, L. E. (1978). "Predicting the Properties of Mixtures. Mixture Rules in Science and Engineering." Dekker, New York.

NOTTINGHAM, P. M. and HUNGATE, R. E. (1968). *J. Bacteriol.* **96,** 2178–2179.

PAYLER, D. K., POMARE, E. W., HEATON, K. W. and HARVEY, R. F. (1975). *Gut* **16,** 209–213.

PERMAN, J. A. and MODLER, S. (1982). *Gastroenterology* **83,** 388–393.

PERMAN, J. A., MODLER, S. and OLSON, A. C. (1981). *J. Clin. Invest.* **67,** 643–650.

REMESY, C. and DEMIGNE, C. (1976). *Rech. Vet.* **7,** 39–55.

ROBERTSON, J. A. and EASTWOOD, M. A. (1981a). *Br. J. Nutr.* **45,** 83–89.

ROBERTSON, J. A. and EASTWOOD, M. A. (1981b). *Br. J. Nutr.* **46,** 247–255.

ROBERTSON, J. A., BRYDON, W. G., TADESSE, K., WENHAM, P., WALLS, A. and EASTWOOD, M. A. (1979). *Am. J. Clin. Nutr.* **32,** 1889–1892.

ROBERTSON, J. A., EASTWOOD, M. A. and YEOMAN, M. M. (1980). *J. Sci. Food Agric.* **31,** 633–638.

ROSS, A. H. Mc L, EASTWOOD, M. A., BRYDON, W. G., ANDERSON, J. R. and ANDERSON, D. M. W. (1983). *Am. Clin. Nutr.* **37,** 368–375.

ROSS, A. H. Mc L., EASTWOOD, M. A., BRYDON, W. G., BUSUTTIL, A., McKAY, L. F., and ANDERSON, D. M. W. (1984). *Br. J. Nutr.* **51,** 47–56.

Royal College of Physicians (1980). "Medical Aspects of Dietary Fibre." Pitman Medical, London.

RUBENSTEIN, R., HOWARD, A. V. and WRONG, O. M. (1969). *Clin. Sci.* **37,** 549–564.

SALYERS, A. A., VERCELLOTTI, J. R., WEST, S. E. H. and WILKINS, T. D. (1977). *Appl. Environ. Microbiol.* **33,** 319–322.

SANDSTEAD, H. H., KELVAY, L. M., JACOB, R. A., MUNOZ, J. M., LOGAN, G. M. JR. and

RECK, S. J. (1979). *In* "Dietary Fibres: Chemistry and Nutrition" (G. E. Inglett and S. I. Falkehag, eds), pp. 147–156. Academic Press, New York.

SAUNDERS, D. R., HEDGES, J. R., SILLERY, J., ESTER, L., MATSUMURA, K. and RUBIN, E. E. (1975). *Gastroenterology* **68**, 1236–1295.

SAVAGE, D. C. (1978). *Am. J. Clin. Nutr.* **31**, S131–S135.

SCHNEEMAN, B. O. (1982). *In* "Dietary Fiber in Health and Disease" (G. V. Vahouny and D. Kritchevsky, eds), pp. 73–83. Plenum, New York.

SCHREZENMEIR, J. and CASPER, H. (1981). *In* "Colon and Nutrition" (H. Casper and H. Goebell, eds), Falk Symp. No. 32, pp. 71–76. M.T.P. Press Ltd., Lancaster, England.

SIEGEL, S. M. (1968). *In* "Comprehensive Biochemistry" (M. Florkin and E. H. Stotz, eds). Vol. 26, pp. 1 Am. Elsevier, New York.

SKUTCHES, C. L., HOLROYDE, C. P., MYERS, R. N., PAUL, P. and REICHARD, G. A. (1979). *J. Clin. Invest.* **64**, 708–713.

SLAVIN, J. L., BRAUER, P. M. and MARLETT, J. A. (1981). *J. Nutr.* **111**, 287–297.

SMITH, A. N., EASTWOOD, M. A. and DRUMMOND, E. (1981). *Am. J. Clin. Nutr.* **34**, 2460–2463.

SMITH-BARBARO, P. A., HANSON, D. and REDDDY, B. S. (1981). *J. Nutr.* **111**, 789–797.

SNOW, P. and ODEA, K. (1981). *Am. J. Clin. Nutr.* **34**, 2721–2727.

SPILLER, G. A. and KAY, R. M. (eds) (1980). "Medical Aspects of Dietary Fiber." Plenum, New York.

SPILLER, G. A., CHERNOFF, M. C., SHIPLEY, E. A., BEIGLER, M. A. and BRIGGS, G. M. (1977). *Am. J. Clin. Nutr.* **30**, 659.

STASSE-WOLTHUIS, M., HAUTVAST, J. G., HERMUS, R. J. J., KATAN, M. B., BAUSCH, J. E., RIEBERG-BRUSSARD, J. H., VELEMA, J. P., ZONDEWAN, J. H., EASTWOOD, M. A. and BRYDON, W. G. (1979). *Am. J. Clin. Nutr.* **32**, 1881–1888.

STEGGARDA, F. R. and DIMMICK, J. F. (1966). *Am. J. Clin. Nutr.* **19**, 120–124.

STEPHEN, A. M. and CUMMINGS, J. H. (1980). *Nature (London)* **284**, 283–284.

TADESSE, K. (1982). *J. Physiol. (London)* **332**, 102–103P.

TADESSE, K. and Eastwood, M. A. (1978). *Br. J. Nutr.* **40**, 393–396.

TADESSE, K., SMITH, D. M. and EASTWOOD, M. A. (1980). *Q. J. Exp. Physiol. Cogn. Med. Sci.* **65**, 85–97.

THORNBER, J. P. and NORTHCOTE, D. H. (1961). *Biochem. J.* **81**, 449–455.

TUCKER, D. M., SANDSTEAD, H. H., LOGAN, G. M., JR., KLEVAY, L. M., MAHALKO, J., JOHNSON, L. K., INMAN, L. and INGLETT, G. E. (1981). *Gastroenterology* **81**, 879–883.

VAHOUNY, G. V. (1982). *In* "Dietary Fiber in Health and Disease" (G. V. Vahouny and D. Kritchevsky, eds), pp. 203–227. Plenum, New York.

VAHOUNY, G. V. and KRITCHEVSKY, D. (eds) (1982). "Dietary Fiber in Health and Disease." Plenum Press, New York.

VAHOUNY, G. V., CASSIDY, M. M., LIGHTFOOT, F., GRAU, L. and KRITCHEVSKY, D. (1981). *Cancer Res.* **41**, 3764–3765.

WIGGINS, H. S. and CUMMINGS, J. H. (1976). *Gut* **17**, 1007–1011.

WILKINS, T. D. (1981). *In* "Gastrointestinal Cancer: Endogenous factors" (C. N. Bruce, P. Correa, M. Lipkin, S. R. Tannenbaum, and T. D. Wilkins, eds), Banbury Rep. No. 7; pp. 33–39. Cold Spring Harbor Lab., Cold Spring Harbor, New York.

WILLIAMS, A. E., EASTWOOD, M. A. and CREGEEN, R. (1978). *Scanning Electron Microsc.* **2**, 707–712.

WILLIAMS, R. D. and OLMSTED, W. G. (1936). *J. Nutr.* **11**, 433–449.

WOLIN, M. J. (1981). *Science* **213**, 1463–1468.

WRONG, O. M., EDMONDS, C. J. and CHADWICK, V. S. (1981). *In* "The Large Intestine", pp. 25–31. M.T.P. Press Ltd., Lancaster, England.

WYMAN, J. B., HEATON, K. W., MANNING, A. P. and WICKS, A. C. B. (1976). *Am. J. Clin. Nutr.* **29**, 1474–1479.

WYMAN, J. B., HEATON, K. W., MANNING, A. P. and WICKS, A. C. B. (1978). *Gut* **19**, 146–150.

YANG, M. G., MANOHARAN, K. and MICHELSON, O. (1970). *J. Nutr.* **100**, 545–550.

Chapter 7

Constipation

ALISON STEPHEN

I. Introduction

Constipation is not a new problem. Throughout this century large numbers have suffered from this disorder, and for decades, ideas have varied about its definition, its aetiology and its treatment. Much of the problem lies in the subjective nature of bowel habits and in disagreement over what is and what is not normal.

II. Definition

Studies of healthy volunteers have shown that the majority of the population in the Western world pass one bowel movement per day with an average daily output of 120 to 130 g of stool (Rendtorft and Kashgarian, 1967). This is true, both for subjects eating their normal diets (Wyman *et al.,* 1978; Kien *et al.* 1981) and for those taking part in dietary studies and consuming metabolically controlled diets that contain typical Western foods (Cummings *et al.,* 1978a; Kelsay *et al.,* 1978). In both types of study, large individual variation is seen, both in frequency and weight of bowel movements, without complaints of either constipation or diarrhoea. Such variability in normal bowel habit makes it difficult to define an abnormal or "constipated" state.

133

Dietary Fibre, Fibre-Depleted Foods
and Disease

There have been four major approaches to a definition of constipation and these differ in the parameter described. Connell *et al.* (1965) suggested that less than three bowel movements per week was abnormal, and hence frequency was the point of focus. However, many people who do not consider themselves constipated would come into this category, as Hinton and Lennard-Jones (1968) have found, and they therefore put forward a slow transit rate as the definition. Transit time is inversely related to stool weight (Burkitt *et al.*, 1972; Cummings, 1978) and those complaining of constipation have been found to have delayed transits (Hinton and Lennard-Jones, 1968; Brocklehurst and Khan, 1969). However, there is considerable controversy over the measurement of transit time itself (Cummings *et al.*, 1976a) and it is not practically feasible to undertake such a measurement in every patient. Moreover, like stool weight, transit shows a large individual variation, even for individuals on identical diets (Cummings *et al.*, 1976b; Stephen, 1980). To define "slow" then becomes the problem. Godding (1980) suggested that the definition should be one based on the consistency of the stool, but this again is difficult to achieve in clinical practice (Devroede, 1978). Finally, Painter (1980) has included a subjective factor to the definition, that any patient who strains to defaecate and does not pass at least one soft stool daily without effort is constipated. This would seem the most satisfactory definition to date, but is impractical in its requirement for a daily stool. Many have bowel movements less frequently, but of a greater weight than those defaecating every day.

III. Incidence of constipation

Individual variability in bowel habit makes an overall definition of constipation almost impossible, and similar problems arise when estimating the incidence of constipation in the community. Studies of random samples have produced very different values for the proportion of the population suffering from constipation. Connell *et al.* (1965) found that 4% of a group of factory workers said they were constipated, while the proportion was 16% for a group attending their medical practitioner. Because the problem is said to be more common in the elderly (Brocklehurst and Khan, 1969; Clark and Scott, 1976), a number of surveys have been conducted with older subjects. Milne and Williamson (1972) found only 3% of a large group of 500 individuals, aged 62–90, who claimed they were constipated, while Johnson *et al.* (1980) more recently reported that 30% of a group of elderly women were bothered by constipation. This wide variation again reflects the subjective nature of this disorder and does not allow a firm statement on the size of the problem in the Western world.

IV. Laxative use

A similarly confused situation is seen in the taking of laxatives where the retail sales are often used as an indicator of the occurrence of constipation. It is true that such sales are enormous. In 1981, $358 million was spent on laxatives in the United States (Annual Report on Consumer Spending, 1982), and the variety of possible formulations available (Curry, 1982) shows that this business is flourishing. However, careful examination of the reasons for taking laxatives suggests that they are not always to alleviate constipation (Cummings, 1976). Many individuals, especially in the older age groups, grew up believing that daily bowel movements are a necessity to cleanse themselves of their bodily toxins, and the advertising media, even today, condones such a belief. A large proportion of those taking laxatives do so as a habit, making laxative intake an unreliable index of constipation.

In summary, information on normal bowel habits, incidence of constipation and intake of laxatives is confused and inconclusive. Although no one would deny that the problem of constipation is large, with great social and economic consequences, data on the actual size of the problem, in numerical terms, are lacking. The major reasons for this are variability in bowel habit and the perception of what is normal. It is likely, therefore, that constipation will continue to be dealt with on an individual basis. In doing so, it is important to recognise that numerous factors influence faecal output, and that one or a number of these may predispose an individual towards becoming constipated.

V. Factors affecting faecal output

A. Disorders that cause constipation

There are a number of diseases that cause constipation, which have been outlined in detail (Devroede, 1978). They are in two general categories, systemic and gastrointestinal, and include metabolic and endocrine disorders, such as diabetes, hypothyroidism and uraemia and bowel abnormalities of either neurogenic origin or from disorders of bowel structures in the colon, rectum or anal canal. In addition, constipation may be induced by a variety of drugs, such as analgesics, antidepressive agents or diuretics (Devroede, 1978). However, the majority of those complaining of constipation are not taking drugs and do not have underlying disease. One or a number of the following factors bring about reduced faecal output and frequency in these people.

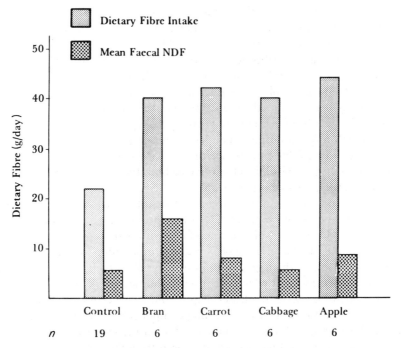

Fig. 7.1. The amount of fibre remaining [as neutral detergent fibre (NDF)] in stools of individuals fed an additional 20 g dietary fibre per day derived from bran, cabbage, carrot and apple. Measurements were made on stools from the third week of each 3-week dietary period. n = Number of subjects on each diet. [Reproduced from Baird and Ornstein (1981) with permission from Kellogg Company of Great Britain Limited.]

B. Diet

During the last decade, a major focus of interest for both gastroenterologists and nutritionists alike has been the relationship between diet and faecal output, particularly the role of dietary fibre. When fed under metabolic conditions, both protein and fat have no effect on faecal weight (Cummings *et al.*, 1978b; 1979), whereas fibre from a number of sources has been shown to increase faecal output on numerous occasions (Southgate and Durnin, 1970; Baird *et al.*, 1977; Farrell *et al.*, 1978; Prynne and Southgate, 1979; Stasse-Wolthius *et al.*, 1980). The extent of the increase in faecal weight varies with the source of fibre and its physical and chemical composition (Cummings *et al.*, 1978a; Heller *et al.*, 1980).

1. Mechanism of faecal bulking by dietary fibre

Until recently, fibre was thought to increase faecal weight according to its water-holding capacity (McConnell *et al.*, 1974), but we have shown that the relationship between water holding and faecal bulking is, in fact, an inverse one (Stephen and Cummings, 1979). The more water a material holds, the less effect it has on faecal weight, not the reverse. To find the mechanism by which fibre increases bulk, we have therefore examined the digestibility of dietary fibre, as shown in Fig. 7.1. When 20 g dietary fibre from one of four sources—bran, apple, cabbage or carrot—was given to healthy individuals for 3 weeks under controlled conditions, it was found that only bran survived to any extent in the stools. The other materials were largely degraded, with very little increase in faecal fibre excretion over the control diet (Stephen, 1980). Cabbage fibre for example, virtually disappeared, yet it had a considerable effect on faecal output when fed, increasing mean daily faecal weight from 117 to 189 g (69%) in six healthy subjects (Cummings et al., 1978a). Since the cabbage itself did not survive to bulk the stool, the increase must have been through some other means.

By examination of the different components of stools, we have found that cabbage, and other vegetable fibre sources, provide carbohydrate substrate which stimulates growth of the microflora within the colon (Stephen and Cummings, 1980). Bacteria are 80% water (Luria, 1960), and their increase in mass in stools with degradable fibre materials largely accounts for the increases in faecal weight which occur when they are fed. On the other hand, bran stimulates bacteria to a lesser degree, but survives itself to hold water. There are, therefore, two water-holding components in the stool with bran, fibre and bacteria, and together these produce larger faecal weights, as in the above study when stool weight was increased from 96 to 197 g/day (127%).

These two different mechanisms for the way fibre increases faecal output are shown schematically in Fig. 7.2, and stress the varied effects that fibre may have. Not only are changes in faecal bulk different, but the greater degradation of fibre with vegetables may have effects elsewhere in the body. For example, volatile fatty acids produced by fibre digestion are now known to be absorbed from the human colon (McNeil et al., 1978; Ruppin et al., 1980), and may have actions in other tissues. These and other metabolic effects of fibre are only beginning to be investigated.

2. *What type of fibre is best?*

It is clear from the foregoing discussion that, to increase faecal bulk, bran and wheat fibre, because of their resistance to degradation, are more effective than fruit and vegetable sources. This is by no means a new finding, but one that needs reiterating. Dimock (1937) stated, ". . . the fibre of green vegetables and ordinary foodstuffs is more readily broken down in the alimentary tract than is that of wheat bran. This explains why the addition of fruit and vegetables to the diet so often fails to prevent constipation." Hence, a diet may seem at first glance adequate enough in fibre to produce satisfactory bowel habits, but may be lacking in cereal fibre constituents. Those suffering from simple constipation tend to have lower fibre intakes (Johnson et al., 1980), but there is considerable overlap with normal individuals. Closer

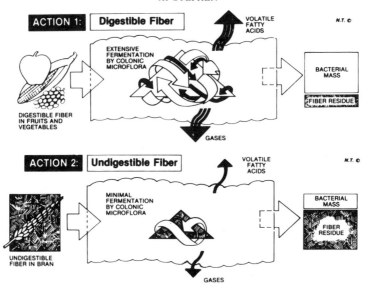

FIG. 7.2. The mechanism of action of dietary fibre in the large intestine. Action 1: Fibre from fruits and vegetables is degraded by the colonic microflora when it enters the colon, providing energy for bacterial growth. Hence the mass of bacteria excreted in the stool increases. The by-products of fibre degradation, the short-chain fatty acids, are absorbed. Very little fibre survives to be excreted in the stool. Action 2: Bran is not degraded well by the colonic microflora and so survives to be excreted in the stool. Faecal bacterial mass is little affected by bran and both production and absorption of short-chain fatty acids is small. (Reproduced with permission of *Nutrition Today* magazine, P.O. Box 1829, Annapolis, Maryland 21404, ©November/December, 1981, with modification.)

examination of the diet, which has not been reported, may indicate that it is the intake of fibre from cereals which is lower in constipated subjects.

C. Transit time

Diet is not the only factor that contributes to the variability in faecal output. When investigating the bacterial component of faeces, we found that there was a range in the daily output of bacteria in the volunteers studied, although they were consuming identical diets with exactly the same fibre content. The mass of bacteria excreted daily was related to the transit time through the intestinal tract, with a greater weight of bacteria with a faster transit time and vice versa (Stephen, 1981). Similar relationships have been shown in other "continuous flow" fermentation systems, such as the rumen (Harrison *et al.*, 1975; Kennedy *et al.*, 1976) or continuous culture (Hobson and Summers, 1967; Isaacson *et al.*, 1975). In these systems, a faster turnover allows for a smaller resident population of bacteria and hence a lesser proportion of the available energy is needed for bacterial cell maintenance, which leaves a larger amount for cell growth (Owens and Isaacson, 1977; Hespell and

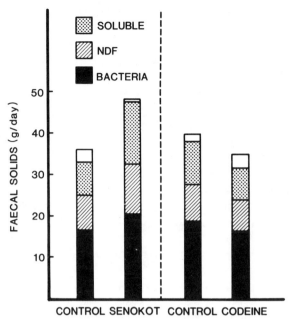

FIG. 7.3. The effect of changing transit time using drugs affecting colonic motility on output of faecal solids. Decreased transit with senokot (2–8 tablets per day) resulted in increased excretion of all components of faecal solids: Solids ($p < 0.005$), NDF, bacteria ($p < 0.05$), soluble ($p < 0.001$). Codeine (30–120 mg/day + 0–8 mg loperamide/day) had the opposite trend: Solids, soluble ($p < 0.05$), NDF, bacterial (NS), four subjects in each group. (From Stephen, 1980).

Bryant, 1979). To test this further, we changed the transit time of healthy individuals using drugs that affect colonic motility, while maintaining a constant diet (Stephen, 1980). Codeine and/or loperamide were used to slow transit and senokot was used to speed it up; doses were adjusted to achieve the desired changes in transit and were maintained for 3-week periods. The changes in transit time resulted in alterations in faecal weight, faecal water and in the components of faecal solids as shown in Fig. 7.3. With a slow transit time, as in constipation, the output of stools and its components decrease, whereas with fast transit, the opposite occurs. Hence, even with a constant diet, faecal output can vary depending on the rate of passage through the gut.

1. *Factors affecting transit time*

(a) *Hormones.* The extent of hormonal influences on gastrointestinal function, including motility and transit time, is as yet uncertain, but there are a number of hormones which are emerging as potentially important in the normal functioning of the intestine. It has frequently been observed, for example, that constipation is more common in women than in men (Connell *et al.*, 1965; Clark and Scott, 1976), and in metabolic studies, women have been found to have smaller faecal outputs than men on similar diets (Stephen, 1980). Moreover, it has been suggested that there may be an effect of the menstrual cycle on faecal output, with a period of constipation before the onset of menstruation, which changes to normality or even mild diarrhoea at the start of the menstrual period (McCance and Pickles, 1960; Rees and Rhodes, 1976). Of all the reproductive hormones, progesterone is the one that increases most in the blood during the second half of the monthly cycle (Thorneycroft *et al.*, 1971). Recent studies examining the effects of progesterone have shown that it inhibits colonic activity *in vitro* (Bruce and Beshudi, 1980) and that *in vivo,* it slows small intestinal transit during the luteal phase of the menstrual cycle (Wald *et al.*, 1981). No conclusive information about progesterone or menstruation and colonic function is yet available, and accurate and continuous measurement over several months would be required to obtain this. Raised progesterone levels may also explain the frequent complaint of constipation in pregnancy (Wald *et al.*, 1982), although since oestrogen has been found to have the opposite effect (Bruce and Beshudi, 1981), the picture remains unclear. Furthermore, aldosterone is also at greater levels in the second half of the menstrual cycle (Katz and Romfh, 1972), and also has effects on the colon, although these are mainly on absorption (Charron *et al.*, 1969; Thompson and Edmonds, 1971).

Faecal output may therefore be influenced by the effect of these hormones on colonic function, and this may, in part, explain the smaller faecal weights in women and their tendency towards constipation. In addition, a vast literature now exists on the effects of gastrointestinal hormones, like motilin, VIP and enteroglucagon on motility in all regions of the intestine (Bloom, 1980). However, their effects at physiological levels and hence their role as regulators of colonic motility remain to be demonstrated.

(b) *Other endogenous compounds.* In addition to hormonal influences, several other endogenous components have been shown to influence colonic motility and hence may play a part in determining faecal output. Some of these, like bile acids (Shiff, 1979), or volatile fatty acids (Yokohura *et al.*, 1977) may alter in concentration as a result of dietary change, whereas others may alter under the influence of other stimuli, as, for example, prostaglandins, shown to influence colonic peristalsis (Bruch *et al.*, 1978) and which are affected by catecholamines and cholinergic stimulation (Bruch *et al.*, 1976). New to the field of intestinal motility are the endogenous opioids (Konturek, 1980). These may also play a regulatory role, as suggested by Kreek *et al.* (1983), who found the opiate antagonist, naloxone, useful in treating constipation.

(c) *Lifestyle.* Since the last century, changes have taken place not only in our diet, but also in our lifestyle, and components of this may also influence transit time and faecal output. The most likely candidate is the level of exercise. Immobility, due to bedrest or travelling, often results in constipation (Jones *et al.*, 1968). Brocklehurst (1980), who has studied constipation in the elderly for many years, believes that it is inactivity which leads to their constipation, not old age itself. Starling (1930) stated that the prevalence of sedentary occupations in civilised communities is as important in producing constipation as a diet lacking in fibre. Indeed, in a recent study in South Africa, the amount of exercise in different populations was related to their faecal output, with the conclusion that exercise does have an influence (Walker *et al.*, 1981). The relationship between personality and stool weight has also been investigated; those who were more socially outgoing, energetic and optimistic produced larger stools (Tucker *et al.*, 1981). Stress has also been shown to influence colonic function (Chaudary and Truelove, 1967).

VI.   Prevention of constipation

The preceding factors affecting stool output have been outlined to indicate the complexity of colonic function and the numerous reasons why constipation may exist. However, prevention of constipation must be the goal, not merely alleviation of the disorder, once it has occurred. Treatment of constipation frequently requires administration of laxatives as well as a high-fibre regimen (Jones and Godding, 1972), whereas constipation can be prevented without the taking of drugs. Education is a key component. An understanding of how the colon functions and the factors that influence it can only help to reduce the incidence of constipation.

Fibre in the diet, particularly wheat fibre, will contribute to a properly functioning colon. This is not to say that vegetable fibre is unnecessary; its degradation products may be essential for other physiological and metabolic actions which fibre is said to have.

Bran supplements have been shown to be effective in preventing constipation in the elderly (Clark and Scott, 1976; Andersson *et al.*, 1979; Smith *et al.*, 1980). One geriatric centre in the United States has initiated a programme of fibre-containing foods for all of its 300 residents (Hull *et al.*, 1980). After 1 year, the use of laxatives in this centre was virtually eliminated, a savings of $44,000. Bowel habits were regular and transient discomfort after beginning the regimen disappeared. However, many find unprocessed bran unpleasant and difficult to tolerate for extended periods. An overall change in dietary pattern to include high-fibre foods in place of refined ones is what is required for the population as a whole. If this was done so that the average intake of dietary fibre was 40 g/day instead of less than 20 g, much of the problem of constipation would be irradicated. In addition, more exercise would be beneficial and women should realise that, as far as bowel habit is concerned they are at a disadvantage, and must compensate.

References

ANDERSSON, H., BOSAEUS, I., FALKHEDEN, T. and MELKERSSON, N. (1979). *Scand. J. Gastroenterol.* **14**, 821–826.

Annual Report on Consumer Spending (1982). *Drug Top.* **126**, 1–79.

BAIRD, I. M. and ORNSTEIN, M. H. (eds.) (1981). "Dietary Fibre: Progress Towards the Future." Kellogg Company of Great Britain Limited, Manchester.

BAIRD, I. M., WALTERS, R. L., DAVIES, P. S., HILL, M. J., DRASER, B. S. and SOUTHGATE, D. A. T. (1977). *Metab.* **26**, 117–128.

BLOOM, S. R. (1980). *J. R. Coll. Physicians,* **14**, 51–57.

BROCKLEHURST, J. C. (1980). *Geriatrics* **35**, 47–54.

BROCKLEHURST, J. C. and KHAN, M. Y. (1969). *Gerontol. Clin.* **11**, 293–300.

BRUCE, L. A. and BESHUDI, F. M. (1980). *Life Sci.* **27**, 427–434.

BRUCE, L. A. and BESHUDI, F. M. (1981). *Proc. Soc. Exp. Biol. Med.* **166**, 355–359.

BRUCH, H. P., SCHMIDT, E. and LAVEN, R. (1976). *Acta Hepato-Gastroenterol.* **23**, 430–434.

BRUCH, H. P., SCHMIDT, E., LAVEN, R., KEHRER, G. and WASNER, K. H. (1978). *Acta Hepato-Gastroenterol.* **25**, 303–307.

BURKITT, D. P., WALKER, A. R. P. and PAINTER, N. S. (1972). *Lancet* **2**, 1408–1412.

CHARRON, R. C., LEME, C. E., WILSON, D. R., ING, T. S. and WRONG, O. M. (1969). *Clin. Sci.* **37**, 151–167.

CHAUDARY, N. A. and TRUELOVE, S. C. (1961). *Gastroenterology,* **40**, 27–36.

CLARK, A. N. G. and SCOTT, J. F. (1976). *Age Ageing* **5**, 149–154.

CONNELL, A. M., HILTON, C., IRVINE, G., LENNARD-JONES, J. E., and MISIEWICZ, J. J. (1965). *Br. Med. J.* **2**, 1095–1099.

CUMMINGS, J. H. (1976). *Recent Adv. Gastroenterol.* **3**, 124–149.

CUMMINGS, J. H. (1978). *J. Plant Foods* **3**, 83–96.

CUMMINGS, J. H., HILL, M. J., JENKINS, D. J. A., PEARSON, J. R. and WIGGINS, H. S. (1976a). *Am. J. Clin. Nutr.* **29**, 1468–1473.

CUMMINGS, J. H., JENKINS, D. J. A. and WIGGINS, H. S. (1976b). *Gut* **17**, 210–218.

CUMMINGS, J. H., SOUTHGATE, D. A. T., BRANCH, W., HOUSTON, H., JENKINS, D. J. A. and JAMES, W. P. T. (1978a). *Lancet* **1**, 5–8.

CUMMINGS, J. H., WIGGINS, H. S., JENKINS, D. J. A., HOUSTON, H., JIVRAJ, T., DRASER, B. S. and HILL, M. J. (1978b). *J. Clin. Invest.* **61**, 953–963.

CUMMINGS, J. H., HILL, M. J., JIVARAJ, T., HOUSTON, H., BRANCH, W. J., and JENKINS, D. J. A. (1979). *Am. J. Clin. Nutr.* **32**, 2086–2093.

CURRY, C. E. (1982). *In* "Handbook of Non-prescription Drugs", 7th edition, pp. 69–83. *Am. Pharm. Assoc.,* Washington, D.C.

DEVROEDE, G. (1978). *In* "Gastrointestinal Disease" (M. H. Sleisenger and J. S. Fordtran, eds), 2nd edition, pp. 368–386. Saunders, Philadelphia, Pennsylvania.

DIMOCK, E. M. (1937). *Br. Med. J.* **1**, 905–908.

FARRELL, D. J., GIRLE, L. and ARTHUR, J. (1978). *Aust. J. Exp. Biol. Med. Sci.* **56**, 469–479.

GODDING, E. W. (1980). *Pharmacology* **20**, Suppl. 1, 88–103.

HARRISON, D. G., BEEVER, D. E., THOMSON, D. J. and OSBOURN, D. F. (1975). *J. Agric. Sci.* **83**, 93–101.

HELLER, S. N., HACKLER, L. R., RIVERS, J. M., VAN SOEST, P. J., ROE, D. A., LEWIS, B. A. and ROBERTSON, J. (1980). *Am. J. Clin. Nutr.* **33**, 1734–1744.

HESPELL, R. B. and BRYANT, M. P. (1979). *J. Anim. Sci.* **49**, 1640–1659.

HINTON, J. M. and LENNARD-JONES, J. E. (1968). *Postgrad. Med. J.* **44**, 720–723.

HOBSON, P. N. and SUMMERS, R. (1967). *J. Gen. Microbiol.* **47**, 53–65.

HULL, C., GRECO, R. S. and BROOKS, D. L. (1980). *J. Am. Geriatr. Soc.* **28**, 410–414.

ISSACSON, H. R., HINDS, F. C., BRYANT, M. P. and OWENS, F. N. (1975). *J. Dairy Sci.* **58**, 1645–1659.

JOHNSON, C. K., KOLASA, K., CHENOWETH, W. and BENNINK, M. (1980). *J. Am. Diet. Assoc.* **77**, 551–557.

JONES, F. A. and GODDING, E. N. (1972). "Management of Constipation". Blackwell, Oxford.

JONES, F. A., GUMMER, J. W. P. and LENNARD-JONES, J. E. (1968). "Clinical Gastroenterology", 2nd edition. Blackwell, Oxford.

KATZ, F. H. and ROMFH, P. (1972). *J. Clin. Endocrinol. Metab.* **34**, 819–821.

KELSAY, J. L., BEHALL, K. M. and PRATHER, E. S. (1978). *Am. J. Clin. Nutr.* **31**, 1149–1153.

KENNEDY, P. M., CHRISTOPHERSON, R. J. and MILLIGAN, L. P. (1976). *Br. J. Nutr.* **36**, 231–242.

KEIN, C. L., CORDANO, A., COOK, D. A. and YOUNG, V. R. (1981). *Am. J. Clin. Nutr.* **34**, 357–361.

KONTUREK, S. J. (1980). *Am. J. Gastroenterol.* **74**, 285–291.

KREEK, M. J., SCHAEFER, R. A., HAHN, E. F. and FISHMAN, J. (1983). *Lancet*, **1**, 261–262.

LURIA, S. E. (1960). *In* "The Bacteria" (I. C. Gunsalus and R. Y. Stainer, eds), Vol. T. pp. 1–34. Academic Press, New York.

McCANCE, R. A. and PICKLES, V. R. (1960). *J. Endocrinol.* **20**, xxvii–xxviii.

McCONNELL, A. A., EASTWOOD, M. A. and MITCHELL, W. D. (1974). *J. Sci. Food Agric.* **25**, 1457–1464.

McNEIL, N. I., CUMMINGS, J. H. and JAMES, W. P. T. (1978). *Gut* **19**, 819–822.

MILNE, J. S. and WILLIAMSON, J. (1972). *Gerontol. Clin.* **14**, 56–60.

OWENS, F. N. and ISAACSON, H. R. (1977). *Fed. Proc., Fed. Am. Soc. Exp. Biol.* **36**, 198–202.

PAINTER, N. S. (1980). *Practitioner* **224**, 387–391.

PHILLIPS, S. F. and STEPHEN, A. M. (1981). *Nutr. Today* **16**(6), 4–12.

PRYNNE, C. J. and SOUTHGATE, D. A. T. (1979). *Br. J. Nutr.* **41**, 495–503.

REES, W. D. W. and RHODES, J. (1976). *Lancet* **2**, 475.

RENDTORFT, R. C. and KASHGARIAN, M. (1967). *Dis. Colon Rectum* **10**, 222–228.

RUPPIN, A., BAR-MEIR, S., SOERGEL, K. U., WOOD, C. M. and SCHMITT, M. G. (1980). *Gastroenterology* **78**, 1500–1507.

SHIFF, S. (1979). *Gastroenterology* **76**, 1307.

SMITH, R. G., ROWE, M. J., SMITH, A. N., EASTWOOD, M. A., DRUMMOND, E. and BRYDON, W. G. (1980). *Age Ageing* **9**, 267–271.

SOUTHGATE, D. A. T. and DURNIN, J. V. (1970). *Br. J. Nutr.* **24**, 517–535.

STARLING, E. H. (1930). "Principles of human physiology", 5th edition. Lea & Febiger, Philadelphia, Pennsylvania.

STASSE-WOLTHIUS, M., ALBERS, H. F. F., VAN JEVEREN, J. G. C., WIL DE JONG, J., HAVTVAST, J. G. A. J., HERMUS, R. J. J., KATA, M. B., BRYDON, W. G. and EASTWOOD, M. A. (1980). *Am. J. Clin. Nutr.* **33**, 1745–1756.

STEPHEN, A. M. (1980). Ph.D. Thesis, University of Cambridge.

STEPHEN, A. M. (1981). *In* "Dietary Fibre: Progress towards the Future" (I. M. Baird and M. N. Ornstein, eds), pp. 14–20. Kellogg Company of Great Britain Limited, Manchester.

STEPHEN, A. M. and CUMMINGS, J. H. (1979). *Gut* **20**, 722–729.

STEPHEN, A. M. and CUMMINGS, J. H. (1980). *Nature* **284**, 283–284.

THOMPSON, B. D. and EDMONDS, C. J. (1971). *J. Endocrinol.* **50**, 163–169.

THORNEYCROFT, I. H., MISHELL, D. R., STONE, D. R., KAHRMA, K. M. and NAKAMURA, R. M. (1971). *Am. J. Obstet. Gynecol.* **111**, 947–951.

TUCKER, D. M., SANDSTEAD, H. H., LOGAN, G. M., KLEVAY, L. M., MAHALKO, J., JOHNSON, L. K., INMAN, S., and INGLETT, G. E. (1981). *Gastroenterology* **81**, 879–883.

WALD, A., VAN THIEL, D. H., HOECHSTETTER, L., GAVALER, J. S., EGLER, K. M., VERNU, R., SCOTT L. and LESTER, R. (1981). *Gastroenterology* **80**, 1497–1500.

WALD, A., VAN THIEL, D. H., HOECHSTETTER, L., GAVALER, J. S., EGLER, K. M., VERNU, R., SCOTT L. and LESTER, R. (1982). *Dig. Dis. Sci.* **27**, 1015–1018.

WALKER, A. R. P., WALKER, B. F., BHAMJEE, D., WALKER, E. J., NCONGWANE, J. and SEGAL, I. (1981). *S. Afr. Med. J.* **62**, 195–199.

WYMAN, J. B., HEATON, K. W., MANNING, A. P. and WICKS, A. C. B. (1978). *Gut* **19**, 146–150.

YOKHURA, T., YAJIMA, T. and HASHIMOTO, S. (1977). *Life Sci.* **21**, 59–62.

Chapter 8

Diverticular disease of the colon

NEIL PAINTER

I.   Introduction

Diverticular disease of the colon is a "new" disease that appeared as a clinical problem as late as the beginning of this century. It is now the most common disorder of the colon in the modern Western world, found in one in three people over 60 years of age. Western communities are the affluent industrial communities of Europe, North America and Australia and comparable groups in South Africa and South America. In Asia, westernization is occurring in Japan and in the cities of India and Pakistan.

It was the first disease to be shown as being caused by a deficiency of fibre in the diet. This claim is based on the epidemiology of the condition, on the

145

Dietary Fibre, Fibre-Depleted Foods
and Disease

history of the emergence of the disease in different populations and on clinical and physiological studies.

The prevalence of the disease varies enormously from one population to another. It may be absent in one yet affect over two-thirds of another group of people. It is still unknown in some parts of the world to this day but has appeared only recently in some peoples who previously were free of the disease. This changing incidence of the disease is discussed first as it provides a clue to its causation.

II.   Prevalence

A.   Western countries

When diverticular disease first appeared as a clinical problem at the turn of this century, it was recognised first as acute diverticulitis because this could be diagnosed clinically. Later the advent of contrast radiology revealed that diverticulosis was common and attempts were made to estimate its prevalence.

Autopsy studies showed that diverticula were an acquired abnormality and rare before the age of 40. It must be remembered that barium enemas are ordered for symptoms and thus are selective, while necropsy studies are performed mainly on older subjects and their results vary with the pathologist's interest in diverticulosis. The true prevalence could be found by giving an annual barium enema to a population sample, but obviously this is not practicable.

Extensive data on the frequency of diverticulosis at necropsy (Table 8.1) and at radiology (Table 8.2) were collected by Painter and Burkitt (1971). The frequency of the disease has been reported in other European countries. In northern Norway, 280 autopsies were performed between 1974 and 1976 at the University of Tromso in patients aged over 20. Diverticula were found in 25% of males and 43% of females, the sigmoid being most commonly

TABLE 8.1. Frequency of diverticulosis: representative selection from necropsy series

Country and author	No.	%	Series	Comments on age (years)
United Kingdom				
Fifield (1927)	22	4.4	10,167	London Hospital, 55% under 30, so higher frequency over 40
Parks (1968)	111	37.0	300	N. Ireland; 50% over 80
United States				
Rankin and Brown (1930)	111	5.6	1,925	All but one over 40
Australia				
Cleland (1968)	78	2.6	3,000	Refers to 1940–1948
	36	6.2	589	Over 70 at that time
Hughes (1969)	90	45.0	200	

TABLE 8.2. Frequency of diverticulosis: representative selection from radiology series, barium enemas

Country and author	No.	%	Series	Comments on age (years)
United Kingdom				
Edwards (1953)	25	16	1,623	For previous 13½ years, all over 35
Manousos et al. (1967)	109	35	109	Over 60
Sweden				
Lunding (1935)	87	4.2	2,090	
France				
Debray et al. (1961)		40.0	500	40% over 70; all had gastrointestinal symptoms
United States				
Rankin and Brown (1930)	1,398	5.7	24,620	Mayo Clinic
Allen (1953)	2,000	30.0	2,000	5% at 45, 66% at older age
Smith and Christensen (1959)		22.0	1,016	Frequency doubled at 80

affected (Eide and Stalsberg, 1979). In Finland, 49.47% of 3125 barium enemas performed between 1951 and 1961 showed diverticula; the average age of the subjects was 49. In Sweden, between 1957 and 1959, diverticula were found in 54.9% of 3563 barium enemas. The average subject age was 55 (Köhler, 1963).

The disease is so rarely seen in Bucharest Medical School, Rumania, that no studies of its prevalence have been made (T. Tincolaeson, personal communication, 1971). The disease is common in Prague, Czechoslovakia where more than half of the barium enemas given to patients over 60 show diverticula (K. T. Vesely, personal communication, 1971).

To sum up, diverticular disease has become very common in affluent Western countries but probably remains rare in the countries of eastern Europe.

B.   Sub-Saharan Africa

Diverticular disease of the colon is very rare in African blacks. This is true in the large modern hospitals and has been confirmed by personal or postal enquiries to over 130 mission and rural hospitals in sub-Saharan Africa. These enquiries showed that diverticular disease was virtually unknown in rural African blacks (Painter and Burkitt, 1971; Painter, 1975). Only recently has it appeared in urban Africans who have adopted Western eating habits (p. 10). It might be suggested that diverticulosis could be missed in small country hospitals, but it is obvious that acute diverticulitis, which is a surgical and often a fatal emergency, would seldom be missed.

The earliest necropsy studies of sub-Saharan blacks reported that colonic diverticula were rare (Keeley, 1958). In Johannesburg, South Africa, only one diverticulum had been found in over 2000 consecutive black necropsies (Higginson and Simson, 1958). In Kampala, Uganda, only two cases of diverticular disease had been reported in 4000 consecutive black necropsies (J. N. P. Davies, personal communication to Trowell, 1960). The latter also noted that other diseases of the large bowel such as constipation, haemor-rhoids, even carcinoma and ulcerative colitis, were likewise rare, and he suggested that African diets might be a protective factor.

In Ethiopia, diverticulosis was infrequent and diverticulitis unknown (Goulston, 1967). In Ghana, Accra, only one case of diverticulitis was seen in 16 years in the Medical School (E. Badoe, personal communication, 1971). This is changing. Sixteen cases were seen in Accra in 3 years from 1974 to 1976, and 10 of them had diffuse diverticulosis (Archampong et al., 1978).

In Monrovia, the capital of Liberia, two cases of diverticular disease were found in 300 barium enemas; both patients came from the high socio-eco-nomic class (J. Diggs, personal communication, 1974). In Freetown, Sierra Leone, O. Williams (personal communication, 1974) saw seven patients with diverticular disease in 20 years of practice; all of them came from the upper classes. In Lagos, Nigeria, Kyle and his associates (1967) reported that only two cases of diverticulitis had been seen in the University Hospital in 3 years. In Salisbury, Zimbabwe (formerly Rhodesia), Wapnick and Levin (1971) reported the first case of diverticular disease in a black African.

South Africa contains both rural and urban African blacks and the disease has only recently appeared in the latter. The 3000-bed Baragwanath Hospi-tal, Johannesburg, serves the most urbanised Africans, but in 2367 autopsies performed between 1954 and 1956, no diverticula were found (Keeley, 1958). At the same hospital, A. Solomon (personal communication, 1971) found six cases in approximately 1000 barium enemas performed in 3 years on black patients. J. I. Levy (personal communication, 1972) who did 100–150 barium enemas annually had seen no cases in 13 years in urbanised blacks. Bremner and Ackerman (1970) stated that the Bantu practically never developed diverticula. Campbell (1967) reported that 4 out of 218 barium enemas performed on urban Zulus showed diverticula but none had been found in rural Zulus. In Pretoria, I. Simpson (personal communication, 1972) meticulously examined 3000 Bantu colons at necropsy and found only five diverticula. In Durban, D. Chapman (personal communication, 1971) saw only one patient with the disease during 14 years at the Surgical Depart-ment of King Edward VIII teaching hospital. In Lesotho, Mokhobo (1975) stated that diverticular disease has not yet been diagnosed in the rural population.

Recently diverticular disease has appeared in black Africans in Johan-nesburg (p. 153). All were educated, had responsible jobs and had adopted Western eating habits (I. Segal, personal communication, 1981).

In Nairobi, Kenya, R. Miller (personal communication, 1971) saw only one case of the disease in a Kenyan during 11 years at the Kenyatta National Hospital. The disease is now more common in this hospital, for Calder and Watsunna (1978) reported five cases in Kenyans in $2\frac{1}{2}$ years. Later, Calder (1979) reported that out of 226 barium enemas performed at the Kenyatta National Hospital, 15 had diverticula, of which 5 were in patients under 40 years of age.

In Kampala, Uganda, A. C. Templeton (personal communication, 1970) studied over 300 autopsies specifically to find diverticula, with no subject being under 30; he found only one case of diverticular disease, which involved the sigmoid colon of an 80-year-old woman. Three caecal diverticula were found but these probably have a different aetiology. Harverson (1979) worked for 17 months during 1972 to 1973 at Kampala, Uganda, and found one diverticulum in a barium enema performed in a 40-year-old government official. His sigmoid was narrow and spastic with a saw-toothed border. This is unusual as Ugandans usually have large colons with a wide diameter.

At the Medical School in Kinshasa, Zaire, A. C. Jain (personal communication, 1971) saw only one case of diverticular disease during 9 years.

C.   India and the Middle East

In these countries the disease is still rare or unknown in rural communities, but it has been found in the cities. In Delhi, India, nine cases were found in 9000 barium enemas (O. U. Bhardwaj, personal communication 1973). In 15 years, A. Bhargave (personal communication, 1973) saw only 12 cases in several thousand barium enemas; all were found in westernized Indians. N. M. Bannergee (personal communication, 1973) had seen less than one case a year, with an annual turnover of 3000 barium enemas. No diverticula were seen in 3 years in the radiological department of the Gauhati Medical College, Assam (G. G. Ahmed, personal communication, 1973).

The disease is hardly ever seen at the Lady Reading Hospital of the University of Peshawar, Pakistan, even in those who eat some western style foods (Mohammed Arif, personal communication, 1981). Only two cases were seen in 15 years at the General Hospital, Colombo, Sri Lanka, where the country population eats a high-fibre diet (K. M. C. de Silva, personal communication, 1971).

In Shiraz, Iran, R. Zarabi and A. Farpour (personal communication, 1971) saw only five cases in 8 years in two University hospitals with a total of 700 beds. The province of Fars includes 2 million people and admission is free to the rural or urban poor. Between 1972 and 1976, 556 barium enemas were performed on adults. The disease was uncommon but increased with age, reaching 4.5% at age 60–69 (Dabestani et al., 1981). In Baghdad University, Iraq, about 1000 barium enemas are performed annually, and only three showed diverticula (Mohamed Abu-Tabikh, personal communication, 1973).

In Israel, Levy and his colleagues (1977) reviewed 1377 barium enemas from two general hospitals. They reported that diverticular disease was very rare in Arabs, both in Israel and in Jordan, but 31% of Ashkenazi Jewish women, who had come from Germany or Poland, had the disease compared with only 3.5% of the male Sephardi Jews who had come from Spain.

To sum up, the disease is still uncommon in India and the Middle East. It is found in the upper socio-economic classes rather than in the rural population.

D.   The Far East

In Singapore, Malaysia, Kyle *et al.* (1967) saw three cases of diverticulitis in 15,000 Europeans but only ten in 1½ million Chinese, Indians and Malays during a 5-year period. They reported only one case in 137,000 Fijian natives but two cases in 7000 local Europeans. M. K. Kutty (personal communication, 1970) found no case at autopsy in 3 years at Kuala Lumpur, Malaysia. In Korea, Kim (1964) found no diverticula in 500 barium enemas.

In Bangkok, Thailand, V. Plengavanit (personal communication, 1972) saw two cases in 91 barium enemas; there had been 150,000 admissions to a Bangkok teaching hospital in 5 years, of which only 0.01% were due to diverticular disease. Over a 6-month period, 4.2% of barium enemas showed diverticula; and of these one-quarter had multiple diverticula confined to the right colon. The distribution of the disease was different: the sigmoid colon was beset with diverticula in only 60% of cases compared with 95% in the West. The incidence rose with age, reaching 10% at 70 (Vajrabukka *et al.*, 1980).

In Japan, diverticular disease formerly was rare but has appeared recently (Sato *et al.*, 1976). Between 1967 and 1971, 131 cases were found in 1987 barium enemas performed at the Tokyo Women's Hospital, a prevalence of 6.6% (C. Yazana, personal communication, 1972).

E.   Mexico and South America

The disease is a major surgical problem in the cities in Mexico, Argentina, Brazil and Uruguay, but it is still uncommon in the rural populations of these countries: This was discussed at the Latin American Proctology Conference, Montevideo in 1981. In Lima, Peru, 6% of barium enemas had shown diverticula in 1972. Subsequently the prevalence had risen; 282 cases were found in 2000 barium enemas during 1977 to 1979, a prevalence of 14%. By contrast in Puno, Peru, the disease is almost non-existent among the local rural population; they have descended from the Incas and have barely changed their diet since the time of the Spanish conquest (O. F. Vellarde, personal communication, 1982).

III. Emergence as a new disease

A. Western countries

Diverticular disease of the colon was virtually unknown to British clinicians in 1900 (Telling, 1908, 1920; Telling and Gruner, 1917). Previously diverticula had been regarded as curiosities. Suddenly this "new" disease appeared on the clinical scene. The term "divertikel" was used by Fleischman in 1815 (Spriggs and Marxer, 1925). Gross (1845), Cruveilhier (1849), Rokitansky (1849), Habershon (1857), and Klebs (1849) all realised that diverticula were acquired and thought that they were caused by constipation. Jones (1859) described a vesico-colic fistula due to diverticulitis. The complications of local and general peritonitis due to diverticulitis were described by Virchow (1853) and Loomis (1870). Peritonitis due to diverticulitis must have been rare at that time as it was still regarded as a surgical curiosity even 30 years later.

Diverticula were merely "collectors' items" until Graser (1899) stressed that infected diverticula could cause peritonitis and perforation. He was soon proved right. Beer (1904) described 18 cases of diverticulitis and the complications of peritonitis, adhesions, fistula and stenosis, but he still believed that diverticula rarely caused symptoms. Diagnoses such as pericolitis sinistra, perisigmoiditis, torsion and inflammation of appendices epiploica lingered on and were still considered respectable by Bland-Sutton (1903), Power (1906), Donaldson (1907), and Roberts (1908). Even in the early years of the present century, Taylor and Lakin (1910) were reluctant to attribute peritonitis to diverticulitis and only did so after seeing two examples of this complication within a few months. The ability of diverticulitis to mimic cancer was still thought newsworthy at this time, both in Britain and America (Mayo et al., 1907; Moynihan, 1907).

Diverticulitis became a common surgical emergency within the first two decades of the present century. Telling of Leeds saw the disease first of all in 1899 when no one was familiar with it, but by 1908 he could describe its complications (Telling, 1908). Subsequently he published his classic paper on diverticulosis in 1917 (Telling and Gruner, 1917). The appearance of diverticulitis early in this century surprised even surgeons of repute. Sir John Bland-Sutton (1920) remarked "in the last ten years, acute diverticulitis is recognised with the same certainty as appendicitis and is a newly discovered bane of elders".

In the United States, Mayo (1930) estimated that 5% of patients over the age of 40 had diverticulosis. Others reported a prevalence of 4 to 10%; Morton (1946), in a review of American autopsies, and Edwards (1953), in a quote on English barium studies, recorded similar figures.

The incidence of diverticulosis has risen dramatically in the United Kingdom, the United States, Australasia and western Europe in the last 30 years. About one-third of those over 60 have diverticulosis. This rises to two-thirds at 80 (Parks, 1968; Hughes, 1969). The disease has become more common in Australia since the 1940s (Cleland, 1968), and is being found more often even under the age of 40 (Painter, 1975).

Thus, diverticular disease was almost unknown in 1900 but is now the most common disorder of the colon in Western man. This change happened in only 70 years, the traditional life span of man.

This affected *only the citizens of the economically developed West*. By contrast, diverticular disease is almost unknown to this day in communities who have not adopted Western habits and have adhered to their traditional eating habits.

B.   Rising incidence following westernization of diet

Only 50 years ago, diverticulosis was much less prevalent in black than in white Americans (Kocour, 1937) but this difference has almost disappeared (Cleave *et al.*, 1969). Similarly, the disease is seen in Asians, Africans and West Indians who have lived in Britain for many years.

The disease was rare in Japan until recently, but, between 1967 and 1971, 1987 barium enemas performed at a Tokyo hospital demonstrated diverticula in 131 patients, an incidence of 6.6% (C. Yazana, personal communication, 1972). By contrast, the disease is as prevalent in American Japanese who were born and bred in Hawaii as it is in white Americans (G. N. Stemmerman, personal communication, 1970). The few cases recorded in India and Iran have been found mostly in the wealthier patients. In Johannesburg, diverticular disease has been found in black patients only in the last 7 years. All were educated and had adopted a Western lifestyle (I. Segal, personal communication, 1976).

The disease, therefore, is not racial but environmental in origin. It appears in those who change their traditional eating habits and eat Western processed foods.

IV.   Dietary factors

A.   Dietary fibre

The dramatic increase in the incidence of diverticular disease in the Western world can theoretically be explained in two ways. First it might be due to observer error and be more apparent than real, but the quality of their writings shows that the clinicians and pathologists of the last century would have recognised diverticulitis had it been common in their day. The second possibility is that the environment of the colon has changed and that diverticula are caused by our modern diet and, in particular, by the low intake of dietary fibre, since this is the fraction of our food which reaches the colon least altered by digestion. The amount of fibre in the diet has a direct effect on the intestinal transit time and on the weight and consistency of the stools (Burkitt *et al.*, 1972, 1974; Painter, 1975). The pressures in the colon are also altered by the amount of fibre in the diet (Srivastava *et al.*, 1976).

Cereal fibre intakes have been falling in Britain during the past 200 years. Wheat flour intakes have declined from an estimated intake of over 400 lb per head per year in 1750 to under 150 lb in 1950 (Hollingsworth and Greaves, 1967). Although there are no data concerning the dietary fibre content of wheat flour in past centuries, it is certain that modern low-fibre white flour slowly replaced the traditional high-fibre coarsely ground wholemeal flour of long ago. At the same time, the consumption of fibre-free sugar and fat have risen during the last 200 years to replace, in terms of energy, the declining intake of both flour and potatoes.

Comparable changes are occurring at the present time among urban black South Africans as their traditional diet, based on a large consumption of home-grown high-fibre maize meal, becomes westernized. This is illustrated in a recent study of diverticular disease at Baragwanath Hospital, Johannesburg. Some 42 black patients, 16 men and 26 women, were admitted during a 3-year period. This University hospital draws patients from a black urban population of 1.5 million. Their average age was 62 years; all came from higher social groups. Their mean daily dietary fibre intake was 26.5 ± 8.5 g. It was significantly lower than sex-age matched urban black controls who ate daily dietary fibre of 32.5 + 11.4 g. Sex-age matched white South Africans ate daily dietary fibre of 22.4 ± 6.0 g (Segal and Walker, 1982). The latter figure is comparable to that reported in England.

In England, Brodribb and Humphreys (1976) compared the crude fibre intake of 40 patients with symptomatic diverticulosis with matched controls. The mean intake was 2.6 g crude fibre daily in patients with diverticulosis and 5.2 g in the control patients. The crude fibre intake was estimated by patients recalling their previous eating habits. The main difference in fibre intake was found to be in the cereal fibre fraction (Gear *et al.*, 1979). Further work using modern methods of estimating dietary fibre intake is required if the connection between diverticulosis and fibre deficiency is to be confirmed.

B. Pathogenesis

Only when cineradiography, coupled with the means of measuring the intra-colonic pressures accurately, became available was it possible to show that diverticula were caused by high localised intraluminal pressures. The living colon can segment to such an extent that it obstructs its lumen intermittently. It then functions not as a tube but as a series of "little bladders" (Fig. 8.1).

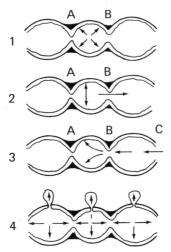

FIG. 8.1. Role of segmentation in colonic physiology and diverticular disease. 1, Segmentation by contraction rings generates local high intracolonic pressures. 2, Contraction ring B relaxes, allowing faeces to pass. 3, Faeces pass relaxed ring B but are halted by tight ring A. 4, Postulates that viscous faeces require extra pressure for propulsion; resultant high intracolonic pressures herniate mucosa to form diverticula.

Segmentation is essential if the colon is to transport or to halt its contents. The colon segments throughout life and, if it has to propel faeces of abnormally high viscosity, these "bladders" become "trabeculated" so that the muscle of the colon wall is thrown into ridges of varying thickness. Between these ridges the muscle is weak and it is here that the mucosal herniation takes place (Edwards, 1934a,b; Painter, 1962, 1963, 1964; Arfwiddson, 1964).

Hence, modern research has confirmed the opinion of Gross (1845) that diverticula are caused by functional obstruction "by which the muscular fibres are separated from each other so as to permit the mucous membranes to protrude". Habershon (1857) blamed constipation for diverticula and Lane (1885) realised that diverticula were caused by a mechanism similar to that which caused bladder diverticula and which involves muscular contraction, an opinion shared by Bristowe (1854) who suggested that costiveness could mimic obstruction.

If fibre deficiency causes diverticulosis, it must be related to colonic segmentation which produces the pressures that drive the mucosa through the muscle coat. Excessive segmentation generates very high localised pressures which cause diverticula (Painter, 1962, 1964; Painter *et al.*, 1965). Whole cereals, such as wholemeal bread and brown rice, and vegetables and fruit, contain an adequate amount of fibre; these prevent diverticulosis in the following manner.

1. The colon that copes with a large volume of faeces is of a wider diameter and does not develop diverticula. This is true of man (Wells, 1949) and experimental animals such as rats (Carlson and Hoelzel, 1949) and rabbits (Hodgson, 1972). A colon that has a wide bore *ab initio* is less able to segment excessively and to obstruct itself than a narrow colon, and so is less prone to diverticulosis (Painter, 1964).

2. The fibre content of food affects profoundly, the transit time, stool weight and consistency. Usually rural Africans, who eat plenty of fibre, have a transit time of less than 40 hours, whereas this may take several days in Englishmen (Burkitt *et al.*, 1972, 1974; Painter, 1975). South African Bantu pass large soft motions at will without straining (Walker *et al.*, 1970). In Africans the colon has to propel soft contents and thus has to segment less and so produces less pressure. Obviously it is less likely to become "trabeculated" and to bear diverticula than the colon that has struggled for many years with the viscous contents which result from a low-fibre diet. In short, the swiftly passed soft stool strains the sigmoid less and does not favour the development of diverticula.

C.   Animal experiments

Rats fed a high-fibre diet by Carlson and Hoelzel (1949) did not develop diverticula, while those fed a low-fibre diet developed diverticula in the colon. Hodgson (1972) fed rabbits on white bread, dairy products and sugar. They gained weight while their health deteriorated and they became constipated. Their intracolonic pressures rose and their colons became narrower. The administration of prostigmine caused reducible diverticula to appear temporarily. These findings are essentially similar to those reported in man by Painter (1962, 1964) and by Painter *et al.* (1965), even though they were produced in animals with a different life span.

V.   Treatment

A.   High-fibre diet

Convinced that uncomplicated diverticulosis was caused by a low-fibre diet, I began treating uncomplicated diverticular disease by fibre replacement in 1966. The high-fibre diet abolished or relieved nearly 90% of the symptoms of 70 patients (Painter *et al.*, 1972). After carcinoma or stenosis of the colon had been excluded, patients were asked to reduce their intake of refined sugar, whether white or brown, and white flour and bread, and to eat 100% wholemeal bread whenever possible. They were advised to eat bran-containing breakfast cereals and plenty of vegetables and fruit. They added miller's bran to each meal and slowly increased this until they passed one or two soft stools daily without straining. The amount of bran needed to achieve this was found by trial and error as there is no "dose" of bran. Most patients required 2 teaspoonfuls of bran three times a day, but some needed several tablespoonfuls. This "bran diet" not only relieved abdominal symptoms, such as the aching, heaviness and distention that are associated with diverticular disease, but also even very severe colic which had been diagnosed erroneously as left renal colic.

Bran improved the appetite of many of these patients and never made it worse. Those who had severe post-prandial distension and discomfort were able to eat normally once the bran diet had taken effect. This shows that the old adage that "roughage irritates the gut" is not true. Bran becomes "softage" when wet (Painter, 1970; Painter et al., 1972). Bran relieved even the severe colic that was once diagnosed as "diverticulitis" and was treated by resection, and thus lessens the need for major surgery in diverticular disease (Painter et al., 1972).

The ability of a high-fibre diet to relieve symptoms has been confirmed by Parks (1973), Srivastava and his colleagues (1976), Tarpila and Miettinen (1978), and by Brodribb and Humphreys (1976). Bran in tablet form (Fybranta) also relieved symptoms, lowered the intracolonic pressures and altered the electrical activity of the diseased colon towards normal (Taylor and Duthie, 1976). Bran in crispbread form relieved symptoms (Plumley and Francis, 1973) and similar biscuits were shown to be effective in a double-blind trial (Brodribb, 1977).

B.   Effect of bran on intracolonic pressures

Bran retains water and renders the stools bulkier and softer and easier to pass. It lowers the intracolonic pressures more effectively than does a pharmaceutical bulk-former (Sterculia). However, when a relaxant is added to sterculia its effect becomes similar to bran. This suggests that bran's effect is not only due to its lowering the viscosity of the stools, but also because it relaxes the colonic musculature (Srivastava et al., 1976).

After myotomy or resection for diverticular disease, only about two-thirds of patients remain symptom-free. Reilly's operation of sigmoid myotomy reduces the intracolonic pressures but these rise again after about 2 years in patients who remain on their usual diet. If, after myotomy or resection, patients change to a high-fibre diet, the intracolonic pressures show no sign of rising after nearly 5 years (Smith et al., 1969, 1971).

These observations suggest that while surgery can deal with the complications of the disease it does not remove its underlying cause, which is fibre deficiency. This view is supported by Hyland and Taylor (1980) who followed up 100 patients who had suffered from the symptoms, or complications of, diverticular disease. Twenty-five had come to surgery. On the high-fibre diet 91% remained free of symptoms over 5 to 7 years. This is in marked contrast to previous reports in which no more than 60% of medically or surgically treated patients remain well (Painter, 1975). All these observations are consistent with the claim that diverticular disease is due to deficiency of fibre in our modern diet.

C. Studies that have questioned the value of the high-fibre diet

The efficacy of bran and fibre supplements and the necessity of prescribing a high-fibre diet in uncomplicated diverticular disease have been questioned recently by Ornstein and his colleagues (1981). In a well-designed, double-blind, cross-over trial they compared the effect of bran biscuits, ispagula and a placebo on bowel function, stool weights and symptoms in 58 patients with diverticular disease. Both fibre regimens altered the frequency of defaecation and the consistency and weight of the stools. They confirmed the well-known ability of bran to relieve constipation but found that the placebo relieved symptoms as effectively as did the fibre supplements. They concluded that fibre supplements were not necessary in diverticular disease unless constipation was a major symptom. Devroede *et al.* (1977) tested six therapeutic regimens and failed to demonstrate that bran was in any way superior to other forms of treatment. Others who have questioned the value of bran have given no less than 30 g daily in biscuit form to patients with irritable bowel syndrome without observing any significant change in the bowel habit (Søltoft *et al.*, 1976).

These trials are open to one or more of the following criticisms:

1. They employed a standard daily "dose" of bran given to each patient regardless of the rest of the diet. This will not give the best results as each patient requires a differing amount of added fibre to render the stools soft and easy to pass. There is no dose of bran that is correct for every patient any more than there is a standard dose of insulin. Each patient must find the amount of bran required by trial and error over a period of at least 3 months.

2. Bran has been given in biscuit and tablet form. It would appear that the processing involved alters the physical properties of bran. How else can one explain the fact that 30 g daily in biscuit form had no significant effect on bowel habit? This amount of miller's bran alters the bulk and consistency of stools profoundly.

3. Some trial periods were too short to allow a steady state to be established.

4. In some trials, patients were switched from one diet to another without a sufficient interval in which the follow-up effects of the previous regimen would disappear.

5. Some patients probably had been given a high-fibre diet by their own doctors before entering the trial. This would lessen the effects of any "fibre" given in the trial.

6. Some patients on the trials had mild symptoms, hence the effect of any

treatment would be minimal. This is in contrast with the trial of Painter *et al.* (1972) and Brodribb and Humphreys (1976), whose patients had significant and often severe symptoms.

7. The inclusion of bagasse, sterculia, ispagula, man-made cellulose, etc. under the term "fibre" is misleading. None of these substances should be termed "dietary fibre" in the sense that it has been used in this chapter.

VI. Conclusion

Diverticular disease of the colon is a "new" disease, which only appeared in the affluent nations of the West at the beginning of the century. Since then it has become the most common affliction of the colon in their populations. It is beginning to appear in other peoples who have recently changed from their traditional foodstuffs and have adopted the Western low-fibre diet. All the evidence suggests that a return to a less refined diet containing more fibre, and especially cereal fibre, not only will relieve the symptoms of the uncomplicated disease but might prevent the emergence of the disease in future generations.

References

ALLEN, A. W. (1953). *Am. J. Surg.* **86,** 545–548.

ARCHAMPONG, E. Q., CHRISTIAN, F. and BADOE, E. A. (1978). *Ann. R. Coll. Surg. Engl.* **60,** 464–470.

ARFWIDSSON, S. (1964). *Acta Chir. Scand. Suppl.* **342,** 5–68.

BEER, E. (1904). *Am. J. Med. Sci.* **128,** 135–145.

BLAND-SUTTON, J. (1903). *Lancet* **2,** 1148–1151.

BLAND-SUTTON, J. (1920). *Proc. R. Soc. Med., Sect. Surg.* **13,** 64–65.

BREMNER, C. G. and ACKERMAN, L. V. (1970). *Cancer* **26,** 991–999.

BRISTOWE, J. S. (1854). *Trans. Pathol. Soc. London* **6,** 191.

BRODRIBB, A. J. M. (1977). *Lancet* **1,** 664–666.

BRODRIBB, A. J. M. and HUMPHREYS, D. M. (1976). *Br. Med. J.* **1,** 424–430.

BURKITT, D. P., WALKER, A. R. P. and PAINTER, N. S. (1972). *Lancet* **2,** 1408–1412.

BURKITT, D. P., WALKER, A. R. P. and PAINTER, N. S. (1974). *JAMA, J. Am. Med. Assoc.* **229,** 1068–1074.

CALDER, J. F. (1979). *Br. Med. J.* **1,** 1465–1466.

CALDER, J. F. and WASUNNA, A. E. (1978). *East Afr. Med. J.* **55,** 579–581.

CAMPBELL, G. D. (1967). *Br. Med. J.* **3,** 243.

CARLSON, A. J. and HOELZEL, F. (1949). *Gastroenterology* **12,** 108–115.

CLEAVE, T. L., CAMPBELL, G. D. and PAINTER, N. S. (1969). "Diabetes, Coronary Thrombosis and the Saccharine Disease", 2nd edition, pp. 128–135. John Wright, Bristol.

CLELAND, J. B. (1968). *Br. Med. J.* **1,** 579.

CRUVEILHIER, J. (1849). "Traité d'anatomie pathologique générale", Vol. I, p. 59. Baillière, Paris.

DABESTANI, A., ALIABADI, P., SHAH-ROOKH, F. D. and BORHANMANESH, F. A. (1981). *Dis. Colon Rectum* **24,** 385–387.

DEBRAY, C., HARDOUIN, J. P., BESANÇON, F. and RAIMBAULT, J. (1961). *Sem. Hôp.* **37,** 1743–1745.

DEVROEDE, C., VOBECKY, J. S., VOBECKY, J. M., BEAUDRY, R., HADDAD, H., NAVERT, H., PEREY, B. and POISSON, J. (1977). *Gastroenterology* **72,** 1157.

DONALDSON, R. (1907). *Br. Med. J.* **2,** 1705–1706.

EDWARDS, H. C. (1934a). *Lancet* **1,** 221–227.

EDWARDS, H. C. (1934b). *Br. J. Surg.* **22,** 88–107.

EDWARDS, H. C. (1953). *Postgrad. Med. J.* **29,** 20–27.

EIDE, T. J. and STALSBERG, H. (1979). *Gut* **20,** 609–615.

FIFIELD, L. R. (1927). *Lancet* **1,** 277–281.

GEAR, J. S. S., WARE, A., FURSDON, P., MANN, J. I., NOLAN, D. J., BRODRIBB, A. J. M. and VESSEY, M. P. (1979). *Lancet* **1,** 511–514.

GOULSTON, E. (1967). *Br. Med. J.* **2,** 378.

GRASER, E. (1899). *Münch. Med. Wochenschr.* **46,** 721.

GROSS, S. (1845). "Elements of Pathological Anatomy", p. 554. Blanchard & Lea, Philadelphia.

HABERSHON, S. O. (1857). "Observations on the Alimentary Canal", p. 297. Churchill, London.

HARVERSON, G. (1979). *Br. Med. J.* **2,** 498–499.

HIGGINSON, J. and SIMSON, I. (1958). *Schweiz. Z. Allg. Pathol. Bakteriol.* **21,** 577–581.

HODGSON, I. (1972). *Br. J. Surg.* **59,** 315.

HOLLINGSWORTH, D. F. and GREAVES, J. P. (1967). *Am. J. Clin. Nutr.* **20,** 65–72.

HUGHES, L. E. (1969). *Gut* **10,** 336–351.

HYLAND, J. M. P. and TAYLOR, I. (1980). *Br. J. Surg.* **67,** 77–79.

JONES, S. (1859). *Trans. Pathol. Soc. London* **10,** 131.

KEELEY, K. J. (1958). *Med. Proc.* **4,** 281–286.

KIM, E. H. (1964). *N. Engl. J. Med.* **271,** 764–768.

KLEBS, E. (1849). "Handbuch der Pathologischen Anatomie", p. 271. Hirschwald, Berlin.

KOCOUR, E. J. (1937). *Am. J. Surg.* **37,** 433–436.

KÖHLER, R. (1963). *Acta Chir. Scand.* **126,** 148–155.

KYLE, J., ADESOLA, A. O., TINCKLER, L. F. and DE BEAUX, J. (1967). *Scand. J. Gastroenterol.* **2,** 77–80.

LANE, A. (1885). *Guy's Hosp. Rep.* **43,** 48.

LEVY, N., LUBOSHITZKI, R., SHIRATZKI, Y. and GHIVARELLO, M. (1977). *Dis. Colon. Rectum* **20,** 477–481.

LOOMIS, A. L. (1870). *N. Y. Med. Rec.* **4,** 497.

LUNDING, E. (1935). *Acta Med. Scand., Suppl.* **72.**

MANOUSOS, O. N., TRUELOVE, S. C. and LUMSDEN, K. (1967). *Br. Med. J.* **3,** 760–762.

MANOUSOS, O. N., VRACHLIOTIS, G., PAPAEVANGELOU, G., DETORAKIS, E., DORITIS, P., STERGIOU, L. and MERIKAS, G. (1973). *Am. J. Dig. Dis.* **18,** 174–176.

MAYO, W. J. (1930). *Ann. Surg.* **92,** 739–743.

MAYO, W. J., WILSON, L. B. and GIFFEN, R. Z. (1907). *Surg. Gynecol. Obstet.* **5,** 8–15.

MOKHOBO, K. P. (1975). *S. Afr. Med. J.* **1,** 1906.

MORTON, J. J. (1946). *Ann. Surg.* **124,** 725–745.

MOYNIHAN, B. G. A. (1907). *Br. Med. J.* **2,** 1381–1385.

ORNSTEIN, M. H., LITTLEWOOD, E. R., BAIRD, I. M., FOWLER, J., NORTH, W. R. S. and COX, A. G. (1981). *Br. Med. J.* **1,** 1353–1356.

PAINTER, N. S. (1962). Master of Surgery Thesis, University of London.

PAINTER, N. S. (1963). *Br. Med. J.* **2,** 309.

PAINTER, N. S. (1964). *Ann. R. Coll. Surg. Engl.* **34,** 98–119.

PAINTER, N. S. (1970). *Proc. R. Soc. Med.* **63,** Suppl., 144–145.

PAINTER, N. S. (1975). "Diverticular Disease of the Colon." Heinemann Medical Books, London.

PAINTER, N. S. and BURKITT, D. P. (1971). *Br. Med. J.* **2**, 450–454.

PAINTER, N. S., TRUELOVE, S. C., ARDRAN, G. M. and TUCKEY, M. (1965). *Gastroenterology* **49**, 169–177.

PAINTER, N. S., ALMEIDA, A. Z. and COLEBOURNE, K. W. (1972). *Br. Med. J.* **2**, 137–140.

PARKS, T. G. (1968). *Proc. R. Soc. Med.* **61**, 932–934.

PARKS, T. G. (1973). *Proc. R. Soc. Med.* **66**, 681–683.

PLUMLEY, P. F. and FRANCIS, B. (1973). *J. Am. Diet. Assoc.* **63**, 527–530.

POWER, D'ARCY (1906). *Br. Med. J.* **2**, 1171–1174.

RANKIN, F. W. and BROWN, P. W. (1930). *Surg. Gynecol. Obstet.* **50**, 836–847.

ROBERTS, J. L. (1908). *Br. Med. J.* **1**, 1174.

ROKITANSKY, C. (1849). "A Manual of Pathological Anatomy" Vol. II. p. 48. Sydenham Society, London.

SATO, T., MATSUZAKI, S., FUJIWARA, Y., TAKAHASHI, J. and SUGURO, T. (1976). *Cancer* **37**, 1316–1321.

SEGAL, I. and WALKER, A. R. P. (1982). *Digestion* **24**, 42–46.

SMITH, A. N., ATTISHA, R. P. and BALFOUR, T. (1969). *Br. J. Surg.* **56**, 895–899.

SMITH, A. N., GIANNOKOS, V. and CLARKE, S. (1971). *J. R. Coll. Surg. Edinburgh* **16**, 276–286.

SMITH, C. C. and CHRISTENSEN, W. R. (1959). *Am. J. Roentgenol., Radium Ther. Nucl. Med.* **82**, 996–999.

SØLTOFT, J., GUDMAND-HØYER, E., KRAG, B., KRISTENSEN, E. and WULFF, H. R. (1976). *Lancet* **1**, 270–272.

SPRIGGS, E. I. and MARXER, O. A. (1925). . *Q. J. Med.* **19**, 1–34.

SRIVASTAVA, G. S., SMITH, A. N. and PAINTER, N. S. (1976). *Br. Med. J.* **1**, 315–318.

TARPILA, S. and MIETTINEN, T. A. (1978). *Gut* **19**, 137–145.

TAYLOR, G. and LAKIN, C. E. (1910). *Lancet* **1**, 495–496.

TAYLOR, I. and DUTHIE, H. L. (1976). *Br. Med. J.* **1**, 988–990.

TELLING, W. H. M. (1908). *Lancet* **1**, 843–850.

TELLING, W. H. M. (1920). *Proc. R. Soc. Med., Sect. Surg.* **13**, 55–64.

TELLING, W. H. M. and GRUNER, O. C. (1917). *Br. J. Surg.* **4**, 468–530.

TROWELL, H. C. (1960). "Non-Infective Disease in Africa", pp. 217–223. Edward Arnold, London.

VAJRABUKKA, T., SAKSORNCHAI, K. and JIMAKORN, P. (1980). *Dis. Colon Rectum* **23**, 151–154.

VIRCHOW, R. (1853). *Virchows Arch. Pathol. Anat. Physiol.* **5**, 335.

WALKER, A. R. P., WALKER, B. F. and RICHARDSON, B. D. (1970). *Br. Med. J.* **3**, 48–49.

WAPNICK, S. and LEVIN, L. (1971). *Br. Med. J.* **4**, 115.

WELLS, C. (1949). *Br. J. Radiol.* **22**, 449–457.

Chapter 9

Cancer of the large bowel

JOHN CUMMINGS

I.   Origins of the fibre–cancer hypothesis

The hypothesis that "dietary fibre prevents large bowel cancer" must be credited largely to Burkitt, who in 1971 described in detail the epidemiology of large bowel cancer and set out its association with dietary fibre intake and with large bowel function. He noted "a close relationship between bowel cancer and other non-infective diseases of the bowel . . . . (and a) close association with the refined diet characteristic of economic development (which) suggests that the removal of dietary fibre may be a causative factor". The strength of Burkitt's hypothesis is that he goes on to suggest a mechanism by which fibre could prevent bowel cancer, through its capacity to "regulate the speed of transit, bulk and consistency of stool . . . .", to dilute carcinogens and to alter microbial metabolism.

Dietary Fibre, Fibre-Depleted Foods
and Disease

The notion that fibre might protect against bowel cancer was not entirely new in 1971, but Burkitt focused and crystallised the idea in a new way. Previously, a number of workers in South Africa had commented on the absence of bowel cancer and other large intestinal diseases in some racial groups and suggested that fibre might hold the key. Walker, working in Johannesburg, pointed out in 1947 that changes in dietary intake could have important effects on large bowel function (Walker, 1947) and he eventually conceded (Walker, 1971), after at first opposing the idea (Walker, 1961), that fibre might be one factor in the aetiology of colonic cancer.

In 1960, Higginson and Oettlé reported their studies of cancer incidence in Bantu and Cape coloured races of South Africa. In order to explain the lack of bowel cancer in Bantu compared to other races they said that it was "difficult to avoid suspecting the diet . . ." and that ". . . in the Bantu a large amount of roughage is normally consumed, and constipation in the Western sense is rare". Oettlé expanded on this in 1964 saying that in the Bantu "stools are bulkier and more frequent, and the complaint of 'constipation' may indicate no more than that the frequency of bowel movements has fallen to 2 or less per day. The use of regular enemas and purges is widespread. These practices would dilute any carcinogens and might shorten the duration of exposure . . .".

Bremner (1964) stated clearly that the roughage content of the Bantu diet, together with their greater use of aperients and greater physical exercise, might explain their low incidence of rectal cancer. Trowell, who also worked in Africa, noted in his book "Non-Infective Disease in Africa" (1960) that the African was rarely constipated, consumed a bulky diet and that this might explain the rarity of Western-type bowel diseases.

In India, Malhotra (1967) was intrigued by the geographical distribution of gut cancer across the continent and felt that diet must have something to do with it. In 1967 he wrote, in relation to the fact that bowel cancer was much more common in South India than in North India, "one explanation that might be likely is the difference in the cellullose and fibre content in the diets of the South Indians as compared to those of the North Indians".

Since 1971 there has been a great deal of interest in the hypothesis and many papers have been written about it (Hill, 1974; Freeman, 1979; Graham and Mettlin, 1979; Royal College of Physicians, 1980; Modan and Lubin, 1980; Cummings, 1981a; Spiller and Freeman, 1981). Where do we stand today? Does the hypothesis remain intact or should it be discarded or modified?

II.   Dietary epidemiology

A.   Population studies

In the past 12 years there have been a further 12 or so studies in which the relation between bowel cancer incidence or mortality and fibre intake has been reported. The results show that there is no general agreement on the protective role of fibre. The papers of Drasar and Irving (1973) and Armstrong and Doll (1975), in which dietary data are derived from FAO food balance sheets, both conclude that there is no evidence for a protective (or other) effect of fibre against large bowel cancer. Similarly Lyon and Sorenson's note (1978) on Seventh Day Adventists points out that fibre intakes were only about two-thirds of those expected despite their significantly lower risk of large bowel cancer. McMichael et al. (1979), however, have related time trends in bowel cancer incidence to fibre intakes in the United States, United Kingdom, Australia and New Zealand and suggest that there is a possible protective effect of fibre.

In these studies fibre intake has been expressed as crude fibre. This chemical determination of fibre derives from animal nutrition and has no numerical or physiological relation to dietary fibre as it is now conceived (Van Soest and McQueen, 1973; Southgate, 1976a). At the time these early studies were carried out, however, crude fibre values were the only ones available.

Recognising the inadequacies of the crude fibre measurement, several investigators have chosen to relate consumption of specific items of food such as cereals, vegetables, fruit, pulses, etc. to colon cancer epidemiology. When Irving and Drasar (1973) did this for 37 countries, again using FAO food intake data, they showed a weakly protective effect [correlation coefficient (r) -0.30] for cereals. Armstrong and Doll (1975) also examined this relationship and were able to confirm a significant simple correlation between cereal consumption in 32 countries and colon cancer incidence (r -0.52 men and -0.51 women) and mortality (r -0.70 men and -0.67 women). However, this relationship was "readily accounted for by the negative association (of cereal consumption) with meat", r' for cereals, controlling for meat or animal protein intake, varying from -0.1 to -0.2 which was not significant. The tendency of one dietary constituent to vary in harmony with another in different populations of the world is a major difficulty in interpreting all epidemiological studies of diet and disease.

Using simple correlations, Schrauzer (1976) found a protective effect of cereal foods (r -0.72) against large bowel cancer in 16 countries as did Howell (1975) also using FAO food balance data. However, Hill et al. (1979) were unable to relate consumption of fibre-containing foods to bowel cancer incidence in various socio-economic groups in Hong Kong. Neither were Liu et al. (1979), using FAO food balance data to calculate consumption of fibre-rich foods in 20 industrialised countries. In the latter study the simple correlation between the proportion of calories supplied by fibre-rich foods and bowel cancer mortality was -0.71, a significant protective effect, yet when partial correlation coefficients were calculated, controlling for cholesterol intake (which was highly and positively correlated with bowel cancer mortality), then the relationship was no longer significant (r' 0.03).

Overall, the results of these studies seem to be evenly balanced with no clear role for fibre emerging. A major difficulty in interpreting such studies, however, relates to the accuracy of the food intake data and the measurement of dietary fibre. Assessment of food intake in individuals or populations is extremely difficult; there are systematic errors in many methods (Mettlin and Graham, 1980; James *et al.*, 1981). Furthermore, accurate information on dietary fibre content of food, or even an agreed definition of fibre, was not available to any of these authors. It is therefore not surprising that their results appear to vary randomly. However, the personal anecdotal knowledge of dietary intake and bowel cancer epidemiology from people who have lived and worked in rural Africa, India and also in the industrialised countries always comes down on the side of the fibre hypothesis (Walker, 1976; Malhotra, 1977; Trowell and Burkitt, 1981).

With an awareness of these problems, the International Association for Research in Cancer (IARC) has co-ordinated two detailed studies in Scandinavia aimed at testing the fibre hypothesis (IARC Intestinal Microecology Group, 1977; Jensen *et al.*, 1982). In the first study, 30 men, randomly selected from population registers in Copenhagen (Denmark) and Kuopio (Finland), were asked to weigh and record all food and drink over a 4-day period and to collect a duplicate 24-h portion of food. Chemical analysis of these diets for fibre was done by the Southgate method (Southgate, 1976a,b). Bowel cancer incidence, derived from good local cancer registries, was almost four times higher in Copenhagen than Kuopio. Total dietary fibre in Copenhagen was 17.2 ± 5.1 g/day and in Kuopio 30.9 ± 11.3 g/day. This difference was statistically significant ($p < 0.001$) and the group concluded that "higher intakes of dietary fibre . . . suggest a possible protective effect". There was also an apparently protective effect of milk.

The IARC decided to extend the study to four further populations in Denmark and Finland and to use newer methods for measuring dietary fibre (Jensen *et al.*, 1982). The areas chosen were rural and urban Denmark (Them and Copenhagen) and rural and urban Finland (Parrikala and Helsinki). Again, 30 men in each area aged 50–59 were randomly selected from population lists and their dietary intake measured by both weighed record and direct chemical analysis of duplicate portions of food. A threefold variation in bowel cancer incidence was present (Table 9.1) and a protective effect was found for total dietary fibre measured as non-starch polysaccharide (NSP) by the method of Englyst *et al.*, (1982). The much lower intakes of "dietary fibre" in this second study are due to recent changes in concepts and techniques for measuring fibre.

Figure 9.1 shows the relationship between average intake of individual foods and cancer incidence for the second Scandinavian study. An association (protective) with cereal consumption and with NSP is clear whilst that with meat and total fat is not significant. The statistical treatment of these results was very detailed and included multivariate analysis; on this occasion no

TABLE 9.1. Large bowel cancer incidence
and non-starch polysaccharide intakes (NSP)
in four Scandinavian populations in 1978[a]

	Cancer incidence[b]	Total NSP (g/day)	Non-cellulosic polysaccharides	Cellulose
Parikkala	14.2	18.5	14.6	4.1
Helsinki	25.7	14.5	11.2	3.4
Them	27.9	18.0	14.3	3.7
Copenhagen	42.1	13.2	10.0	3.2

[a] Data from Jensen *et al.*, 1982.

[b] Age standardised rates for colon and rectal cancer for men (per 100,000 men annually).

relation with milk consumption was found but that with cereal foods and total fibre remained significant. Surprisingly there were also negative (protective) associations with saturated fatty acids, available carbohydrates, starch and protein. Alcohol consumption was the only variable positively correlated with large bowel cancer (Fig. 9.1). The apparently protective effect of saturated

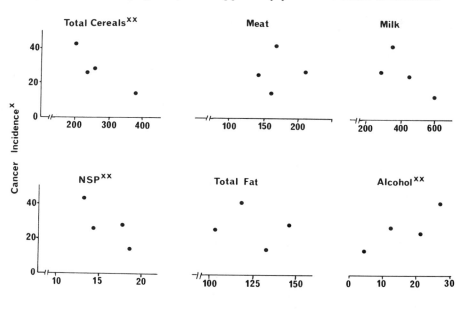

Food Intake (g or ml per day)

FIG. 9.1. Average daily intakes of selected foods and nutrients by 50- to 59-year-old men in four areas in Denmark and Finland in relation to large bowel cancer incidence. (Data from Jensen *et al.*, 1982.) X = Average annual age-standardized (world population) incidence rates per 100,000 men for colon + rectal cancer in four areas of Denmark and Finland; XX = significantly associated with large bowel cancer incidence; NSP = non-starch polysaccharide.

fat and protein is in disagreement with other dietary epidemiological studies. Possible sources of error in the study were discussed by the investigators but none was thought to invalidate the findings. Overall, the conclusions were that a "complex interaction of varying dietary components determines colon cancer risk". Cereals were felt to be the main determinant through a protective effect of fibre. The IARC studies illustrate the complexities of dietary epidemiological data in which a number of foods and nutrients may interact to produce the final experience of cancer in a particular population.

Scandinavia is, of course, a small part of the world and the IARC findings may not be relevant to populations with different genetic and cultural backgrounds. In the United Kingdom, Bingham et al. (1979) obtained food intake data from the British National Food Survey for the nine Registrar General regions, calculated nutrient intakes using the food composition tables of McCance and Widdowson (Paul and Southgate, 1978), and related these to colon and rectal cancer mortality using multivariate analysis. No association with consumption of fat, animal protein or total dietary fibre intake was found, but intakes of the pentose fraction of dietary fibre and of vegetables were protective (r -0.94 and r -0.96) (Fig. 9.2). When, however, more accurate and detailed figures for the dietary fibre composition of foods subsequently became available (Englyst et al., 1982), Bingham and colleagues (1985) recalculated the association with bowel cancer mortality. The new data showed that total dietary fibre intakes (measured as non-starch polysaccharides) were significantly inversely correlated with colon cancer (r -0.72). Of the individual components of fibre, cellulose and uronic acids were inversely correlated with cancer risk but no significant relation with fibre-pentose was found.

The Japanese are a much-studied population because their cancer risks are unlike those of other industrial societies. In particular they have a very low mortality from large bowel cancer. It might therefore be expected that their fibre intake would be high, especially in view of their large intake of rice. Minowa et al. (1983) have now reported bowel cancer mortality data and fibre intakes in Japanese using food consumption data derived from the National Nutrition Survey. Dietary fibre intakes in 1979 were estimated to be 19.4 g/person/day, an amount as low as that found in many Western countries such as the United Kingdom and Denmark where colon cancer is common.

Another population which may not fit neatly into the fibre hypothesis is the New Zealand Maori (Table 9.2). In the studies of Pomare and colleagues (1981), Maori death rates from large bowel cancer were found to be only half those of New Zealand Europeans, yet intakes of dietary fibre were very similar in the two groups, and comparable with those of the United Kingdom or urban Denmark. Interestingly, Maori death rates from gastric, lung and pancreatic cancer are two to four times the New Zealand European rates.

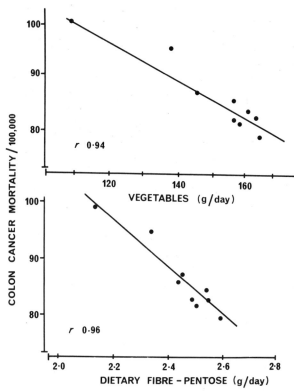

FIG. 9.2. Five-year age- and sex-standardized truncated death rates per 100,000 persons for colon cancer in the nine Registrar General regions of England, Wales and Scotland, in relation to average dietary intake of fibre–pentose and of vegetables (excluding potatoes), 1969–1973. (From Bingham *et al.*, 1979.)

TABLE 9.2. Dietary fibre intake and bowel cancer in Maoris and Europeans in New Zealand[a]

	Maoris	Europeans
Cancer death rate[b]		
Age 45–64	22	49
Age 65+	120	200
Dietary fibre intake (g/day)	16.1	18.1
Stool weight (g/day)	119 ± 48	113 ± 46
Transit time (h)	56 ± 27	52 ± 23

[a] Data from Pomare, 1980, and Pomare *et al.*, 1981.
[b] Rates per 100,000 population for males and females for colon + rectal cancer in 1975.

The picture to emerge from epidemiological studies is anything but clear. It is certainly not possible to use it to argue for a simple protective effect of fibre against large bowel cancer. This is partly because of the great methodological difficulties in measuring food intake, the lack of agreement as to what constitutes fibre and the lack of a widely accepted method to measure it. Problems in interpretation are compounded by the association of dietary constituents with one another in food consumption patterns such as high fat, high cholesterol with low fibre, or high fibre with high starch. Moreover it is becoming apparent that fibre is not a single uniform substance but contains a variety of polysaccharides and cell-wall components that have varying physiological effects. The ultimate development of colon cancer is likely to be the result of many interacting processes which include those promoting and inhibiting tumor growth. Since fibre is thought to be protective, it is possible for a population to have a low-fibre intake yet little bowel cancer, provided the tumour-causing agents are not present. This is probably the situation in Japan. Furthermore, bowel cancer may have different causes in different parts of the world. The problem in interpreting epidemiological studies of diet and cancer are therefore considerable.

B.   Case control studies

Faced with these difficulties a number of epidemiologists have compared patients and controls as a means of testing the fibre–bowel cancer hypothesis. About 12 such studies have been published in which the consumption of fibre-containing foods such as fruit, vegetables and cereals or of constituents such as fibre are compared in cases and controls.

The most striking feature of these studies is their lack of unanimity. Three papers report values for crude fibre intakes, two of which show that it is similar in cases and controls (Dorfman et al., 1976; Jain et al., 1980a) whilst that of Bjelke (1974) indicates that cancer cases ate less crude fibre. Of these studies, those of Bjelke (1974) and Jain et al. (1980a) are very comprehensive, involve many hundreds of subjects and use dietary methods whose validity was tested. Bjelke (1974) ascertained the frequency of food use 1 year prior to interview using a questionnaire administered by a trained person in over 600 cases of colorectal cancer and about 3000 hospital controls in Norway and in Minnesota, U.S.A. Although the interview gave higher values for food consumption than did the same questionnaire when self-administered through the post, Bjelke felt able to conclude that colorectal cancer patients consumed less fruit, vegetables, vitamin A, cereals and crude fibre than controls. One food that was particularly protective against colon cancer was carrot.

Jain et al. (1980a) studied 542 cases and 1077 controls in Canada. Their aim was to assess, by an interview in the subject's home 2–4 months after surgery (in the cases) and by means of food models, the amount and frequency of consumption of assorted foods. Aware of the criticisms levelled at dietary methods, they had previously published a detailed evaluation of their questionnaire (Jain et al., 1980b). The subjects were asked to recall food intake for a 2-month period 6 months prior to this interview. The cases showed greater overall energy intake than controls but no difference in crude fibre. The authors did point out, however, that dietary fibre values might be more relevant and hoped to re-analyse their data when appropriate food tables were available.

Other case control studies have looked simply at the consumption of foods rather than of food constituents. Those of Higginson (1966) and Wynder and Shigematsu (1967) antedate the Burkitt hypothesis and do not mention fibre as such. Both studies used many hundreds of cases and controls and looked retrospectively at consumption of foods such as bread, cereals, fruit, green-yellow vegetables, and potatoes. No differences emerged from either study but Higginson says, and Wynder and Shigematsu agree, that "the retrospective method may be unsatisfactory for demonstrating etiological factors in a relatively homogeneous population . . .".

Haenzel et al. (1973) used a diet history method to measure frequency of food use prior to the onset of symptoms. The method had been evaluated in previous studies (Haenzel et al., 1972). Their result in 179 cases and 357 controls was that meat intake (especially beef) and intake of legumes (especially string beans) were risk factors for bowel cancer (relative risks 2.2–2.6). The suggestion that a vegetable may cause bowel cancer goes somewhat against the tide of other studies and has never been fully explained. The population in question were Japanese living in Hawaii and in the process of transition from a Japanese to Western diet. Probably the real risk identified in Haenzel's study was transfer to Western-style food.

Modan et al. (1975), who were the first to write specifically about fibre, Graham et al. (1978), Dales et al. (1978), and Phillips (1975) all show a protective effect of fruit, vegetables or high-fibre foods against bowel cancer. Modan et al. (1975), using dietary methods developed with Graham (Graham et al., 1967; Modan et al., 1974), attempted to estimate the frequency of consumption of a large number of foods 1 year prior to interview. They showed, for colon but not rectal cancer, a significantly lower consumption of fibre-containing foods such as beans, cabbage, melon, pickle and cucumbers. Similarly, Graham et al. (1978) in a study of over 3000 subjects, showed that the consumption of raw vegetables, especially cabbage and other members of the brassica family, were protective against bowel cancer. Cereal foods were not enquired about in this study.

One population study stands out from the others because it is so enormous, involving 265,118 adult subjects, is prospective and has been going on for 15 years (Hirayama, 1981). This study involves 94.8% of the Japanese population over 40 years of age in 29 districts of Japan. Already there have been 726 cases of bowel cancer, despite a low incidence in that country, and Hirayama reports that the consumption of meat, rice and wheat protects against bowel cancer but that consumption of green and yellow vegetables does not. These findings, particularly in relation to meat and green-yellow vegetables, are at variance with many other studies but the fact that this one is prospective overcomes many potential criticisms. Fibre as such has not been measured and the dietary method is a questionnaire that has not been subjected to extensive checks of validity, as have the questionnaires of Graham et al. (1967) and of Miller's group (Jain et al., 1980b).

Overall, therefore, despite the considerable effort that has gone into them, these studies do not identify a clear role for fibre. There are numerous possible reasons for this, apart from the possibility that fibre is unrelated to bowel cancer risk. In no study published to date has dietary fibre, as opposed to crude fibre or fibre-containing foods, been measured. The problem of assessing food intake in case control studies has been extensively discussed by Graham and colleagues (Graham and Mettlin, 1979; Mettlin and Graham, 1980). These difficulties are magnified in bowel cancer cases because the diet is likely to be modified when this cancer first causes symptoms. Subjects who develop abdominal pain due to obstruction in their gut and whose bowel habits change are likely to eat less fruit, vegetables and cereal foods since these are known to stimulate large bowel activity. This has led some investigators to try and assess dietary intake before the onset of symptoms (Bjelke, 1974; Haenzel et al., 1973; Modan et al., 1975; Dales et al., 1978; Graham et al., 1978; Jain et al., 1980a). In the study of Dales et al. (1978), the reference time for diet questions was 3 or 5 years prior to the interview. Even this may not be early enough since the latent period for large bowel cancer, that is the period between initiation and clinical presentation, may be 5–10 years or longer (Morson, 1976). Considering the vagueness of people's memory for their food consumption even a week ago, it is difficult to see how accurate information can be obtained retrospectively. A number of studies have been reported in which the accuracy of retrospective assessment of dietary intake was determined (Byers et al., 1983; Jensen et al., 1985; Rohan and Potter, 1984). The principal, and the most striking, finding in these studies is the observation that the best correlation of past diet is with present diet, i.e. in trying to recall their diet of years ago people are probably strongly influenced by their present dietary intake. Prospective studies will overcome these problems, but, like population studies, they will be partly confounded by the close interrelation in people's diets of one foodstuff with another. It is only when all these problems are solved in a single study that the fibre hypothesis will be really tested.

III.   Mechanisms and metabolic epidemiology

It is unrealistic to expect epidemiology alone to provide the definitive answer to bowel cancer aetiology. At their best, geographical studies point to associations between environmental or other agents and cancer, thus allowing the development of hypotheses which can be tested experimentally in laboratory, animal or human studies. To be credible such hypotheses should not be just a simple re-statement of an observation, such as "high fat diets lead to bowel cancer", but should include a postulated mechanism or chain of events compatible with known human physiology which links cause and effect. For example, it may be suggested that "high fat diets lead to bowel cancer by stimulating bile acid secretion leading to increased colonic bile acid levels which promote tumour growth in the presence of carcinogens". Such an hypothesis can be tested epidemiologically since it predicts that bowel cancer patients have higher colonic bile acid levels than non-cancer patients. Testing such ideas in the field has led to the science of metabolic epidemiology, which has been widely used in bowel cancer studies.

What then are the proposed mechanisms for the cause of bowel cancer and how does fibre fit in? There is no shortage of ideas. Dietary fat, animal protein (especially beef), cholesterol, potassium, vitamins C and E have all been implicated in the bowel cancer story, in addition to genetic factors. Pre-existing abnormalities such as colonic polyps, ulcerative colitis, ureterosigmoidostomy and cholecystectomy are widely accepted as relevant. It has been suggested that the diet may contain naturally occurring mutagens or that mutagens may develop in the gut from more benign precursors. These substances include the aromatic amines, N-nitroso compounds, protein breakdown products like volatile phenols and ammonia, fecapentaenes and products of cooking such as pyrolysates of tryptophan. Anti-cancer substances may also be present in the diet and may be naturally occurring, e.g. vitamin E, vitamin C, retinoids, protease inhibitors, selenium salts and sterols, or may be products of microbial metabolism, e.g. lignans.

In addition, bile acids have been implicated either as promoters of tumour growth or as precursor carcinogens or possibly through direct morphological effects. The colonic microflora almost certainly play a part, either through specific reactions like the nuclear dehydrogenating clostridia, the production of microbial enzymes like nitro- and azo-reductase, steroid dehydrogenase and β-glucuronidase, or through the products of fermentation such as butyric acid (Bruce et al., 1981; Malt and Williamson, 1982; Bruce and Gustafsson, 1981).

From this it will be evident that no single, generally accepted mechanism for the development of large bowel cancer has emerged. Faced with this diversity it is difficult to be sure exactly where fibre fits in as a preventive agent. How and what it prevents can only be surmised at present. Nevertheless there are already a number of proposed mechanisms.

A.   Stool weight

It was an early observation in the development of the fibre–cancer hypothesis that populations with low cancer risk passed large amounts of faeces (Burkitt,

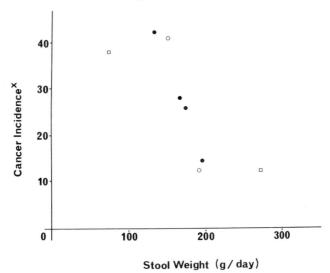

FIG. 9.3. Mean daily stool weight and large bowel cancer incidence in Scandinavia. ○ = IARC Intestinal Microecology Group, 1977; ● = Cummings *et al.*, 1982; □ = Reddy *et al.*, 1978; X = age-standardised (world population) incidence rates for colon + rectal cancer (ICD 153 + 154) in men. (Cancer incidence data for New York State obtained from Waterhouse *et al.*, 1976, p. 496.)

1971; Burkitt *et al.*, 1972). The most detailed exposition of this idea was by Burkitt, Walker and Painter who in 1972 reported stool weights in 10 racially very different groups of people, amounting to over 1000 subjects in all. They noted that low fibre intakes corresponded with low stool weights and high bowel cancer incidence. Information on bowel cancer was obtained by personal enquiry of around 200 hospitals in more than 20 countries. Whilst the results of these enquiries are not given in the paper the authors say they point clearly to an association of low fibre, low stool weight with high risk of bowel cancer.

Several investigators have sought to test this association further. In the two IARC-sponsored studies, stool weight in groups of middle-aged men, measured as stool output over a single 24-h period, and bowel cancer incidence in Scandinavia have been correlated (Fig. 9.3) (IARC, 1977; Cummings *et al.*, 1982). Within this geographically and culturally defined area, a high stool weight appears to protect against large bowel cancer.

Reddy *et al.* (1978) also measured stool output in relation to bowel cancer in 15 middle-aged male Finns from Kuopio and 20 age-matched men from metropolitan New York. Data from this study are also given in Fig. 9.3, and fit the general pattern.

However Pomare *et al.* (1981) reported stool weights in Maoris and New Zealand Europeans. Although Maori death rates from bowel cancer are half

TABLE 9.3. Effects of fibre on large intestine which may be important in determining large bowel cancer incidence

1. Physical dilution of contents through water-holding capacity.
2. Provision of a surface for adsorption.
3. Decreased transit time (more rapid turnover rate) of contents.
4. Consequences of fermentation.
    Production of acetate, propionate, butyrate
    Lower pH
    Stimulation of microbial cell growth
    Lower NH_4 levels
    ? mucus sparing
5. Altered bile acid metabolism (many possible mechanisms).

those of the New Zealand Europeans, their stool weights and fibre intakes are the same (Table 9.3). These data do not appear to fit the general hypothesis.

It is conceivable that as further data are collected on other populations, especially those with low risk, a simple relationship between stool weight and bowel cancer will not exist. Perhaps the hypothesis should be that a high faecal weight protects against bowel cancer but that a low faecal weight is not necessarily causative. We should, therefore, ask the question: how might a large stool output protect against large bowel cancer?

Passing a large stool as such is unlikely to be a vital factor. More likely a large stool is indicative of some other colonic event. It could simply reflect dietary fibre intake which undoubtedly influences stool weight. The benefit of passing large stools could lie in more effective emptying of the left colon since the majority of cancers of the large bowel in high-risk areas occur in the sigmoid and rectum. Alternatively, a large stool weight may reflect dilution of colonic contents.

B. Dilution of colonic contents

The evidence that dietary fibre leads to dilution of colonic contents has been reviewed in detail elsewhere (Cummings and Branch, 1982). It is likely that the bulk of colonic contents is increased by fibre although the difficulties in sampling from the colon mean that most of the evidence is indirect, by examination of faeces. Since the precise nature of the substances causing bowel cancer have yet to be identified, it is not possible to say exactly how dilution affects their physical state. Moreover, different sources of fibre have varying effects on the colon so that generalisations about fibre–carcinogen interactions may be misleading.

The increased bulk of colonic contents due to fibre has several components (Fig. 9.4). On an average U.K. diet, about 75% of total stool weight is water. This is not free water that can be poured off the top of a sediment of solid

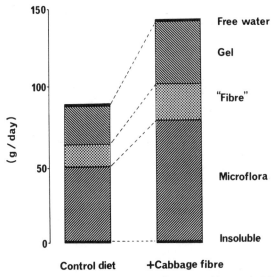

FIG. 9.4. Proposed faecal weight and composition of person taking typical Western-type diet (control) and then the same diet with the addition of 18 g dietary fibre from cabbage. Data calculated from Stephen and Cummings (1980a) assuming the extent of hydration of all cellular material (bacteria and plant cells) in a given stool is similar (69.4% control diet; 74.6% with added cabbage fibre). It is unlikely that there will be measurable free water if overall hydration is less than 80% since competition for water by the bacteria will be considerable.

matter. Most of it is intracellular either in bacteria which make up the major component of the stool (Stephen and Cummings, 1980a) or in the remnants of plant cells, which measure as dietary fibre. All these cells are enmeshed in a gell consisting of free water with mucus secreted into the gut and microbial polysaccharides (Eastwood *et al.,* 1980). Centrifugation of such stool, even at high *g* forces, usually produces very little free water (Wrong *et al.,* 1965; Tarlow and Thom, 1974). When fibre is added to the diet the stool becomes wetter (Cummings *et al.,* 1976; Stephen and Cummings, 1980a) and it is generally easier to remove free water from it by centrifugation. However, the majority of the water, probably 80–90%, is intracellular. With added fibre in the diet (from mixed sources), the microbial cell mass will increase and so will excretion of plant cell material and the gel. This complex interaction of physical and metabolic changes in the colon with fibre means that it is not easy to predict, or even define, what the concentration of a particular substance will be. More direct measurements are needed.

C.   Transit time

Both Burkitt (1971) and Walker *et al.* (1970) suggested that one mechanism by which fibre might protect against large bowel cancer is through reducing transit time. Several studies in man have shown that fibre speeds up transit, i.e. the time it takes for material to pass through the gut (Harvey et al., 1973; Kirwan et al., 1974; Cummings, 1978). Do high-risk populations in fact have slow transit through the gut and, if so, how does this affect colonic function?

In Burkitt and Walker's original observations (Burkitt et al., 1972), transit through the gut was measured using carmine markers or single doses of radio-opaque pellets in African, Indian and U.K. population groups. In the low-risk areas (African villagers, Indian nurses, Ugandan school children), transit was between 33 and 47 h on average whilst in the high-risk group (U.K. naval ratings, boarding school pupils and students) it was 48–83 h.

Since these original observations, four reports of transit in relation to bowel cancer in other populations of the world have appeared, not one of which shows the expected differences. Glober et al. (1974) measured transit with a single dose of radio-opaque pellets in Japanese and in Japanese living in Hawaii, as well as in Hawaii Caucasians. The Japanese and Caucasian inhabitants of Hawaii have a high large bowel cancer risk which is six times that of Japanese living in Japan. Nevertheless, transit times in the two Japanese groups were similar, about 30 h, whilst for the Caucasians it was 54 h.

The two IARC studies in Scandinavia (IARC, 1977; Cummings et al., 1982) used the single stool method for measuring transit time and found no difference between high- and low-risk populations. Mean transit time was identical at 37 ± 1 h in Copenhagen, where large bowel cancer incidence was highest at 42.1/100,000, and in rural Finland, where cancer risk was lowest at 14.2/100,000. Similarly, the study of Pomare et al. (1981; see Table 9.2) revealed no difference in transit time between the low-risk Maori population and the high-risk New Zealand Europeans.

These data show clearly that the rate of transit through the gut is not of overriding importance in determining the risk of bowel cancer. However, population averages like these do not exclude the possibility that in individuals there is a specific risk of very slow transit or that, other risk factors being equal, transit may be a determining factor.

What may keep the transit debate alive is the fact that, in man, transit rate does affect colonic metabolism. The details of this have been reviewed elsewhere (Cummings, 1978; Stephen and Cummings, 1980b; Cummings and Branch, 1982). Changes in transit rate are associated with alterations in stool weight, faecal microbial cell excretion, ammonia concentrations in stool and urinary volatile phenol excretion. Equally important is the evidence from ruminant studies that transit rate is an important determinant of microbial cell metabolism in the gut (Hespell, 1979).

D. Microbial metabolism

The key to any protective effect of fibre probably lies in its capacity to influence colonic microbial metabolism. The problem here lies in methodology. One approach to identifying microbial involvement has been to apply the techniques of classical bacteriology to culturing the stools from populations with different risks of bowel cancer, and from cases and controls. Early studies by Aries *et al.* (1969) and Hill *et al.* (1971) reported that the faeces of low-risk populations (Uganda, India and Japan) contained fewer *Bacteroides* sp. and Bifidobacteria than British and American stools. Conversely, the Indian and Japanese had more aerobic bacteria (Streptococci and Enterobacteria) than those living on Western diets. The $\log_{10}$ ratio of total anaerobes to total aerobes in the stool was lower in the Ugandans (1.1), Japanese (0.5) and Indians (1.5) than in those of the United Kingdom (2.1 and 2.5) and North America (2.7). These findings were confirmed by Koornhof *et al.* (1979) in South Africans and North Americans, although not in their Japanese population. However, Finegold *et al.* (1974) were unable to detect significant differences in the flora of two groups of Japanese Americans living in Los Angeles, one eating traditional Japanese food and the other principally Western diets.

A number of other studies have failed to show differences in the faecal flora of high- and low-risk populations including Seventh Day Adventists (Goldberg *et al.*, 1977; Finegold *et al.*, 1977; Finegold and Sutter, 1978), other vegetarians (Aries *et al.*, 1971b), various Scandinavian groups (IARC, 1977; Schwan *et al.*, 1982) and in colonic polyp patients when compared with controls (Finegold *et al.*, 1975).

One way in which the microflora may be associated with the development of bowel cancer is through their ability to produce potential carcinogens in the gut. Clostridia are important gut bacteria and one strain, *Clostridium paraputrificum,* has a steroid dehydrogenase which performs a key reaction in the production of aromatic steroids (Aries *et al.*, 1971a). Drasar *et al.* (1975) were able to show in faeces from healthy people in the United Kingdom, North America, Japan, Uganda and Hong Kong that there was a relationship between the carriage rate of the population for *Clostridium paraputrificum* and the risk of bowel cancer. Hong Kong in fact did not fit neatly into this relationship. The same group also showed in a case control study (Hill *et al.*, 1975) that the carriage rate of these nuclear dehydrogenating Clostridia was higher amongst cases than controls. However, their case control findings were not confirmed by Vargo *et al.* (1980), nor were there any such differences in the IARC studies (Schwan *et al.*, 1982).

The failure to demonstrate consistent differences in the faecal flora of populations with contrasting risks of large bowel cancer may be related partly to the many technical problems of anaerobic culture. Despite this, several groups have tried to see if feeding dietary fibre to man altered the flora. However, Drasar *et al.* (1976) feeding bran, Fuchs *et al.* (1976) with All-Bran, Walters *et al.* (1975) with bagasse, and Drasar and Jenkins (1976) with guar gum or plantain bananas have not shown any great differences in faecal flora with these diets in short-term studies. Changes in the ratio of anaerobes to aerobes were registered by Fuchs *et al.* (1976) and by Doyle *et al.* (1981) feeding pectin. Generally, however, the faecal flora appears to be remarkably stable in the face of large changes in diet using current techniques.

E. Faecal enzymes

Faced with the complexities of the flora and the failure to show changes with diet, some investigators have felt that more sensitive means are needed to measure microbial metabolism. One such method is to look at the metabolism of the faecal flora by measuring the activity in the faeces of enzymes thought to be mainly microbial in origin. These enzymes include β-glucuronidase, which will hydrolyse glucuronide conjugates such as diethyl stilboestrol β-D glucuronide and thus allow reabsorption of the steroid (Clark *et al.*, 1969), nitro- and azo-reductase, which may be involved in the generation of potentially mutagenic N-nitroso compounds (Balish *et al.*, 1981), and a variety of enzymes active on the ring structure of steroids (Eriksson and Gustafsson, 1970a,b; Eriksson *et al.*, 1968, 1969; Bjorkhem *et al.*, 1971; Aries *et al.*, 1969).

In animals dietary change can lead to alterations in faecal enzyme activity. Goldin and Gorbach (1976) showed a twofold increase in nitro- and azo-reductase and in β-glucuronidase in rats when they changed from a high-grain diet to one containing 72% lean beef. Bauer *et al.* (1979), however, who fed wheat bran, carrot fibre and pectin to rats together with a standard Western-type diet found changes only in β-glucuronidase activity, which increased tenfold. Epidemiological studies in man have shown differences between high- and low-risk populations. Reddy and Wynder reported in 1973 that β-glucuronidase activity in the faeces of Americans was higher than in vegetarian Americans, Seventh Day Adventists, Japanese and Chinese. In 1978 the same group (Mastromarino *et al.*, 1978) showed that the activities of steroid 7-α-dehydroxylase and cholesterol dehydrogenase were higher in bowel cancer patients and polyp patients than in healthy controls but they were unable to show differences in β-glucuronidase activity. MacDonald *et al.* (1978) measured several steroid dehydrogenases in the faeces of bowel cancer patients, controls and Seventh Day Adventists. 7-α-Hydroxy steroid dehydrogenase was highest in the cancer patients and lowest in the Adventists. In the studies of Goldin *et al.* (1980), Americans eating their usual diet had higher levels of β-glucuronidase, nitro-reductase, azo-reductase and steroid 7-α-dehydrogenase than vegetarians.

It is more difficult to show changes in faecal enzymes with fibre supplementation. Drasar *et al.* (1976) and Goldin *et al.* (1980) were unable to alter β-glucuronidase activity in faeces on feeding wheat bran although Bourke and Neale (1980) have been more successful in this respect. Goldin's group

(Goldin *et al.*, 1980) showed a small change in steroid 7-α-dehydrogenase activity but not in nitro- or azo-reductase.

There are difficulties in interpreting these studies in relation to the fibre–cancer hypothesis apart from their inconsistency. The colonic microflora are highly active metabolically and readily induce enzymes in response to substrate availability. Their enzyme activity at any particular moment may be the result of many interacting dietary and endogenous factors. Furthermore, the significance of these particular enzymes in the cancer process has yet to be established. Neither is it known whether the differences between populations and between diet groups are significant in determining product formation in the gut. Nevertheless there is other evidence that dietary fibre has significant effects on the metabolism of the microflora in man.

F.   Importance of fermentation

What was probably not appreciated by early proponents of the fibre–bowel cancer hypothesis was the importance of fibre in determining colonic metabolism. This has been developed only recently and has many implications.

Substantial amounts of dietary fibre are broken down in the colon by the anaerobic flora (Cummings, 1982). The principal events in this process are shown in Fig. 9.5. The major component of fibre is non-starch polysaccharide (NSP). This is fermented by the flora with the production of short-chain fatty acids (acetic, propionic and butyric acids), various gases (carbon dioxide, hydrogen and methane) and the release of energy which bacteria use for growth, cell division and maintenance requirements. This fermentation process is subject to a number of controls including the water solubility of the polysaccharides, their degree of lignification, particle size and the amount ingested. The polysaccharides in wheat bran are fermented much less than those in cabbage (Wiggins, unpublished data). Host factors are also important, such as transit time and the range and constituents of a person's microflora. There is marked variation from person to person in the fermentation of polysaccharides (Stephen, 1980). It is not possible to generalise about the effect of NSP in the colon and it is probably important in epidemiological studies to identify as precisely as possible the type and composition of any NSP being consumed.

G.   Short-chain fatty acids

There is little information at present concerning the amount of NSP consumed by people (see Chapter 5) and still less on the amount fermented in the large intestine. On the basis of what is known, however, it can be calculated that about 20 g/day of dietary polysaccharide is fermented in the large bowel of people consuming Western style diets. This would lead to the production of around 200 mmol of short-chain fatty acids comprising 120

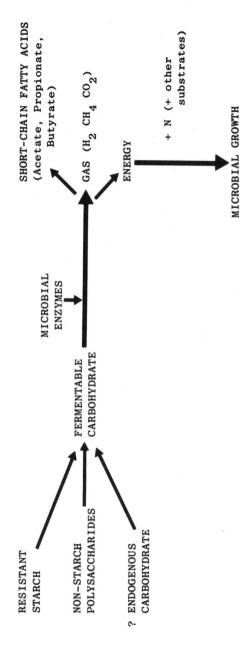

FIG. 9.5. Consequences of the fermentation of carbohydrate in the human large intestine.

mmol of acetate, 50 mmol propionate and 30 mmol butyrate (Cummings, 1981b).

Butyrate is an important intermediate in colonic metabolism. It has been shown recently to be a substrate for energy metabolism by colonic epithelial cells (Roediger, 1980; von Engelhardt and Rechkemmer, 1983) and is known from extensive cancer cell biology studies to be a potent differentiating agent. It will reversibly change the *in vitro* properties of human colorectal cancer cell lines by prolonging doubling time and generally slowing down growth rate (Kim *et al.*, 1982). It affects a wide range of cellular enzymes (Prasad, 1980), induces the accumulation of acetylated histones in cell culture and may stabilise chromatin structure during cell division. Low concentrations of butyrate have been shown to reduce DNA synthesis *in vitro* and suppress cell proliferation in a variety of cells (Hagopian *et al.*, 1977). Virus-induced cellular differentiation can be reversed by butyrate (Leder and Leder, 1975); whilst in rat hepatoma cells butyrate leads to a reversal of the cell to more normal appearance and to their becoming anchorage-dependent for growth, a characteristic of non-transformed cells (Borenfreund *et al.*, 1980). The concentration of butyrate used in these studies is well within the range found in the human colon, which is around 10 to 25 mmol/litre.

The potential for butyrate to inhibit tumour growth in the colon seems to be great; since NSP is at present thought to be the only major source for butyrate, this provides a ready link between fibre and bowel cancer.

H. pH

pH in the large intestine may fall as a result of fermentation. In studies of the fermentable disaccharide lactulose, Bown *et al.* (1974) showed that pH in the right colon fell from 6.0 (range 5.5–7.5) to 4.85 (range 3.5–6.1) in 10 subjects who took 30–40 g of this substrate daily. No comparable studies have been done with fibre in man. Faecal pH has been measured in adults and children after ingestion of bran (Walker *et al.*, 1979; Stephen and Cummings, 1981) and no significant changes were observed.

pH may play an important role in the regulation of cell growth in the colon and in the control of absorption and secretion. In Pikovski's studies (1954), an alkaline medium was shown to provide selective growth conditions for epithelial tumour cells in tissue culture. Cancer cells grow over a wide pH range and are not susceptible to growth inhibitory effects of pH (Ceccarini and Eagle, 1971). Contact inhibition between cells is pH dependent.

Bile acid degradation is also pH dependent. In an acid environment the initial conversion step of primary to secondary bile acids, 7-α-dehydroxylation, is inhibited (Midtvedt and Norman, 1968). It has been argued by Thornton (1981) that this is a key step in the development of bowel cancer. Low luminal pH may also trap ammonia in the bowel lumen and so reduce absorption into epithelial cells (Bown *et al.*, 1975).

The importance of these findings lies in the observation that patients with bowel cancer have higher faecal pH than controls (MacDonald *et al.*, 1978). Furthermore, in epidemiological studies of high- and low-risk populations for bowel cancer, Malhotra (1982) has reported that pH in the high-risk group is 7.8 ± 1.14 (SD) compared to 6.5 ± 1.02 ($p<0.001$) in the low-risk group.

As with many links between bowel cancer and gut function, a direct causal association has not been established. However, the effect of fibre on pH through its fermentation is a possible protective mechanism.

I. *Microbial growth and nitrogen metabolism*

When dietary fibre intake is increased, faecal nitrogen excretion also increases. Both animal and human studies have shown that this is largely attributable to greater microbial mass in faeces (Mason, 1969; Mason and Palmer, 1973; Stephen and Cummings, 1979). Although bacteria are able to use free amino acids for protein synthesis the nitrogen available to them is mainly in the form of ammonia. This is generated by microbial breakdown of urea, protein and other non-urea sources. Ammonia produced in the large intestine may be used by the microflora for protein synthesis or it may be absorbed, transported to the liver, reformed into urea and excreted in urine. The amount of nitrogen which bacteria require for growth and cell division will depend on the energy available to them. This energy is derived largely from fermentation, so the amount of fermentable substrate available to the microflora will directly influence nitrogen utilisation by bacteria. Feeding dietary fibre stimulates microbial cell growth and increases microbial requirements for nitrogen. More ammonia is used for protein synthesis and thus less should be absorbed. Animal studies have shown that portal blood ammonia levels fall in these circumstances (Demigne and Remesy, 1979). Overall faecal nitrogen excretion increases but ammonia concentrations fall (Cummings and Branch, 1982).

Ammonia is an important regulator of cell metabolism and cell growth. Visek (1972, 1978) has shown that it alters the susceptibility of cells to virus-induced tumour changes. Low concentrations alter DNA synthesis, reduce the life span of cells and induce faster cell turnover. In general, healthy epithelial cells are more susceptible to the toxic effects of ammonia than transformed cells and therefore high concentrations in the bowel lumen may select for neoplastic growth. Ammonia, by increasing cell turnover, increases the probability of genetic damage occurring in the presence of tumour-promoting agents. Rapidly dividing cell populations are more susceptible to chemical carcinogenesis (Warwick, 1971).

Although direct evidence linking nitrogen metabolism to tumour pathology in the human large intestine is not available, the increased risk of colonic tumours in ureterosigmoidostomy patients may be related to their high luminal ammonia concentrations (McConnell *et al.*, 1979; Tank *et al.*,

1973). *N*-nitroso compounds have also been implicated in the large bowel cancer hypothesis (Bruce *et al.*, 1977) and these may be derived in the bowel from nitrite (Tannenbaum *et al.*, 1978). The potential for dietary fibre to alter colonic nitorgen metabolism is therefore a possible protective mechanism.

J. Bile acids and mutagens

It is a widely held view that the immediate cause of bowel cancer is the presence in the colonic lumen of a substance or substances capable of transforming healthy epithelial cells into malignant tissue. There is considerable effort being directed into identifying these carcinogens or mutagens. An important group of substances to be discussed in this context is the bile acids which Hill and colleagues first suggested were related to bowel cancer (Aries *et al.*, 1969; Hill *et al.*, 1971; Drasar and Hill, 1974). They noted that bile acids were present in higher concentrations in the stools of people from high-risk populations than in those from low-risk areas. The same group went on to show that faecal bile acid concentrations were also higher in bowel cancer patients than controls (Hill *et al.*, 1975) and more recently have confirmed in the IARC Scandinavian studies these epidemiological associations (Hill *et al.*, 1982). Other confirmatory data were reported by Reddy and co-workers (Reddy and Wynder, 1973; Reddy *et al.*, 1978).

Hill postulated (1977) that bile acids are converted in the large intestine of man to unsaturated steroid structures which closely resemble known carcinogens (Aries *et al.*, 1971a; Goddard *et al.*, 1975).

Where does fibre fit into this scheme? Experimental studies in man have shown, in general, that fibre increases faecal excretion of bile acids. This is true for pectin (Kay and Truswell, 1977a; Miettinen and Tarpila, 1977; Cummings *et al.*, 1979; Ross and Leklem, 1981), for guar gum (Jenkins *et al.*, 1979), for cellulose (Shurpalekar *et al.*, 1971; Stanley *et al.*, 1973), for psyllium (Forman *et al.*, 1968; Stanley *et al.*, 1973) and for bagasse (Walters *et al.*, 1975). The results of studies with wheat bran, however, have not been consistent. Some investigators have demonstrated an increase in total bile acid excretion (Cummings *et al.*, 1976, 1979; McDougall *et al.*, 1978) whilst others have not (Eastwood *et al.*, 1973; Walters *et al.*, 1975; Kay and Truswell, 1977b) or have felt that the effects were unclear due to variation amongst individuals in bile acid outputs (Bell *et al.*, 1981). Where diets containing mixed sources of fibre have been fed faecal bile acid, excretion has increased (Antonis and Bersohn, 1962; Kretsch *et al.*, 1979; Ullrich *et al.*, 1981), although not always (Raymond *et al.*, 1977).

Epidemiologically, however, it is the concentration, not the total output, of bile acids in faeces that has been related to bowel cancer risk. Concentration has been defined by Hill's group as the amount of bile acid per gram of dry faecal material. This complicates the situation since some forms of fibre, such as pectin, increase bile acid excretion without greatly affecting stool solids excretion (Cummings *et al.*, 1979), whereas wheat bran leads to a great increase in solids excretion and a lesser increase in bile acids and thus, overall, to a decrease in faecal bile acid concentration. Moreover, the role of bile acids in promoting bowel cancer must depend on their physiological state in colonic contents. Presumably it is the concentration of bile acids intracellularly or in the water phase of luminal contents which is critical in determining their effects. At the present time this information is unavailable.

In the light of the proposition that it is bile acid metabolites, not bile acids themselves, which cause cancer, some people have looked at bile acid metabolism in relation to fibre. Ullrich *et al.* (1981) showed a reduction in the proportion of secondary bile acids in faeces from 98 to 68% in healthy young men after only 4 days on a high-fibre diet. However, Ross and Leklem (1981) fed pectin for 18 days and were unable to show any change in secondary bile acid excretion nor in the activity in faeces of steroid 7-α-dehydroxylase. An alternative approach is that used by Pomare and Heaton (1973) who examined bile composition in women before and after consuming wheat bran for 6 to 10 weeks. They found evidence of reduced 7-α-dehydroxylation in that deoxycholic acid levels in bile fell. Similar findings were reported from healthy subjects with supersaturated bile by Watts *et al.* (1978), but Brydon *et al.* (1979) were unable to change biliary bile composition in gallstone patients by feeding psyllium. Overall there is clearly a physiological interaction between some fibres and bile acids and, in light of the epidemiological associations, the possibility should not be excluded that this is one link between fibre and large bowel cancer.

There is little if any evidence relating fibre to the metabolism of other potential mutagens in the colon. The role of faecal mutagens in the determination of large bowel cancer has been well reviewed by Venitt (1982), who concludes

> The finding that most people's faeces contain substances which are mutagenic . . . should not be altogether surprising bearing in mind the enormous variety of chemicals ingested in normal diets in the form of foodstuffs, alcoholic and non-alcoholic beverages, food additives, drugs and contaminants and the influence of diet on the composition or metabolic activity of the intestinal flora.

IV.   Conclusions

The hypothesis that dietary fibre will prevent large bowel cancer is an intriguing one and worthy of consideration. For a variety of reasons, however, many current published epidemiological findings, either population or case control studies, do not support it. Physiological studies have shown quite clearly that dietary fibre alters large bowel function in a number of ways which could be protective against cancer (Table 9.3), although in the absence of a proven mechanism for the cause of large bowel cancer it is difficult to judge the significance of such studies. Similarly, the value of metabolic epidemiological findings in relation to bile acids, faecal mutagens, microbial metabolism and bowel habit cannot be judged in light of our present ignorance of the ultimate cause of bowel cancer.

Given the complexities of the bowel cancer story, it is unrealistic to believe that dietary fibre is *the* only important determinant of this disease. Provided it is acknowledged, however, that there may not be one universal aetiology for bowel cancer in all parts of the world and that many dietary, genetic and environmental factors contribute to the eventual experience of a community of this cancer, then in the context of Europe, America and possibly other industrialised countries, a case can be made that dietary fibre is protective. Nevertheless, we are a long way from being able to determine which sort of fibre and how much.

References

ANTONIS, A. and BERSOHN, I. (1962). *Am. J. Clin. Nutr.* **11**, 142–155.

ARIES, V. C., CROWTHER, J. S., DRASAR, B. S., HILL, M. J. and WILLIAMS, R. E. O. (1969). *Gut* **10**, 334–335.

ARIES, V. C., GODDARD, P. and HILL, M. J. (1971a). *Biochim. Biophys. Acta* **248**, 482.

ARIES, V. C., CROWTHER, J. S., DRASAR, B. S., HILL, M. J. and ELLIS, F. R. (1971b). *J. Pathol.* **103**, 54–56.

ARMSTRONG, B. and DOLL, R. (1975). *Int. J. Cancer* **15**, 617–631.

BALISH, E., WITTER, J. P. and GATLEY, S. (1981). *In* "Gastrointestinal Cancer: Endogenous Factors" (W. R. Bruce, P. Correa, M. Lipkin, S. R. Tannenbaum and T. D. Wilkins, eds.), Banbury Rep. No. 7, pp. 305–319. Cold Spring Harbor Lab., Cold Spring Harbor, New York.

BAUER, H. G., ASP, N.-G., OSTE, R., DAHLQVIST, A. and FREDLUND, P. E. (1979). *Cancer Res.* **39**, 3752–3756.

BELL, E. W., EMKEN, E. A., KLEVAY, L. M. and SANDSTEAD, H. H. (1981). *Am. J. Clin. Nutr.* **34**, 1071–1076.

BINGHAM, S., WILLIAMS, D. R. R., COLE, T. J. and JAMES, W. P. T. (1979). *Br. J. Cancer* **40**, 456–463.

BINGHAM, S. A., WILLIAMS, D. R. R. and CUMMINGS, J. H. (1985). *Br. Med. J.* (in press).

BJELKE, E. (1974). *Scand. J. Gastroenterol.* **9**, Suppl. 31, 1–235.

BJORKHEM, I., ERIKSSON, H. and GUSTAFSSON, J. A. (1971). *Eur. J. Biochem.* **20**, 340–343.

BORENFREUND, E., SCHMID, E., BENDICH, A. and FRANKE, W. W. (1980). *Exp. Cell Res.* **127**, 215–235.

BOURKE, G. and NEALE, G. (1980). *Ir. J. Med. Sci.* **149**, 38.

BOWN, R. L., GIBSON, J. A., SLADEN, G. E., HICKS, B. and DAWSON, A. M. (1974). *Gut* **15**, 999–1004.

BOWN, R. L., GIBSON, J. A., FENTON, J. C. B., SNEDDEN, W., CLARK, M. L. and SLADEN, G. E. (1975). *Clin. Sci. Mol. Med.* **48**, 279–287.

BREMNER, C. G. (164). *S.-Afr. Tydskr. Chir.* **2**, 119–123.

BRUCE, A. and GUSTAFSSON, J.-A. (eds) (1981). "Dietary Factors Influencing the Risk of Cancer", Var Foeda, Vol. 33, Suppl. 1. Statens Livsmedelsverk, Uppsala, Sweden

BRUCE, W. R., VARGHESE, A. J., FURRER, R. and LAND, P. C. (1977). *In* "Origins of Human

Cancer" (H. H. Hiatt, J. D. Watson and J. A. Winsten, eds), pp. 1641–1646. Cold Spring Harbor Lab., Cold Spring Harbor, New York.

BRUCE, W. R., CORREA, P., LIPKIN, M., TANNENBAUM, S. R. and WILKINS, T. D. (eds) (1981). "Gastrointestinal Cancer: Endogenous Factors", Banbury Rep. No. 7. Cold Spring Harbor Lab., Cold Spring Harbor, New York.

BRYDON, W. G., BORUP-CHRISTENSEN, S., VAN DER LINDEN, W. and EASTWOOD, M. A. (1979). Z. Ernährungswiss. 18, 77–80.

BURKITT, D. P. (1971). Cancer 28, 3–13.

BURKITT, D. P., WALKER, A. R. P. and PAINTER, N. S. (1972). Lancet 2, 1408–1412.

BYERS, T. E., ROSENTHAL, R. I., MARSHALL, J. R., RZEPKA, T. F., CUMMINGS, K. M. and GRAHAM, S. (1983). Nutr. Cancer 5, 69–77.

CECCARINI, C. and EAGLE, H. (1971). Proc. Natl. Acad. Sci. U.S.A. 68, 229–233.

CLARK, A. G., FISCHER, L. J., MILBURN, P., SMITH, R. L. and WILLIAMS, R. T. (1969). Biochem. J. 112, 17.

CUMMINGS, J. H. (1978). J. Plant Foods 3, 83–95.

CUMMINGS, J. H. (1981a). Proc. Nutr. Soc. 40, 7–14.

CUMMINGS, J. H. (1981b). Gut 22, 763–779.

CUMMINGS, J. H. (1982). In "Colon and Nutrition" (H. Kasper and H. Goebell, eds), pp. 91–104. M.T.P. Press Ltd., Lancaster, England.

CUMMINGS, J. H. and BRANCH, W. J. (1982). In "Dietary Fiber in Health and Disease" (G. V. Vahouny and D. Kritchevsky, eds), pp. 313–325. Plenum, New York.

CUMMINGS, J. H., HILL, M. J., JENKINS, D. J. A., PEARSON, J. R. and WIGGINS, H. S. (1976). Am. J. Clin. Nutr. 29, 1468–1473.

CUMMINGS, J. H., SOUTHGATE, D. A. T., BRANCH, W. J., WIGGINS, H. S., HOUSTON, H., JENKINS, D. J. A., JIVRAJ, T. and HILL, M. J. (1979). Br. J. Nutr. 41, 477–485.

CUMMINGS, J. H., BRANCH, W. J., BJERRUM, L., PAERREGAARD, A., HELMS, P. and BURTON, R. (1982). Nutr. Cancer 4, 61–66.

DALES, L. G., FRIEDMAN, G. D., URY, H. K., GROSSMAN, S. and WILLIAMS, S. R. (1978). Am. J. Epidemiol. 109, 132–143.

DEMIGNE, C. and REMESY, C. (1979). Ann. Biol. Anim., Biochim., Biophys. 19, 929–935.

DORFMAN, S. H., ALI, M. and FLOCH, M. H. (1976). Am. J. Clin. Nutr. 29, 87–89.

DOYLE, R. B., WOLFMAN, M., VARGO, D. and FLOCH, M. H. (1981). Am. J. Clin. Nutr. 34, 635.

DRASAR, B. S. and HILL, M. J. (1974). "Human Intestinal Flora." Academic Press, London.

DRASAR, B. S. and IRVING, D. (1973). Br. J. Cancer 27, 167–172.

DRASAR, B. S. and JENKINS, D. J. A. (1976). Am. J. Clin. Nutr. 29, 1410–1416.

DRASAR, B. S., GODDARD, P., HEATON, S., PEACH, S. and WEST, B. (1975). J. Med. Microbiol. 9, 63–71.

DRASAR, B. S., JENKINS, D. J. A. and CUMMINGS, J. H. (1976). J. Med. Microbiol. 9, 423–431.

EASTWOOD, M. A., KIRKPATRICK, J. R., MITCHELL, W. D., BONE, A. and HAMILTON, T. (1973). Br. Med. J. 4, 392–394.

EASTWOOD, M. A., BRYDON, W. G. and TADESSE, K. (1980). In "Medical Aspects of Dietary Fiber" (G. A. Spiller and R. M. Kay, eds), pp. 1–26. Plenum, New York.

ENGLYST, H. N., WIGGINS, H. S. and CUMMINGS, J. H. (1982). Analyst 107, 307–318.

ERIKSSON, H. and GUSTAFSSON, J. A. (1970a). Eur. J. Biochem. 16, 252–260.

ERIKSSON, H. and GUSTAFSSON, J. A. (1970b). Eur. J. Biochem. 16, 268–277.

ERIKSSON, H., GUSTAFSSON, J. A. and SJÖVALL, J. (1968). Eur. J. Biochem. 6, 219–226.

ERIKSSON, H., GUSTAFSSON, J. A. and SJÖVALL, J. (1969). Eur. J. Biochem. 9, 550–554.

FINEGOLD, S. M. and SUTTER, V. L. (1978). Am. J. Clin. Nutr. 31, S116–S122.

FINEGOLD, S. M., ATTEBERY, H. R. and SUTTER, V. L. (1974). Am. J. Clin. Nutr. 27, 1456–1469.

186   J. CUMMINGS

FINEGOLD, S. M., FLORA, D. J., ATTEBERY, H. R. and SUTTER, V. L. (1975). *Cancer Res.*
   35, 3407–3417.
FINEGOLD, S. M., SUTTER, V. L., SUGIHARA, P. T., ELDER, H. A., LEHMANN, S. M. and
   PHILLIPS, R. L. (1977). *Am. J. Clin. Nutr.* **30**, 1781–1792.
FORMAN, D. T., GARVIN, J. E., FORESTNER, J. E. and TAYLOR, C. B. (1968). *Proc. Soc.
   Exp. Biol. Med.* **127**, 1060–1063.
FREEMAN, H. J. (1979). *Can. Med. Assoc. J.* **121**, 291–296.
FUCHS, H.-M., DORFMAN, S. and FLOCH, M. H. (1976). *Am. J. Clin. Nutr.* **29**, 1443–1447.
GLOBER, G. A., KLEIN, K. L., MOORE, J. O. and ABBA, B. C. (1974). *Lancet* **2**, 80–81.
GODDARD, P., FERNANDEZ, F., WEST, B., HILL, M. J. and BARNES, P. (1975). *J. Med.
   Microbiol.* **8**, 429–435.
GOLDBERG, M. J., SMITH, J. W. and NICHOLS, R. L. (1977). *Ann. Surg.* **186**, 97–100.
GOLDIN, B. R. and GORBACH, S. L. (1976). *J. Natl. Cancer Inst. (U.S.)* **57** (2), 371–375.
GOLDIN, B. R., SWENSON, L., DWYER, J., SEXTON, M. and GORBACH, S. L. (1980). *JNCI,
   J. Natl. Cancer Inst.* **64** (2), 255–261.
GRAHAM, S. and METTLIN, C. (1979). *Am. J. Epidemiol.* **109**, 1–20.
GRAHAM, S., LILIENFELD, A. and TIDINGS, J. (1967). *Cancer* **20**, 2224–2234.
GRAHAM, S., DAYAL, H., SWANSON, M., MITTELMAN, A. and WILKINSON, G. (1978).
   JNCI, J. Natl. Cancer Inst. **61**, 709–714.
HAENZEL, W., KURIHARA, M., SEGI, M. and LEE, R. K. C. (1972). *J. Natl. Cancer Inst.
   (U.S.)* **49**, 969–988.
HAENZEL, W., BERG, J. W., SEGI, M., KURIHARA, M. and LOCKE, F. B. (1973). *J. Natl.
   Cancer Inst. (U.S.)* **51**, 1765–1779.
HAGOPIAN, H. K., RIGGS, M. G., SWARTZ, L. A. and INGRAM, V. M. (1977). *Cell* **12**, 855–
   860.
HARVEY, R. F., POMARE, E. W. and Heaton, K. W. (1973). *Lancet* **1**, 1278–1280.
HESPELL, R. B. (1979). *Fed. Proc., Fed. Am. Soc. Exp. Biol.* **38**, 2707–2712.
HIGGINSON, J. (1966). *J. Natl. Cancer Inst. (U.S.)* **37**, 527–545.
HIGGINSON, J. and OETTLÉ, A. G. (1960). *J. Natl. Cancer Inst. (U.S.)* **24**, 589–671.
HILL, M. J. (1974). *Digestion* **11**, 289–306.
HILL, M. J. (1977). *In* "Origins of Human Cancer" (H. Hiatt, J. Watson and J. Winsten, eds),
   pp. 1627–1640. Cold Spring Harbor Lab., Cold Spring Harbor, New York.
HILL, M. J., DRASAR, B. S., ARIES, V., CROWTHER, J. S., HAWKSWORTH, G. and WIL-
   LIAMS, G. (1971). *Lancet* **1**, 95–100.
HILL, M. J., DRASAR, B. S., WILLIAMS, R. E. O., MEADE, T. W., COX, A. G., SIMPSON, J.
   E. P. and Morson, B. C. (1975). *Lancet* **1**, 535–539.
HILL, M. J., MacLENNAN, R. and NEWCOMBE, K. (1979). *Lancet* **1**, 436.
HILL, M. J., TAYLOR, A. J., THOMPSON, M. H. and WAIT, R. (1982). *Nutr. Cancer* **4**, 67–
   73.
HIRAYAMA, T. (1981). *In* "Gastrointestinal Cancer: Endogenous Factors" (W. R. Bruce, P.
   Correa, M. Lipkin, S. R. Tannenbaum and T. D. Wilkins, eds)., Banbury Rep. No. 7, pp.
   409–429. Cold Spring Harbor Lab., Cold Spring Harbor, New York.
HOWELL, M. A. (1975). *J. Chronic Dis.* **28**, 67–80.
IARC Intestinal Microecology Group (1977). *Lancet* **2**, 207–211.
IRVING, D. and DRASAR, B. S. (1973). *Br. J. Cancer* **28**, 462–463.
JAIN, M., COOK, G. M., DAVIS, F. G., GRACE, M. G., HOWE, G. R. and MILLER, A. B.
   (1980a). *Int. J. Cancer* **26**, 757–768.
JAIN, M., HOWE, G. R., JOHNSON, K. C. and MILLER, A. B. (1980b). *Am. J. Epidemiol.* **111**,
   212–219.
JAMES, W. P. T., BINGHAM, S. A. and COLE, T. J. (1981). *Nutr. Cancer* **2**, 203–212.
JENKINS, D. J. A., REYNOLDS, D., LEEDS, A. R., WALLER, A. C. and CUMMINGS, J. H.
   (1979). *Am. J. Clin. Nutr.* **32**, 2430–2435.

JENSEN, O. M., MACLENNAN, R. and WAHRENDORF, J. (1982). *Nutr. Cancer* **4**, 5–19.

JENSEN, O. M., WAHRENDORF, J., ROSENQVIST, A. and GESER, A. (1985). *Am. J. Epidemiol.* (in press).

KAY, R. M. and TRUSWELL, A. S. (1977a). *Am. J. Clin. Nutr.* **30**, 171–175.

KAY, R. M. and TRUSWELL, A. S. (1977b). *Br. J. Nutr.* **37**, 227–235.

KIM, Y. S., TSAO, D., MORITA, A. and BELLA, A. (1982). *In* "Colonic Carcinogenesis" (R. A. Malt and R. C. N. Williamson, eds), Falk Symp. No. 31, pp. 317–323. M.T.P. Press Ltd., Lancaster, England.

KIRWAN, W. O., SMITH, A. N., MCCONNELL, A. A., MITCHELL, W. D. and EASTWOOD, M. A. (1974). *Br. Med. J.* **4**, 187–189.

KOORNHOF, H. J., RICHARDSON, N. J., WALL, D. M. and MOORE, W. E. C. (1979). *Isr. J. Med. Sci.* **15**, 335–340.

KRETSCH, M. J., CRAWFORD, L. and CALLOWAY, D. H. (1979). *Am. J. Clin. Nutr.* **32**, 1492–1496.

LEDER, A. and LEDER, P. (1975). *Cell* **5**, 319–322.

LIU, K., MOSS, D., PERSKY, V., STAMLER, J., GARSIDE, D. and SOLTERO, I. (1979). *Lancet* **2**, 782–785.

LYON, J. L. and SORENSON, A. W. (1978). *Am. J. Clin. Nutr.* **31**, S227–S230.

MCCONNELL, J. B., MORISON, J. and STEWARD, W. K. (1979). *Clin. Sci.* **57**, 305–312.

MACDONALD, I. A., WEBB, G. R. and MAHONY, D. E. (1978). *Am. J. Clin. Nutr.* **31**, S233–S238.

MCDOUGALL, R. M., YAKYMYSHYN, L., WALKER, K. and THURSTON, O. G. (1978). *Can. J. Surg.* **21**, 433.

MCMICHAEL, A. J., POTTER, J. D. and HETZEL, B. S. (1979). *Int. J. Epidemiol.* **8**, 296–303.

MALHOTRA, S. L. (1967). *Gut* **8**, 361–372.

MALHOTRA, S. L. (1977). *Med. Hypotheses* **3**, 122–126.

MALHOTRA, S. L. (1982). *J. R. Soc. Med.* **75**, 709–714.

MALT, R. A. and WILLIAMSON, R. C. N. (eds) (1982). "Colonic Carcinogenesis", Falk Symp. No. 31. M.T.P. Press Ltd., Lancaster, England.

MASON, V. C. (1969). *J. Agric. Sci.* **73**, 99–111.

MASON, V. C. and PALMER, R. (1973). *Acta Agric. Scand.* **23**, 141–150.

MASTROMARINO, A. J., REDDY, B. S. and WYNDER, E. L. (1978). *Cancer Res.* **38**, 4458–4462.

METTLIN, C. J. and GRAHAM, S. (1980). *Nutr. Cancer* **1**, 46–55.

MIDTVEDT, T. and NORMAN, A. (1968). *Acta Pathol. Microbiol. Scand.* **72**, 313–329.

MIETTINEN, T. A. and TARPILA, S. (1977). *Clin. Chim. Acta* **79**, 471–477.

MINOWA, M., BINGHAM, S. and CUMMINGS, J. H. (1983). *Hum. Nutr.: Appl. Nutr.* **37A**, 81–82.

MODAN, B. and LUBIN, F. (1980). *In* "Medical Aspects of Dietary Fiber" (G. A. Spiller and R. M. Kay, eds), pp. 119–136. Plenum, New York.

MODAN, B., LUBIN, F., BARELL, V., GREENBERG, R. A., MODAN, M. and GRAHAM, S. (1974). *Cancer* **34**, 2087–2092.

MODAN, B., BARELL, V., LUBIN, F., MODAN, M., GREENBERG, R. A. and GRAHAM, S. (1975). *J. Natl. Cancer Inst. (U.S.)* **55**, 15–18.

MORSON, B. C. (1976). *Clin. Gastroenterol.* **5** (3), 505–525.

OETTLÉ, A. G. (1964). *J. Natl. Cancer Inst. (U.S.)* **33**, 383–439.

PAUL, A. A. and SOUTHGATE, D. A. T. (1978). *In* "McCance and Widdowson's The Composition of Foods". H. M. Stationery Office, London.

PHILLIPS, R. L. (1975). *Cancer Res.* **35**, 3513–3522.

PIKOWSKI, M. A. (1954). *Exp. Cell Res.* **7**, 52–57.

POMARE, E. W. (1980). "Maori Standards of Health", Med. Res. Counc. N. Z. Spec. Rep. Ser. No. 7. M.R.C., Wellington, New Zealand.

POMARE, E. W. and HEATON, K. W. (1973). *Br. Med. J.* **4**, 262–264.

POMARE, E. W., STACE, N. H. and FISHER, A. (1981). *Aust. N.Z. J. Med.* **11**, 221.

PRASAD, K. N. (1980). *Life Sci.* **27**, 1351–1358.

RAYMOND, T. L., CONNOR, W. E., LIN, D. S., WARNER, S., FRY, M. M. and CONNOR, S. L. (1977). *J. Clin. Invest.* **60**, 1429–1437.

REDDY, B. S. and WYNDER, E. L. (1973). *J. Natl. Cancer Inst. (U.S.)* **50**, 1437–1442.

REDDY, B. S., HEDGES, A. R., LAAKSO, K. and WYNDER, E. L. (1978). *Cancer* **42**, 2832–2838.

ROEDIGER, W. E. W. (1980). *Gut* **21**, 793–798.

ROHAN, T. E. and POTTER, J. D. (1984). *Am. J. Epidemiol.* **120** 876–887.

ROSS, J. K. and LEKLEM, J. E. (1981). *Am. J. Clin. Nutr.* **34**, 2068–2077.

Royal College of Physicians (1980). "Medical Aspects of Dietary Fibre." Pitman Medical, London.

SCHRAUZER, G. N. (1976). *Med. Hypotheses* **2**, 39–49.

SCHWAN, A., RYDEN, A.-C. and LAURELL, G. (1982). *Nutr. Cancer* **4**, 74–79.

SHURPALEKAR, K. S., DORAISWAMY, T. R., SUNDARAVALLI, O. E. and NARAYANA, R. M. (1971). *Nature (London)* **232**, 554–555.

SOUTHGATE, D. A. T. (1976a). *In* "Fiber in Human Nutrition" (G. A. Spiller and R. J. Amen, eds), pp. 73–107. Plenum, New York.

SOUTHGATE, D. A. T. (1976b). "Determination of Food Carbohydrates." Applied Science Publishers, London.

SPILLER, G. A. and FREEMAN, H. J. (1981). *Am. J. Clin. Nutr.* **34**, 1145–1152.

STANLEY, M. M., PAUL, D., GACKE, D. and MURPHY, J. (1973). *Gastroenterology* **65**, 889–894.

STEPHEN, A. M. (1980). "Dietary Fibre and Human Colonic Function." Ph.D. Thesis, University of Cambridge.

STEPHEN, A. M. and CUMMINGS, J. H. (1979). *Proc. Nutr. Soc.* **38**, 141A.

STEPHEN, A. M. and CUMMINGS, J. H. (1980a). *Nature (London)* **284**, 283–284.

STEPHEN, A. M. and CUMMINGS, J. H. (1980b). *Gut* **21**, A420.

STEPHEN, A. M. and CUMMINGS, J. H. (1981). *Gastroenterology* **80**, 1294.

TANK, E. S., KARSCH, D. N. and LAPIDES, J. (1973). *Dis. Colon Rectum* **16**, 300–304.

TANNENBAUM, S., TETT, D., YOUNG, V., LAND, P. and BRUCE, W. (1978). *Science* **200**, 1487–1489.

TARLOW, M. J. and THOM, H. (1974). *Gut* **35**, 608–613.

THORNTON, J. R. (1981). *Lancet* **1**, 1081–1083.

TROWELL, H. C. (1960). "Non-Infective Disease in Africa", pp. 217–220. Edward Arnold, London.

TROWELL, H. C. and BURKITT, D. P. (1981). "Western Diseases: Their Emergence and Prevention." Edward Arnold, London.

ULLRICH, I. H., LAI, H.-Y., VONA, L., REID, R. L. and ALBRINK, M. J. (1981). *Am. J. Clin. Nutr.* **34**, 2054–2060.

VAN SOEST, P. J. and McQUEEN, R. W. (1973). *Proc. Nutr. Soc.* **32**, 123–130.

VARGO, D., MOSKOVITZ, M. and FLOCH, M. H. (1980). *Gut* **21**, 701–705.

VENITT, S. (1982). *In* "Colonic Carcinogenesis" (R. A. Malt and R. C. N. Williamson, eds), Falk Symp. No. 31, pp. 59–72. M.T.P. Press Ltd., Lancaster.

VISEK, W. J. (1972). *Fed. Proc., Fed. Am. Soc. Exp. Biol.* **31**, 1178–1193.

VISEK, W. J. (1978). *Am. J. Clin. Nutr.* **31**, S216–S220.

VON ENGELHARDT, W. and RECHKEMMER, G. (1983). *Bull.—R. Soc. N.Z.* **20**, 149–155.

WALKER, A. R. P. (1947). *S. Afr. Med. J.* **21**, 590–596.

WALKER, A. R. P. (1961). *S. Afr. Med. J.* **35**, 114–115.

WALKER, A. R. P. (1971). *S. Afr. Med. J.* **45**, 377–379.

WALKER, A. R. P. (1976). *Am. J. Clin. Nutr.* **29**, 1417–1426.

WALKER, A. R. P., WALKER, B. F. and RICHARDSON, R. D. (1970). *Br. Med. J.* **3**, 48–49.

WALKER, A. R. P., WALKER, B. F. and SEGAL, I. (1979). *S. Afr. Med. J.* **55**, 495–498.

WALTERS, R. L., BAIRD, I. M., DAVIES, P. S., HILL, M. J., DRASAR, B. S., SOUTHGATE, D. A. T., GREEN, J. and MORGAN, B. (1975). *Br. Med. J.* **2**, 536–538.

WARWICK, G. P. (1971). *Fed. Proc., Fed. Am. Soc. Exp. Biol.* **30**, 1760–1765.

WATERHOUSE, J., MUIR, C., CORREA, P. and POWELL, J. (1976). "Cancer Incidence in Five Continents", Vol. III, I.A.R.C. Sci. Publ. No. 15. I.A.R.C., Lyon.

WATTS, J. McK., JABLONSKI, P. and TOOULI, J. (1978). *Am. J. Surg.* **135**, 321–324.

WRONG, O., METCALFE-GIBSON, A., MORRISON, R. B. I., NG, S. T. and HOWARD, A. V. (1965). *Clin. Sci.* **28**, 357–375.

WYNDER, E. L. and SHIGEMATSU, T. (1967). *Cancer* **20**, 1520–1561.

Chapter 10

Appendicitis

ALEXANDER WALKER and DENIS BURKITT

I.   The problem: to what extent is appendicitis related to the fibre depletion of diets?

A century ago, appendicitis was rare in Western populations. In the United Kingdom, appendicectomy is now the fifth most common surgical operation. The rise in frequency occurred simultaneously with a number of dietary changes which included a decrease in the intake of fibre-containing foods, with associated changes in bowel behaviour and *milieu intérieur*. Accordingly, some have reasoned and advanced that these two variables are aetiologically related. Others consider an aetiological relationship to be wholly unproven and based on simplistic thinking. The problem is—to what extent does evidence support the dietary hypothesis?

Dietary Fibre, Fibre-Depleted Foods
and Disease

II. Epidemiology

A. Appendicitis in Western populations

Between 1820 and 1840, 33 cases of abscesses in the right iliac fossa were reported in the literature, and between 1840 and 1860, 102 cases; these were widely distributed in Europe and North America (Short, 1920). Although Melier (1827) suggested that such abscesses were derived from perforation of the appendix, the term "perityphitis" was generally used. The designation "appendicitis" was adopted after what Short (1920) called "the epoch-making treatise" of Fitz in 1886.

In the United Kingdom before 1880, appendicitis was a rare disease even making allowance for the change in nomenclature (Leading Article, 1906). From figures obtained from St. Bartholomew's and St. Thomas's hospitals, and also from certain large provincial hospitals, Watson (1906) showed that a spectacular sixfold rise in incidence occurred between 1876 and 1880 and 1896 and 1900. From 1901 to 1918, deaths from the disease doubled (Short, 1920). In Oxford, Elliot-Smith (1971) noted that from 1900 to 1970, the incidence there had risen from 5 to 10 cases to 500 cases annually.

In the United States, the incidence rose earlier than in most European countries. The increase was considerably slower in black compared with white populations. At the turn of the century, Matas (1896) remarked on the relative rarity of appendicitis in blacks. Much later, Boland (1942) made the same observation. Short (1946) related that "many doctors practising in the 'black belt' of Alabama can scarcely recall a case in a negro". In the early 1930s in New Orleans, appendicitis was four times more common in white than in black communities, but by 1950 the difference had fallen to twofold (Boyce, 1951). This racial disparity has now become narrower for, where both races live in a similar environment, as in the armed forces, operations for appendicitis appear to be almost equally common (Editorial, 1949). Notwithstanding, even as late as 1968, appendicectomy was still less *prevalent* in blacks (especially in males) than in whites (Hyams and Wynder, 1968).

In the United Kingdom, prevalences vary regionally (West and Carey, 1978; Barker and Liggins, 1981) as they do also in the United States (Hyams and Wynder, 1968). As to the overall situation in the United Kingdom, Ashley (1967) calculated that "some 15% of males and 18% of females are subjected to appendicectomy". Using data on the age distribution of appendicectomies prevailing in the United Kingdom (Wright, 1963), calculations indicate that in South Africa prevalence of the operation for the *total* white population is about 17% (Walker *et al.*, 1973). This figure resembles that given for New Zealanders (Ludbrook and Spears, 1965), about 16%. Prevalence, however, would seem higher in the United States (Hyams and Wynder, 1968) and in Germany (Lichtner and Pflanz, 1971). As to annual incidence, in the United Kingdom appendicectomy ranked fifth amongst surgical operations performed during 1977, the total for the year being 74,230 (Donaldson, 1981–1982).

The frequency of the operation may now be decreasing, according to reports from the United Kingdom (Howie, 1966), United States (White *et al.*, 1975; Mendeloff, 1975), Norway (Noer, 1975), and Canada (Mindell *et al.*, 1982). In two Norwegian cities "the number of operations for acute appendicitis per 5 year period has decreased by more than 50% during these 30 years". This could be accounted for by better diagnosis of mimicking conditions, such as gynaecological disorders and spastic colon.

In some countries, appendicectomy is slightly more common in females than males, as in the United Kingdom (Ashley, 1967) and South Africa (Walker *et al.*, 1973); the converse is true in New Zealand (Ludbrook and Spears, 1965). Peak occurrence is in adolescence at 18 to 20 years in New Zealand (Ludbrook and Spears, 1965) and, in Wales, at 15 to 19 years in girls but at 10 to 14 years among boys (West and Roberts, 1974).

B.   Appendicitis in Third World populations

One or two generations ago, clinicians and other observers testified unanimously to the rarity of appendicitis in Third World populations. In Africa, where the disease attracted most attention, it was deemed extremely uncommon in former Rhodesia (Gelfand, 1956), in territories in tropical Africa (Trowell, 1960; Janssens and De Muynck, 1966; Burkitt, 1971) and in South Africa (Erasmus, 1939). Its former rarity in other parts of the world has also been reported (Hallilay, 1924; Schaefer, 1979).

Recently, however, the indications are that increases have occurred. This has been noted in Accra (Badoe, 1971), Nairobi (Ochola-Abila, 1979), Khartoum (Osman, 1974), rural Kenya (Branicki, 1981), Dar-es-Salaam (Shija, 1975), and in urban areas in Nigeria (Taiwo *et al.*, 1977; Onuigbo, 1977) and Botswana (Bhattacharyya and Durrani, 1974). Increases have also been reported in South Africa (Moore and Robbs, 1979; Nel and Theron, 1979; Griffiths, 1981; Blumberg, 1981; Walker *et al.*, 1982). Despite these increases, there is still a wide difference in *prevalence* of appendicectomy between developed and developing populations. For example, in South Africa, in a study on 16,939 high school pupils, 16–18 years old, mean prevalences of appendicectomy were rural blacks, 0.6%; urban blacks, 0.7%; Eur-African-Malays, 1.7%; Indians, 2.9%; but whites, 10.5%. Percentages were similar in boys and girls. Only in Eur-African-Malays and Indians did *prevalence,* as distinct from *incidence,* appear to have significantly increased (Walker *et al.*, 1973, 1982).

How valid are these data indicating very low frequencies in African and other Third World populations?

C. Validity of appendicectomy data

1. Accuracy of diagnosis of appendicitis

According to White *et al.* (1975) working in the United States, "Removal of up to 20 per cent of normal appendices has been considered acceptable". In black patients at Pelonomi Hospital, Bloemfontein, in 1975–1978, the diagnosis was confirmed histologically in 82% of appendicectomies (Nel and Theron, 1979).

2. Confounding factors

Could not the lower prevalence of appendicectomy among less privileged populations be due in part (1) to the cost of the operation being a deterrent, or (2) to medical services being less accessible (de Dombal and Hedley, 1979; Rose and Barker, 1978)? As to charges for the operation, in South African black rural dwellers, the chief cost is for transport to and from the hospital. At Baragwanath Hospital, Johannesburg, the charge for blacks is R1 ($1.3), which is 0.3 to 0.6% of average monthly wages. For Indians and Eur-African-Malays (most of whom are urban dwellers), the charge at Coronation Hospital, Johannesburg, is under R2, or 0.5–2% of average monthly wages. Accordingly, costs of the operation are unlikely to explain the far lower frequencies of appendicectomy found in black, Indian and Eur-African-Malay adolescents. As to accessibility of facilities, in rural Mission Hospitals surgical emergencies such as ruptured uterus or ectopic pregnancies are not uncommon, whereas acute appendicitis is extremely rare. In urban areas, black residents have in our experience always been ready to seek medical attention when seriously sick. It is therefore considered that the low prevalence data reported are valid.

III.   Dietary characteristics

A. Dietary changes in Western populations

Concerning cereal intake in the United Kingdom, in 1880 a change began to occur in the character of the national loaf (Drummond and Wilbraham, 1939; Cruickshank, 1946). Formerly, it had been made from stone-ground flour from which bran was incompletely removed, if at all. The introduction of roller mills resulted in bran-free white flour, yielding a loaf that won immediate popularity. Wheat flour consumption in Britain varied little during most of the last century and was about 350 g/person/day; the level started falling in the last years of that century to about 250 g/person/day in the 1930s and has continued to fall (Hollingsworth and Greaves, 1967). Cereal dietary fibre in Britain fell from 12.2 g/person/day in 1880 to 8.1 g/person/day in 1970 (Southgate *et al.*, 1978). While consumption of certain vegetables and fruits has risen, total mean dietary fibre intake remains low, being about 20 g/day (Gear *et al.*, 1979).

In the United States, similar dietary changes occurred. According to Riley (1948), "the mass of the food of our fathers and grandfathers . . . . was subjected to the simplest and most necessary processing only"; and he then referred to the changes in milling that took place when Benjamin Harrison was President.

As described by Cleave (1974), Hollingsworth (1975), Lowenberg *et al.* (1979), den Hartog (1980b) and others, associated changes in diet included rises in intakes of total energy, animal protein and fat, and sugar.

In brief, in the more prosperous of Western populations, the combination of the lower cereal extraction rate, the fall in bread consumption, the lesser effectiveness in laxation of the increased consumption of fruit and vegetables (other than potatoes), and the rise in sugar consumption has greatly reduced the stool-bulking capacity of the diet, with major implications in bowel physiology (Walker, 1947).

B. Diet in Third World populations

In Third World populations, with minor exceptions, diets are composed mainly of plant products, principally cereals and their products, also legumes, tubers and a variety of wild and cultivated vegetables and fruits. Such a diet is low to moderate in energy value and animal protein; it is very low in fat, and low in certain mineral salts such as calcium, and in certain vitamins such as vitamin D. It is high in dietary fibre (McCarrison, 1936; Gelfand, 1956; Trowell, 1960; Lowenberg *et al.*, 1979; Walker and Segal, 1979).

With urbanization, a measure of westernization of diet occurs, slight in socio-economically poor countries, but marked in more prosperous countries (Manning *et al.*, 1974; den Hartog, 1980a; Fatma and Kies, 1981). The tendency is toward a lower dietary fibre intake, associated with partial refinement of cereal products, and a higher intake of fat, sugar and sugar-containing foods.

IV. The role of altered bowel behaviour

Historically, from ancient times until as late as the turn of this century, disorder of bowel movement, constipation and purging took a considerable toll of physicians' time and art. Hippocrates held that, for the maintenance of good health, defaecation should occur "twice or thrice" daily (Adams, 1939).

There seems to have been general agreement over the primary cause of the commonness of constipation. Cheadle (1886) listed the chief reason as consumption of "food which leaves little residue; very completely digested food . . . . . faecal matter too small to duly excite peristalsis". Sir Lauder

Brunton (1896) of St. Bartholomew's Hospital blamed fine wheaten bread and thoroughly cooked vegetables. Up to the time of Cheadle and Brunton, diets were high in bulk-forming capacity. But, as already indicated, this situation changed. Goodhart (1910) affirmed "that with advancing civilization aperients would always be with us", but lamented "the change from the occasional pill of our forefathers to the excess of the present day". In the United States, an editorial (1928) in *Journal of the American Medical Association* drew attention to the "imperative need that millions of persons feel for something that will assist in the regulation of the bowel". Currently, the huge numbers of prescriptions for laxatives, as well as the extent of sales over the counter, speak for themselves (Christopher and Crooks, 1974).

Nowadays, among most Western populations, the great majority defaecate once daily (Taylor, 1975). In contrast, in those Third World populations on which we have information, a frequency of twice a day or more is usual (Ekwueme, 1978; Walker and Segal, 1979). The difference is believed to be due almost wholly to the difference in consumption of fibre-containing foods. Among Western compared with Third World populations, transit time is longer: double or more. The dry weight of faeces voided daily is smaller, 20–25 g versus 40–60 g or more. A far higher proportion of faeces are formed in consistency, and concentrations of faecal bile acids and steroids are higher (Walker and Segal, 1979; Reddy, 1979).

What is the evidence that altered bowel behaviour is associated with proneness to appendicitis? Certainly, early observers considered that intestinal stasis was associated with appendicitis or promoted its occurrence (Bell, 1880; MacEwen, 1904). Charles Mayo (1924), referring to appendicitis, maintained that "a soil has become engendered and has become susceptible to diseases by changes in food that have been developed within a few decades", a view that was shared by Ogilvie (1938). Lately, however, the association has been regarded as unproven (Current Comment, 1939; Hyams and Wynder, 1968; Royal College of Physicians, 1980). One factor that hinders the search for a link is people's rather poor recollection of their bowel behaviour, including frequency of defaecation and stool consistency (Manning *et al.*, 1974; Walker *et al.*, 1982). Recall is frequently at variance with records of bowel movements.

V.   Can dietary changes reduce frequency of the disease?

Our knowledge of the relationship between bowel behaviour and appendicitis remains defective. The practical question is—if individuals or segments of Western populations elected to alter their habitual diets and reverted in measure to diets of the past, *inter alia,* by markedly increasing their consumption of fibre-containing foods (e.g. by eating more of wholemeal bread, legumes, vegetables)—would the frequency of bowel diseases, particularly appendicitis, decrease?

. Unfortunately, there is a lack of telling evidence in this area. Long-term intervention studies have not yet been undertaken. However, in short-term studies some suggestive results have been obtained. For example, on changing the diet of volunteers from low- to high-fibre containing foods, the changes noted in faecal steroid concentrations were so rapid that the authors regarded them as having "implications for the prevention of arteriosclerosis and cancer of the colon" (Ullrich et al., 1981). The pH value of faeces, postulated as being of relevance to the development of colon cancer (Thornton, 1981), is also readily altered by changing the fibre content of diets (Walker et al., 1979).

Of particular interest are results of *involuntary* dietary changes that occurred during World Wars I and II, when restriction of imports and food rationing forced diets to revert, to some extent, to those of the past. The energy content fell, as did the intake of animal protein, total fat (especially animal fat), cholesterol and sugar. Simultaneously, intakes of cereal foods (less refined), legumes and vegetables increased, as consequently did intakes of dietary fibre. Some data are available on populations that experienced marked changes, i.e. in the Channel Islands (Banks and Magee, 1945), Switzerland (Fleisch, 1946) and the Netherlands (Van Ouwerkerk, 1951), Norway (Strom and Jensen, 1951) and post-war Germany (Pezold, 1959; Schettler, 1979). Defaecation became more frequent and incidences of constipation and appendicitis fell. Such epidemiological evidence, with that already cited, may be regarded as supporting a causal relationship between level of intake of fibre foods, bowel behaviour, *milieu intérieur,* and degree of proneness to appendicitis.

But is it likely that *voluntary* rises in intakes of fibre-containing foods could reduce the incidence of appendicitis? Young and Russell (1939) considered that "under existing conditions of modern life, it seems improbable that a sufficient change in dietary habits will be introduced to influence to an appreciable extent the incidence of appendicitis". This view is supported by the results of a number of studies. In a community study in Cardiff, Westlake et al. (1980) noted that those who ate wholemeal bread daily had a lower frequency of appendicitis than those who ate it rarely or never, but the difference was not significant. Analogous unpublished studies undertaken on white students in Johannesburg and Bloemfontein have led us to the same conclusion. Additionally, it was found that, although higher compared with lower fibre-consuming moieties had greater frequencies of defaecation, the differences were not significant, which suggested that substantially higher fibre intakes are necessary to alter bowel behaviour enough to prevent appendicitis.

VI. Possible mechanisms

While no definite mechanism has been demonstrated, the following considerations seem relevant.

As emphasised by Burkitt (1975), fibre is the only dietary constituent which markedly affects the consistency, bulk and speed of transit of faeces. Fibre can also lower the pressure within the colon (see Chapter 8).

Clinical and pathological evidence suggest that the initial change is raised pressure within the appendix, which leads to devitalization of the mucosa, bacterial invasion being secondary. Increased pressure could be the result of muscular spasm or of obstruction to the appendiceal lumen by faecoliths. Faecoliths are lumps of inspissated faecal material containing calcium and magnesium phosphates and carbonates. The presence of a faecolith implies appendicular stasis.

Early in this century, Van Zwalenburg (1904, 1905) demonstrated that the viability of bowel mucosa could be impaired by increasing the pressure on it, and he postulated that inflammation could follow bacterial invasion. He believed that faecal concretions could exert a valve-like action and thus lead to raised intraluminal pressures; Wilkie (1914) agreed. In 1937, Wangensteen and Bowers wrote, "Obstruction and infection are the two causative factors important in bringing about a picture of acute appendicitis". In 1938, a leading article on the aetiology of appendicitis concluded ". . . it seems possible that in most cases of appendicitis the infecting organisms are those normally present in the appendix; that obstruction by faecoliths is a predisposing cause; and that the precipitating factor is a complete obstruction of the lumen with injury to the mucosa". Possibly the lesser bowel motility and more common stasis in susceptible populations could favour formation of concretions. Also, the stagnation would, according to Aschoff's theory (Leading Article, 1938), raise the virulence of a normal inhabitant of the alimentary tract enabling it to break down the natural defenses of the mucosa. In 1940, Fantus et al. reported that, when healthy young Americans added bran to their diet, a previously unvisualised appendix was sometimes seen on barium follow-through X-rays. Otherwise, experimental support for these ideas is lacking.

A factor that could contribute to obstruction of the appendix is the width of the lumen. Lymphoid tissue in the appendix begins to atrophy in the second decade of life; this atrophy would seem likely to increase the diameter of the lumen, making obstruction less likely. This could account for the maximum prevalence of the disease in childhood and adolescence. It could also account for increased prevalence during epidemics of infectious disease.

To summarise the suggested chain of events:

1. Faecoliths or spasm obstruct the lumen and cause stasis.
2. Pressure rises within the lumen.

3. The mucosa becomes infected and inflamed. Inflammatory changes affect the whole appendix distal to a line of demarcation, and rarely if ever extend into the caecum.

Unfortunately, little progress has been made in testing this hypothesis which in essence was put forward early in this century. The Royal College of Physicians (1980), in its report on dietary fibre, concluded that there was much evidence of a causal environmental agent in appendicitis and that a low intake of dietary fibre should be considered. However, it stated that recent studies of the coincidence of faecoliths with appendicitis reported a far lower incidence than previous investigations (Horton, 1977). It pointed out that little is known concerning the viscosity of caecal contents on different diets or of intraluminal pressures within the appendix. To this may be added ignorance concerning the size of the lumen in different ethnic groups or in groups that have different diets.

As to causative or promotive factors other than changes in diet and altered bowel behaviour, Ashley (1967) considered that vascular disorders and non-specific viral infections may be important. More recently, Creed (1981) provided evidence that a stressful life, emotional problems and depression may be influential. A further factor could be familial predisposition (Andersson *et al.*, 1979).

As to *precipitating* causes, it was maintained by Cope (1950) that knowledge on this aspect is little beyond what Fitz (1886) taught 100 years ago, and this still appears to be true.

VII.   Effect of appendicectomy on future health

Increasing although sporadic interest is being shown in possible delayed ill-effects associated with appendicectomy and, interestingly, tonsillectomy.

A study conducted in the United States indicated that hospitalized women aged 40 years had a more than twofold prevalence of previous appendicectomy compared with a non-hospitalized control population (Friskey, 1968). In another American study "men with Hodgkin's disease evidence . . . had significantly higher rates of past appendicectomy than the appropriate control group" (Hyams and Wynder, 1968). In an investigation on a Greek population, "in patients with cancer of the breast and ovaries, the incidence of appendicectomy was found to be very high" (Cassimos *et al.*, 1973). In another study it was noted that, in patients with non-Hodgkin's lymphomas, the prevalence of previous appendicectomy was higher than that in a control group (Wilson, 1981). Regarding tonsillectomy, in a series of children diagnosed as having acute myelocytic leukaemia, frequency of previous tonsillectomy was considerably higher than that among non-affected children (Cuneo, 1972). Tonsillectomy has been stated to be associated with proneness to

Hodgkin's disease: "Tonsillectomized children appear to have 2.7 to 3.2 times the risk of Hodgkin's disease as their non-tonsillectomized sibs" (Vianna *et al.*, 1980). In a study in Scotland "the incidence of prior tonsillectomy was higher in 200 patients with lymphomas than in control subjects" (Dawson *et al.*, 1979). However, greater liability to any of the diseases mentioned was not observed in a study carried out in Greece (Cassimos *et al.*, 1973).

A recent investigation revealed that "the rate of prior appendicectomy was higher with men with colon cancer . . . A previous hemorrhoidectomy was also found more common . . . Long standing constipation was present more often in patients with cancer" (Vobecky *et al.*, 1983).

None of the investigations on appendicectomy and tonsillectomy and subsequent health was definitive but, taken together, they strongly suggest that those who have had their appendix or tonsils removed are at greater risk of certain serious diseases.

The current belief that the lymphoid aggregates present in the tonsils, Peyer's patches and vermiform appendix may have an important immunological function corresponding to that of the bursa of Fabricius in birds is consistent with the above observations.

Prevalences of appendicectomy and tonsillectomy among South African blacks (Walker *et al.*, 1981, 1982) are only one-tenth or so of those among whites; in consonance, all the associated diseases referred to remain very uncommon among these people.

Obviously, more research is required in this important area.

VIII.   Summary and conclusions

Epidemiologically, appendicitis was rare in Western populations until 1870 to 1880, when its frequency began to increase. At present, in the United Kingdom appendicectomy is the fifth most common surgical operation and is undergone by about one-sixth of the population. Although the frequency of appendicectomy is falling, the extent to which acute appendicitis is decreasing is not known with certainty.

In Third World countries, appendicitis is virtually absent in rural areas. In big cities, although the disease does occur and is increasing, it is still only one-tenth or so as common as in White populations.

Concurrently with the rise in frequency of appendicitis in Western populations, there have been major changes in diet. These have included increased intakes of energy, protein (especially animal protein) and fat (especially animal fat). Decreases have occurred in the stool-bulking capacity of the diet. In particular, there has been a decreased intake of dietary fibre from cereal foods. Associated dietary changes include increased intakes of refined carbohydrate foods, principally sugar.

The evidence suggests that the primary influencing factor is the intake of fibre, with its many effects on bowel behaviour and physiology and on the chemical and microbiological makeup of faeces. In consonance with this suggestion, there is epidemiological evidence that when national diets involuntarily reverted towards diets of the past, including, *inter alia,* a much higher fibre intake, as occurred in certain countries during World War II, the frequency of constipation and appendicitis decreased. Notwithstanding, it is judged unlikely that Western peoples will voluntarily change their diet enough to reduce their proneness to appendicitis.

While a link between reduced stool output or constipation and proneness to appendicitis seems plausible, a step-by-step mechanism has not been worked out and would be difficult to prove. A sequence of stasis, obstruction by faecoliths, rise in intraluminal pressure, infection and inflammatory changes seems reasonable, but direct evidence is still required.

Other aetiological factors may include certain infections, life events, and possibly a familial predisposition.

As to *precipitating* factors, they remain quite unknown.

There is some evidence that appendicectomy, possibly through the role of the appendix in the immune and other physiological systems, may increase the risk of development of certain malignant tumours.

References

ADAMS, F. (1939). "The Genuine Works of Hippocrates." Williams and Wilkins, Baltimore.
ANDERSSON, N., GRIFFITHS, H., MURPHY, J., ROLL, J., SERENYI, A., SWANN, I., COCKCROFT, A., MYERS, J. and ST. LEGER, A. (1979). *Br. Med. J.* 2, 697–698.
ASHLEY, D. J. B. (1967). *Gut* 8, 533–538.
BADOE, E. A. (1971). *Ghana Med. J.* 10, 265–269.
BANKS, A. L. and MAGEE, H. E. (1945). *Mon. Bull. Minist. Health. Public Health Lab. Serv.* (*G.B.*) 4, 184–187.
BARKER, D. J. P. and LIGGINS, A. (1981). *Br. Med. J.* 2, 1083–1085.
BELL, R. (1880). *Lancet* 1, 243–244.
BHATTACHARYYA, S. K. and DURRANI, A. M. (1974). *J. Med. Dent. Assoc. Botswana* 4, 5–7.
BLUMBERG, L. (1981). *S. Afr. Med. J.* 60, 648.
BOLAND, F. K. (1942). *Ann. Surg.* 115, 939–944.
BOYCE, F. F. (1951). *Ann. Surg.* 133, 631–641.
BRANICKI, F. J. (1981). *Ann. Coll. Surg.* 63, 348–352.
BRUNTON, T. L. (1896). *In* "Allbutt's System of Medicine" (T. C. Allbutt, ed.), Vol. III, p. 696. Macmillan, New York.
BURKITT, D. P. (1971). *Br. J. Surg.* 58, 695–699.
BURKITT, D. P. (1975). *In* "Refined Carbohydrates and Disease" (D. P. Burkitt and H. C. Trowell, eds), pp. 87–97. Academic Press, New York and London.
CASSIMOS, C., SKLAVUNU-ZURUKZOGLU, S., CATRIU, D. and PANAJIOTIDU, C. (1973). *Cancer* 32, 1374–1379.
CHEADLE, W. B. (1886). *Lancet* 2, 1063–1064.
CHRISTOPHER, L. and CROOKS, J. (1974). *World Health,* April Issue, pp. 16–21.
CLEAVE, T. L. (1974). "The Saccharine Disease." John Wright, Bristol.

COPE, V. Z. (1950). *Br. Med. J.* **1**, 1242.

CREED, F. (1981). *Lancet* **1**, 1381–1385.

CRUICKSHANK, E. W. A. (1946). "Food and Nutrition." Livingstone, Edinburgh.

CUNEO, J. M. (1972). *Lancet* **1**, 846–847.

Current Comment (1939). *JAMA, J. Am. Med. Assoc.* **112**, 2606.

DAWSON, A. A., FORMAN, K. M. and ENTRICAN, J. H. (1979). *Clin. Oncol.* **3**, 221–226.

DE DOMBAL, F. T. and HEDLEY, A. J. (1979). *Br. Med. J.* **1**, 820.

DEN HARTOG, A. P. (1980a). *Voeding* **41**, 292–302.

DEN HARTOG, A. P. (1980b). *Voeding* **41**, 334–342, 348–357.

DONALDSON, L. J. (1981-1982). In "The Medical Annual" (R. B. Scott and J. Fraser, eds), pp. 293–302. John Wright, Bristol.

DRUMMOND, J. C. and WILBRAHAM, A. (1939). "The Englishman's Food." Jonathan Cape, London.

Editorial (1928). *JAMA, J. Am. Med. Assoc.* **90**, 206–207.

Editorial (1949). *U.S. Nav. Med. Bull.,* **49**, 1180–1181.

EKWUEME, O. (1978). *Trop. Geogr. Med.* **30**, 247–251.

ELLIOT-SMITH, A. (1971). In "Just Consequences" (R. Waller, ed.), p. 149. Knight, London.

ERASMUS, J. F. P. (1939). *S. Afr. Med. J.* **13**, 601–606.

FANTUS, B., KOPSTEIN, G. and SCHMIDT, H. R. (1940). *JAMA, J. Am. Med. Assoc.* **114**, 404–408.

FATMA, M. and KIES, C. (1981). *Nutr. Rep. Int.* **23**, 437–446.

FITZ, R. H. (1886). *Am. J. Med. Sci.* **92**, 321–323.

FLEISCH, A. (1946). *Schweiz. Med. Wochenschr.* **76**, 889–893.

FRISKEY, R. W. (1968). *J. Chronic Dis.* **21**, 383–385 (Editorial).

GEAR, J. S. S., WARE, A., FURSDON, P., MANN, J. I., NOLAN, D. J., BRODRIBB, A. J. M. and VESSEY, M. P. (1979). *Lancet* **1**, 511–514.

GELFAND, M. (1956). "The Sick African", 3rd edition, p. 720. Juta, Cape Town.

GOODHART, J. F. (1910). *Lancet* **2**, 468–471.

GRIFFITHS, M. L. (1981). *S. Afr. Med. J.* **59**, 983–986.

HALLILAY, H. (1924). *Ind. Med. Gaz.* **59**, 403.

HOLLINGSWORTH, D. (1975). *Commun. Health* **7**, 21–27.

HOLLINGSWORTH, D. and GREAVES, J. C. (1967). *J. Am. Clin. Nutr.* **20**, 67–72.

HORTON, L. W. L. (1977). *Br. Med. J.* **4**, 1672–1673.

HOWIE, J. G. R. (1966). *Lancet* **2**, 1334–1337.

HYAMS, L. and WYNDER, E. L. (1968). *J. Chronic Dis.* **21**, 391–415.

JANSSENS, P. G. and DE MUYNCK, A. (1966). *Trop. Geogr. Med.* **18**, 81–96.

Leading Article (1906). *Br. Med. J.* **1**, 815–816.

Leading Article (1938). *Lancet* **1**, 559–560.

LICHTNER, S. and PFLANZ, N. (1971). *Med. Care* **9**, 311–315.

LOWENBERG, M. E., TODHUNTER, E. N., WILSON, E. D., SAVAGE, J. R. and LUBAWSCI, J. L. (1979). "Food and People", 3rd edition. Wiley, New York.

LUDBROOK, J. and SPEARS, G. F. S. (1965). *Br. J. Surg.* **52**, 856–858.

McCARRISON, R. (1936). "Nutrition and National Health." Faber and Faber, London.

MacEWEN, W. (1904). *Br. Med. J.* **2**, 873–878.

MANNING, A. P., WYMAN, J. B. and HEATON, K. W. (1974). *Br. Med. J.* **3**, 213–214.

MATAS, R. (1896). *Trans. Am. Surg. Assoc.* **14**, 483.

MAYO, C. H. (1924). *JAMA, J. Am. Med. Assoc.* **83**, 592–593.

MELIER, F. (1827). *J. Gen. Med. Chir. Pharm. Fr. Etrangeres* **100**, 317.

MENDELOFF, A. I. (1975). In "Fiber Deficiency and Colonic Cancer" (R. W. Reilly and J. B. Kirsner, eds), pp. 145–146. Plenum, New York.

MINDELL, W. R., VAYDA, E. and CARDILLO, B. (1982). *Can. Med. Assoc. J.* **127**, 23–27.

MOORE, S. W. and ROBBS, J. V. (1979). *S. Afr. Med. J.* **55**, 700.

NEL, C. J. C. and THERON, E. J. (1979). *S. Afr. Med. J.* **55**, 939–941.

NOER, T. (1975). *Acta Chir. Scand.* **141**, 431–432.

OCHOLA-ABILA, P. (1979). *East Afr. Med. J.* **56**, 368–374.

OGLIVIE, W. H. (1938). *Br. Med. J.* **1**, 1193–1198.

ONUIGBO, W. I. B. (1977). *S. Afr. J. Surg.* **15**, 67–69.

OSMAN, A. A. (1974). *Int. Surg.* **59**, 218–221.

PEZOLD, F. A. (1959). "Atherosclerosis and Nutrition." Steinkopff, Darnstadt.

REDDY, B. S. (1979). *Adv. Nutr. Res.* **2**, 199–218.

RILEY, R. H. (1948). *JAMA, J. Am. Med. Assoc.* **138**, 333–335.

ROSE, G. and BARKER, D. J. P. (1978). *Br. Med. J.* **2**, 1483–1484.

Royal College of Physicians (1980). "Medical Aspects of Dietary Fibre", Report of a Working Party. Pitman, Tunbridge Wells.

SCHAEFER, O. (1979). *Br. Med. J.* **1**, 1215.

SCHETTLER, G. (1979). *Prev. Med.* **8**, 581–590.

SHIJA, J. K. (1975). *Med. J. Zambia* **9**, 48–52.

SHORT, A. R. (1920). *Br. J. Surg.* **8**, 171–178.

SHORT, A. R. (1946). "The Causation of Appendicitis." John Wright, Bristol.

SOUTHGATE, D. A. T., BINGHAM, S. and ROBERTSON, J. (1978). *Nature (London)* **274**, 51–52.

STROM, A. and JENSEN, R. A. (1951). *Lancet* **1**, 126–129.

TAIWO, O., ITAYEMI, S. O. and SERIKI, O. (1977). *Trop. Geogr. Med.* **29**, 35–40.

TAYLOR, I. (1975). *Br. J. Clin. Pract.* **29**, 289–291.

THORNTON, J. R. (1981). *Lancet* **1**, 1081–1082.

TROWELL, H. C. (1960). "Non-Infective Disease in Africa", pp. 220–222. Edward Arnold, London.

ULLRICH, I. H., LAI, H. Y., VONA, L., PERD, R. L. and ALBRINK, M. J. (1981). *Am. J. Clin. Nutr.* **34**, 2054–2060.

VAN OUWERKERK, L. W. (1951). *Arch. Chir. Neerl.* **3**, 164.

VAN ZWALENBURG, C. (1904). *JAMA, J. Am. Med. Assoc.* **42**, 820–827.

VAN ZWALENBURG, C. (1905). *Ann. Surg.* **41**, 437–450.

VIANNA, N. J., DAVIES, J. N. P., HARRIS, S., LAWRENCE, C. E., ARBUCKLE, J., MARANI, W. and WILKINSON, J. (1980). *Lancet* **2**, 338–342.

VOBECKY, J., CARO, J. and DEVROEDE, G. (1983). *Cancer* **51**, 1958–1963.

WALKER, A. R. P. (1947). *S. Afr. Med. J.* **21**, 590–596.

WALKER, A. R. P. and SEGAL, I. (1979). *Isr. J. Med. Sci.* **15**, 309–313.

WALKER, A. R. P., WALKER, B. F., RICHARDSON, B. D. and WOOLFORD, A. (1973). *Postgrad. Med. J.* **49**, 243–249.

WALKER, A. R. P., WALKER, B. F. and SEGAL, I. (1979). *S. Afr. Med. J.* **55**, 495–498.

WALKER, A. R. P., WALKER, B. F., DUVENHAGE, A., JONES, J., NCONGWANE, J. and SEGAL, I. (1981). *Trop. Geogr. Med.* **33**, 383–386.

WALKER, A. R. P., WALKER, B. F., DUVENHAGE, A., JONES, J., NCONGWANE, J. and SEGAL, I. (1982). *Digestion* **23**, 274–278.

WANGENSTEEN, O. H. and BOWERS, W. F. (1937). *Arch. Surg. (Chicago)* **34**, 496.

WATSON, C. (1906). *Br. Med. J.* **1**, 947.

WEST, R. R. and CAREY, M. J. (1978). *Br. Med. J.* **1**, 1662–1664.

WEST, R. R. and ROBERTS, C. J. (1974). *Int. J. Epidemiol.* **3**, 351–357.

WESTLAKE, C. A., ST. LEGER, A. S. and BURR, M. L. (1980). *J. Hum. Nutr.* **34**, 267–272.

WHITE, J. J., SANTILLANA, M. and HALLER, J. A. (1975). *Am. Surg.* **41**, 793–798.

WILKIE, D. P. D. (1914). *Br. Med. J.* **2**, 959–962.

WILSON, J. M. G. (1981). *Lancet* **1**, 895–896.

WRIGHT, R. B. (1963). *Lancet* **2**, 475–479.

YOUNG, M. and RUSSELL, W. T. (1939). *Med. Res. Counc. (G.B.)*, *Spec. Rep. Ser.* **233**, 58–64.

Chapter 11

Crohn's disease and ulcerative colitis

KENNETH HEATON

I. Introduction

Crohn's disease and ulcerative colitis are often discussed together under the title of non-specific inflammatory bowel disease because they have many features in common, including a maximum incidence in young adults and an unknown aetiology. With both diseases there is a weak but definite hereditary tendency. Up to one-third of patients have a relative with the same disease and ulcerative colitis is not uncommon in the relatives of patients with Crohn's disease (Farmer *et al.*, 1980). The two diseases have very similar systemic or non-intestinal complications and very similar treatment. Howev-

205

Dietary Fibre, Fibre-Depleted Foods
and Disease

er, their pathology and clinical features are very different and quite characteristic except for occasional cases of unclassifiable colitis (Kirsner and Shorter, 1982).

II.   Current views on pathogenesis and aetiology

The intensive research of the last 20 years has concentrated on two aspects—
altered immunological mechanisms and infection by microorganisms.

A.   Immunology

A host of papers has appeared on this complex subject and numerous abnormalities of humoral and especially cellular immunity have been described.
However, the conclusions of expert reviewers show that even they are confused and uncertain of the significance of their findings. Undoubtedly, there
must be interactions between ingested and other intraluminal antigens (some
of which share antigenicity with colonic mucosal cells, histocompatibility
antigens and other normal body components) on the one hand, and "the rich
immunologic resources and immunological responsiveness of the gastrointestinal tract" on the other (Kraft, 1979; Kirsner and Shorter, 1982). Nevertheless, most if not all of the immunological phenomena noted in inflammatory bowel disease "are not demonstrable as antecedents of the disease;
they may be epiphenomena, although they may contribute secondarily to the
tissue reaction" (Kirsner and Shorter, 1982).

   Immunological differences may help us to understand why, in a given
community at a given time, one person develops inflammatory bowel disease
and another does not, but they are unlikely to explain dramatic variations in
disease incidence in different places or at different times.

B.   Infection by micro-organisms

New bacterial causes of enteritis and colitis in the form of *Yersinia entero-
colitica* and *Campylobacter fetus* sp. *jejuni,* have been described in recent
years, and there are many bacterial causes of chronic enteritis and colitis in
animals, but there is little support for the idea that typical ulcerative colitis
and Crohn's disease are bacterial infections of man (Mayberry *et al.,* 1980a;
Sachar *et al.,* 1980; Kirsner and Shorter, 1982). One intriguing possibility is
that cell-wall defective variants of *Pseudomonas*-like bacteria which grow
only in hypertonic media may be involved in Crohn's disease. Parent forms
(bacterial revertants) were isolated from the intestine or a mesenteric lymph
node in each of 8 patients with Crohn's disease but not from any of 9 patients
with ulcerative colitis nor from 20 controls (Parent and Mitchell, 1978), and
an antibody against these organisms was discovered in the sera of 22 of 25

patients with Crohn's disease but not in patients with ulcerative colitis nor controls (Shaafi *et al.*, 1981). However, it is possible that cell-wall defective pseudomonads are merely secondary invaders of an already damaged intestinal mucosa.

Viral causes have been sought intensively since the 1970 report of a filter-passing agent transmissible to mice from Crohn's disease tissue (Mitchell and Rees, 1970), but many subsequent attempts to find the virus have been negative (Heatley *et al.*, 1975; Whorwell *et al.*, 1976; Phillpotts *et al.*, 1980; Moráin *et al.*, 1981).

Infective theories for Crohn's disease are rendered less attractive by the lack of any evidence for transmission of the disease to close contacts (D. S. Miller *et al.*, 1976). There have been two reports of Crohn's disease in husband and wife (Whorwell *et al.*, 1981) but this could have a number of interpretations.

Infective theories, like immunological ones, fail to explain the major facts about the epidemiology of these two diseases.

III.   Epidemiology

A.   *Geographical variations*

Thorough surveys of the incidence and prevalence of inflammatory bowel disease have been carried out mainly in Britain and Scandinavia and, to a lesser extent, the United States. Between 1951 and 1977, similar annual incidence rates for Crohn's disease of 1 to 2 per 100,000 population were recorded in England, Scotland, United States, Switzerland, Denmark, Norway and Israel, and slightly higher rates of 4 to 5 per 100,000 in Sweden and South Wales (Langman, 1979; and see Table 11.1). For ulcerative colitis, including proctitis, incidence rates are somewhat higher at 4 to 7 per 100,000 in the same areas (Langman, 1979; Mendeloff, 1980).

Estimates of disease frequency from other areas are little more than guesses (Langman, 1979). However, clinical impressions are strong that Crohn's disease is rare or non-existent in most of India, China, Africa and South America (Kyle, 1972; Trowell, 1975). Series of only three cases have been published from Sudan (Masri and Satir, 1975) and the Transvaal (Davis *et al.*, 1974). The West Indies may have an intermediate place, since 14 cases of Crohn's disease were seen in Trinidad in 10 years (Bartholomew and Butler, 1979). The incidence of ulcerative colitis is probably very low in most tropical areas, and in southern Europe (Trowell, 1975) but it is possible that cases are missed because of the high frequency of infective bowel disease (Langman, 1979). Similarly, Crohn's disease could easily be confused with ileocaecal tuberculosis.

TABLE 11.1. Incidence and prevalence of Crohn's disease per 100,000 population

Location	Years	Incidence	Prevalence	Reference
Oxford, England	1951–1960	0.8	9	Evans and Acheson (1965)
Baltimore, U.S.A.	1960–1963	1.8		Monk et al. (1967)
Aberdeen, Scotland	1955–1968	2.0	32.5	Kyle (1971)
Nottingham, England	1958–1972	2.0	26.5	Miller et al. (1974)
Norway	1964–1969	1.1		Myren et al. (1971)
Basle, Switzerland	1960–1969	1.6		Fahrländer and Baerlocher (1971)
Copenhagen, Denmark	1960–1970	1.3		Höj et al. (1973)
Malmö, Sweden	1958–1973	4.8	75.2	Brahme et al. (1975)
Uppsala and Västmanland, Sweden	1968–1973	5.0	50.0	Bergman and Krause (1975)
Tel-Aviv, Israel	1970–1976	1.3	12.3	Rozen et al. (1979)
Cardiff, Wales	1971–1975	4.8		Mayberry et al. (1979)

B. Ethnic variations

Both Crohn's disease and ulcerative colitis are relatively uncommon in the blacks of the United States. Of 1557 patients treated for inflammatory bowel disease in Chicago, only 58 were black (Rogers et al., 1971). In Baltimore, the annual hospitalisation rate for Crohn's disease per 100,000 population in 1973 was 3.65 for white males and only 0.83 for non-white males. For ulcerative colitis, the figures were 3.92 and 0.84, respectively (Mendeloff, 1980). In New Zealand, ulcerative colitis is much less common in Maoris than in whites (Wigley and MacLaurin, 1962). In South Africa, the whites seem to suffer from Crohn's disease as often as Europeans (Walker and Segal, 1979), but in the blacks it is rare. Baragwanath Hospital serves a huge population of blacks in Central Transvaal as well as Johannesburg but has records of only 18 black patients with Crohn's disease in the 22-year period from 1958 to 1979, despite a high index of suspicion among the gastroenterologists (Segal et al., 1981). Jews have had a greater prevalence of ulcerative colitis and Crohn's disease than non-Jews in Baltimore (Monk et al., 1967) and amongst U.S. veterans (Acheson, 1960). In Israel itself, the incidence of inflammatory bowel disease is not particularly high, but there is an interesting difference between Ashkenazi Jews, who are mostly immigrants from Europe and America and their descendants, and the others. In Ashkenazis the prevalence of Crohn's disease is four times higher (Rozen et al., 1979).

C. Secular trends

It is generally accepted that Crohn's disease is a product of the twentieth century. It was first described in detail in 1913 (Dalziel, 1913) and was not generally recognised until after the classic paper of Crohn et al. (1932). Since the 1950s there has been a remarkable rise in the incidence of Crohn's disease in every country in which it has been looked for. This applies to England

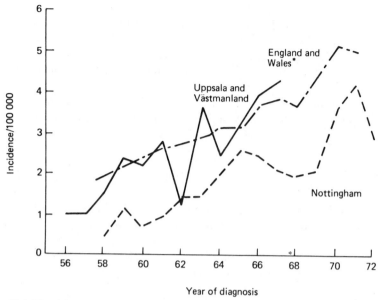

FIG. 11.1 The rising incidence of Crohn's disease in England and in Sweden. (From Bergman and Krause, 1975.)

(Miller *et al.*, 1974), Wales (Mayberry *et al.*, 1979), Scotland (Kyle, 1971; Smith *et al.*, 1975), Sweden (Norlén *et al.*, 1970; Brahme *et al.*, 1975), Denmark (Höj *et al.*, 1973), Switzerland (Fahrländer and Baerlocher, 1971) and the United States (Mendeloff, 1980). The recorded increase has varied between two- and five-fold (Fig. 11.1). It may be due in part to better diagnosis but it is unlikely to be due to reclassification of cases of ulcerative colitis since the incidence of colitis has stayed the same. This inexorable rise may at last have stopped, at least in Wales (Harries *et al.*, 1982), while in Scotland it may even have reversed (Kyle and Stark, 1980). Nevertheless, it remains the best-documented and most provocative fact in the epidemiology of inflammatory bowel disease.

In contrast to Crohn's disease, ulcerative colitis has not been recorded as increasing in incidence since the 1950s (Langman, 1979). It was well described in the nineteenth century (Wilks, 1859) and one can only speculate as to whether it has increased since then.

IV. Dietary hypotheses

A. Food additives

The idea has long been entertained that Crohn's disease represents an immunological reaction to a toxic substance or pathogenic agent in the lumen of the intestine. The marked increase in the use of food additives, natural and synthetic, during the twentieth century has led to suspicions that one or a combination of these could be the causative agent (Carstensen and Poulsen, 1971) but no additive has been shown experimentally to cause Crohn's-like lesions (though certain metals can cause granulomas). Carrageenans, sulphated polysaccharides derived from seaweed and used widely in the food industry as filling agents, can (in their degraded form) produce colonic ulcers in guinea-pigs (Marcus and Watt, 1969), but, unlike ulcerative colitis, the lesions are chiefly in the right colon. In any case, ulcerative colitis occurred before carrageenans were introduced.

B.   Cow's milk

Cow's milk intolerance has been suggested as a factor in ulcerative colitis. Patients with colitis are more likely than controls to have been bottle-fed as babies (Whorwell *et al.*, 1979) but they do not have an increased frequency of positive skin tests to milk protein (Jewell and Truelove, 1972). In babies, cow's milk intolerance can certainly cause a colitis (Jenkins *et al.*, 1982). The hypothesis merits further testing.

C.   Refined foods

The increasing use of refined foods in the twentieth century led some to speculate that Crohn's disease could be related to refined carbohydrates (Heaton, 1973; Painter, 1975; Trowell, 1975) but supporting evidence was not available until case-control studies were published.

D.   Case—control studies in Crohn's disease

In Marburg, Germany, Martini and Brandes (1976) used a postal questionnaire to ascertain the eating and drinking habits of 63 patients with Crohn's disease and of 63 controls matched for age, sex and social class. The patients admitted to eating substantially more cakes, pastries, and other sugar-containing foods as well as more table sugar (Table 11.2). In all other respects their eating habits were unremarkable. Shortly after this report, another German group, using personal interviews and even closer matching of controls, found that Crohn's patients ate twice as much sugar as healthy people (B. Miller *et al.*, 1976). In both these studies, the abnormally high sugar intake was claimed to precede the symptoms of the disease. In the following year, James (1977) reported the curious finding that 34 patients with Crohn's disease ate cornflakes for breakfast significantly more often than 68 matched controls.

   These papers evoked much interest and led to several more studies of the eating habits of patients with Crohn's disease. Five groups looked at breakfast

TABLE 11.2. Refined sugar intake in patients with Crohn's disease and in matched controls: results of eight studies

	Number of patients	Mean sugar intake (g/24 h)		
		Patients		Controls
		Pre-illness	Illness	
Martini and Brandes (1976)	63	177	116	74
B. Miller et al. (1976)	34	150	115	55
Graham et al. (1978)	68	—	10 tsp[b]	7 tsp[b]
Thornton et al. (1979)	30	122[a]	—	65[a]
Kasper and Sommer (1979)	35	156	—	91
Mayberry et al. (1980b)	120	—	10.6 tsp[b]	6.0 tsp[b]
Silkoff et al. (1980)	27	—	35[b]	16[b]
Penny et al. (1983)	70	—	65[b]	29[b]

[a] Median value.
[b] Visible sugar only; tsp, teaspoons.

habits and all five failed to confirm James's findings (Mayberry et al., 1978; Rawcliffe and Truelove, 1978; Archer and Harvey, 1978; Graham et al., 1978; Thornton et al., 1979). The intake of visible or added sugar was assessed by Graham et al. (1978) and twice by Mayberry et al. (1978, 1980b) and it was consistently greater in the Crohn's patients.

Two groups in Bristol and Würzburg have tried to collect more detailed nutritional information, including data on dietary fibre intake, and have tried to overcome an important limitation of Martini and Brandes' (1976) original study: that their patients were diagnosed several years previously and were being asked to recall eating habits of long ago. Thus, Thornton and colleagues (1979) limited their study to newly diagnosed patients, most of whom had had symptoms for only a few months. Thirty such patients and 30 controls who were obtained from a fracture clinic and were matched for marital status as well as age, sex, social class, height and weight, were questioned by a single dietitian about their habitual diets. There was no difference in the intake of protein, fat or starch. However, the median intake of refined sugar was nearly twice as high in the Crohn's patients as in the controls (122 versus 65 g/day, $p < 0.002$). An equally striking finding was the low intake of raw fruit and vegetables in the Crohn's patients, many of whom hardly ate any (Fig. 11.2). Similar findings were reported by Kasper and Sommer (1979) in 35 patients with disease of fairly recent onset and 70 controls. The patients ate 71% more sugar and less fruit, but they also ate slightly more starch and their total energy intake was higher.

Thus, all studies agree that patients with Crohn's disease have been habitually heavy consumers of refined sugar and, when it has been recorded, their intake of fresh fruit and vegetables has been poor. There is no consistent

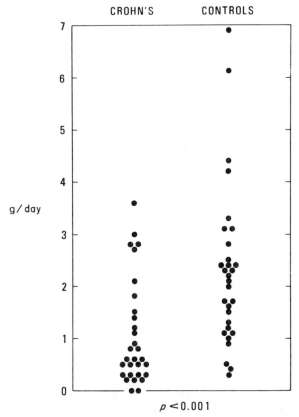

FIG. 11.2 Habitual intake of dietary fibre from raw fruit and vegetables in 30 patients with Crohn's disease before their illness and in 30 healthy controls. (From Thornton *et al.*, 1979.)

difference in total dietary fibre intakes (Thornton *et al.*, 1979; Kasper and Sommer, 1979).

E.　Interpretation of case–control studies

Some authors have considered that this dietary pattern could have aetiological significance (Martini and Brandes, 1976; Thornton *et al.*, 1979) while others have been uncertain. The Bristol group's attitude was coloured by the fact that, on empirical grounds, Heaton had advised an unrefined, fibre-rich diet to his patients with Crohn's disease for 7 years. Thirty-two patients had been advised in this way and, over a mean follow-up period of $4\frac{1}{2}$ years, they had between them required only one intestinal resection and 111 days in the hospital, compared with five resections and 533 days in the hospital in a control group of Crohn's patients who had been given no dietary advice

(Heaton *et al.*, 1979). A randomised, prospective trial is essential to confirm or disprove these findings and this is in progress at centres throughout Britain. Meanwhile, a small prospective trial in Germany has suggested that patients with active disease do indeed fare better on an unrefined diet than on a sugar-rich diet (Brandes and Lorenz-Meyer, 1981).

Recall of eating habits is imperfect and the technique of estimating dietary intake by interview is inaccurate. However, inaccurate methods would not be expected to result in a systematic difference between patients and controls. On the contrary, they would tend to obscure a trend. In any case, better methods of assessing past eating habits are not available.

Some gastroenterologists have suspected that the abnormal eating habits of Crohn's patients are the result of the disease—the patient eating more sugar to combat weight loss and less raw fruit to try and counteract loose stools. However, the data do not support this idea. Patients either deny that their eating habits have changed at all (Thornton *et al.*, 1979) or state that their sugar intake has decreased since they have had symptoms (Martini and Brandes, 1976; B. Miller *et al.*, 1976). Furthermore, when patients with ulcerative colitis, who also suffer diarrhoea and weight loss, have been questioned they have been found to have no consistent difference from controls in their dietary intake (Martini *et al.*, 1980; Thornton *et al.*, 1980).

Another possible interpretation of the high sugar intake is that a liking for sweetness is genetically linked with the predisposition to Crohn's disease. This is rendered less likely by the observation that the taste threshold for sweetness is normal in patients with Crohn's disease (Kasper and Sommer, 1980).

F. Possible mechanisms

The weakness of any dietary hypothesis for the aetiology of Crohn's disease lies in our ignorance of the pathogenesis of the disease and hence the impossibility of fitting a diet into an accepted scheme. However, a high sugar intake can be fitted into one possible scheme. As noted on p. 206, there is evidence to implicate cell-wall defective *Pseudomonas*-like bacteria whose growth requires a hypertonic medium. Sugar more than any other part of the diet is responsible for rendering the gastric contents hypertonic. Hence, sugar could promote the survival of these bacteria.

A diet rich in refined sugar and poor in fresh fruit and vegetables is almost certain to contain sub-optimal amounts of some vitamins and minerals (Heaton *et al.*, 1983). According to Horrobin *et al.* (1979), inadequate supplies of vitamin C, pyridoxine or zinc could lead to impaired function of T lymphocytes. There is considerable evidence that the function of T lymphocytes is abnormal in Crohn's disease (Kraft, 1979).

V. Future research

The absence of an adequate animal model for Crohn's disease makes it difficult to perform controlled dietary experiments. Prospective epidemiological studies are difficult because of the relative rarity of the disease. However, it might be worth looking for a reduced incidence of the disease in vegetarians and also in people, like diabetics, who have avoided refined sugar since childhood.

VI. Summary

Crohn's disease and ulcerative colitis are probably rare in developing countries. The incidence of Crohn's disease has increased markedly in Europe and America in the last 30 years. Immunological reactions are involved in both diseases but what provokes them is unknown. Case–control studies consistently show that Crohn's disease is preceded by a heavy consumption of refined sugar and possibly by a low intake of fruit and vegetables.

References

ACHESON, E. D. (1960). *Gut* 1, 291–293.
ARCHER, L. N. J. and HARVEY, R. F. (1978). *Br. Med. J.* 2, 540.
BARTHOLOMEW, C. and BUTLER, A. (1979). *Br. Med. J.* 2, 824–825.
BERGMAN, L. and KRAUSE, U. (1975). *Scand. J. Gastroenterol.* 10, 725–729.
BRAHME, F., LINDSTRÖM, C. and WENCKERT, A. (1975). *Gastroenterology* 69, 342–351.
BRANDES, J. W. and LORENZ-MEYER, H. (1981). *Z. Gastroenterol.* 19, 1–12.
CARSTENSEN, J. and POULSEN, E. (1971). *In* "Regional Enteritis (Crohn's Disease)" (A. Engel and T. Larsson, eds), pp. 283–299. Nordiska Bokhandelns Förlag, Stockholm.
CROHN, B. B., GINSBURG, L. and OPPENHEIMER, G. D. (1932). *JAMA, J. Am. Med. Assoc.* 99, 1323–1329.
DALZIEL, T. K. (1913). *Br. Med. J.* 2, 1068–1070.
DAVIS, R., SCHMAMAN, A. and COSMAN, B. (1974). *S. Afr. Med. J.* 48, 580–586.
EVANS, J. G. and ACHESON, E. D. (1965). *Gut* 6, 311–324.
FAHRLÄNDER, H. and BAERLOCHER, C. (1971). *Scand. J. Gastroenterol.* 6, 657–662.
FARMER, R. G., MICHENER, W. M. and MORTIMER, E. A. (1980). *Clin. Gastroenterol.* 9, 271–277.
GRAHAM, W. B., TORRANCE, B. and TAYLOR, T. V. (1978). *Br. Med. J.* 2, 768.
HARRIES, A. D., BAIRD, A., RHODES, J. and MAYBERRY, J. F. (1982). *Br. Med. J.* 284, 235.
HEATLEY, R. V., BOLTON, P. M., OWEN, E., JONES WILLIAMS, W. and HUGHES, L. E. (1975). *Gut* 16, 528–532.
HEATON, K. W. (1973). *Nutrition (London)* 27, 170–183.
HEATON, K. W., THORNTON, J. R. and EMMETT, P. M. (1979). *Br. Med. J.* 2, 764–766.
HEATON, K. W., EMMETT, P. M., HENRY, C. L., THORNTON, J. R., MANHIRE, A. and HARTOG, M. (1983). *Hum. Nutr. Clin. Nutr.* 37C, 31–35.
HÖJ, L., BRIX JENSEN, P., BONNEVIE, O. and RIIS, P. (1973). *Scand. J. Gastroenterol.* 8, 381–384.
HORROBIN, D. F., MANKU, M. S., OKA, M., MORGAN, R. O., CUNNANE, S. C., ALLY, A. I., GHAYUR, T., SCHWEITZER, M. and KARMALI, R. A. (1979). *Med. Hypotheses* 5, 969–985.

JAMES, A. H. (1977). *Br. Med. J.* **1**, 943–945.

JENKINS, H. R., MILLA, P. J., PINCOTT, J. R., SOOTHILL, J. F. and HARRIES, J. T. (1982). *Gut* **23**, A924.

JEWELL, D. P. and TRUELOVE, S. C. (1972). *Gut* **13**, 903–906.

KASPER, H. and SOMMER, H. (1979). *Am. J. Clin. Nutr.* **32**, 1898–1901.

KASPER, H. and SOMMER, H. (1980). *J. Hum. Nutr.* **34**, 455–456.

KIRSNER, J. B. and SHORTER, R. G. (1982). *N. Engl. J. Med.* **306**, 775–785, 837–848.

KRAFT, S. C. (1979). *In* "Immunology of the Gastrointestinal Tract" (P. Asquith, ed), pp. 95–128. Churchill-Livingstone, Edinburgh and London.

KYLE, J. (1971). *Gastroenterology* **61**, 826–833.

KYLE, J. (1972). "Crohn's Disease." Heinemann, London.

KYLE, J. and STARK, G. (1980). *Gut* **21**, 340–343.

LANGMAN, M. J. S. (1979). "The Epidemiology of Chronic Digestive Disease", pp. 80–102. Edward Arnold, London.

MARCUS, R. and WATT, J. (1969). *Lancet* **2**, 489–490.

MARTINI, G. A. and BRANDES, J. W. (1976). *Klin. Wochenschr.* **54**, 367–371.

MARTINI, G. A., STENNER, A. and BRANDES, W. J. (1980). *Br. Med. J.* **1**, 1321.

MASRI, S. H. E. and SATIR, A. A. (1975). *East Afr. Med. J.* **52**, 284–293.

MAYBERRY, J. F., RHODES, J. and NEWCOMBE, R. G. (1978). *Br. Med. J.* **2**, 1401.

MAYBERRY, J. F., RHODES, J. and HUGHES, L. E. (1979). *Gut* **20**, 602–608.

MAYBERRY, J. F., RHODES, J. and HEATLEY, R. V. (1980a). *Gastroenterology* **78**, 1080–1084.

MAYBERRY, J. F., RHODES, J. and NEWCOMBE, R. G. (1980b). *Digestion* **20**, 323–326.

MENDELOFF, A. I. (1980). *Clin. Gastroenterol.* **9**, 259–270.

MILLER, B., FERVERS, F., ROHBECK, R. and STROHMEYER, G. (1976). *Verh. Dtsch. Ges. Inn. Med.* **82**, 922–924.

MILLER, D. S., KEIGHLEY, A. C. and LANGMAN, M. J. S. (1974). *Lancet* **2**, 691–693.

MILLER, D. S., KEIGHLEY, A., SMITH, P. G., HUGHES, A. O. and LANGMAN, M. J. S. (1976). *Gastroenterology* **71**, 385–387.

MITCHELL, D. N. and REES, R. J. W. (1970). *Lancet* **2**, 168–171.

MONK, M., MENDELOFF, A. I., SIEGEL, C. I. and LILIENFELD, A. (1967). *Gastroenterology* **53**, 198–210.

MORÁIN, C. Ó., PRESTAGE, H., HARRISON, P., LEVI, A. J. and TYRRELL, D. A. J. (1981). *Gut* **22**, 823–826.

MYREN, J., GJONE, E., HERTZBERG, J. N., RYGVOLD, O., SEMB, L. S. and FRETHEIM, B. (1971). *Scand. J. Gastroenterol.* **6**, 511–514.

NORLÉN, B. J., KRAUSE, U. and BERGMAN, L. (1970). *Scand. J. Gastroenterol.* **5**, 385–390.

PAINTER, N. S. (1975). "Diverticular Disease of the Colon", pp. 285–286. Heinemann, London.

PARENT, K. and MITCHELL, P. (1978). *Gastroenterology* **75**, 368–372.

PENNY, W. J., MAYBERRY, J. F., AGGETT, P. J., GILBERT, J. O., NEWCOMBE, R. G. and RHODES, J. (1983). *Gut* **24**, 288–292.

PHILLPOTTS, R. J., HERMON-TAYLOR, J., TEICH, N. M. and BROOKE, B. N. (1980). *Gut* **21**, 202–207.

RAWCLIFFE, P. M. and TRUELOVE, S. C. (1978). *Br. Med. J.* **2**, 539–540.

ROGERS, B. H. G., CLARK, L. M. and KIRSNER, J. B. (1971). *J. Chronic Dis.* **24**, 743–773.

ROZEN, P., ZONIS, J., YEKUTIEL, P. and GILAT, T. (1979). *Gastroenterology* **76**, 25–30.

SACHAR, D. B., AUSLANDER, M. O. and WALFISH, J. S. (1980). *Clin. Gastroenterol.* **9**, 231–257.

SEGAL, I., OU TIM, L., HAMILTON, D. G. and MANNELL, A. (1981). *In* "Crohn's Workshop. A Global Assessment of Crohn's Disease" (E. C. G. Lee, ed), pp. 107–115. H.M. & M. Publishers, London.

SHAAFI, A., SOPHER, S., LEV, M. and DAS, K. M. (1981). *Lancet* **2**, 332–334.

SILKOFF, K., HALLAK, A., YEGENA, L., ROZEN, P., MAYBERRY, J. F., RHODES, J. and NEWCOMBE, R. G. (1980). *Postgrad. Med. J.* **56,** 842–846.

SMITH, I. S., YOUNG, S., GILLESPIE, G., O'CONNOR, J. and BELL, J. R. (1975). *Gut* **16,** 62–67.

THORNTON, J. R., EMMETT, P. M. and HEATON, K. W. (1979). *Br. Med. J.* **2,** 762–764.

THORNTON, J. R., EMMETT, P. M. and HEATON, K. W. (1980). *Br. Med. J.* **280,** 293–294.

TROWELL, H. (1975). *In* "Refined Carbohydrate Foods and Disease: Some Implications of Dietary Fibre". (D. P. Burkitt and H. C. Trowell eds), pp. 138–139. Academic Press, London.

WALKER, A. R. P. and SEGAL, I. (1979). *Isr. J. Med. Sci.* **15,** 309–313.

WHORWELL, P. J., BALDWIN, R. C. and WRIGHT, R. (1976). *Gut* **17,** 696–699.

WHORWELL, P. J., HOLDSTOCK, G., WHORWELL, G. M. and WRIGHT, R. (1979). *Br. Med. J.* **1,** 382.

WHORWELL, P. J., HODGES, J. R., BAMFORTH, J. and WRIGHT, R. (1981). *Lancet* **1,** 334.

WIGLEY, R. D. and MACLAURIN, B. P. (1962). *Br. Med. J.* **2,** 228–231.

WILKS, S. (1859). "Lectures on Pathological Anatomy." Longman, Brown, Green, Longmans & Roberts, London.

Chapter 12

Functional gastrointestinal disorders: irritable bowel and other syndromes

RICHARD F. HARVEY

I. Syndromes of functional gastrointestinal disorder

Before considering the relevance of dietary factors to the irritable bowel syndrome, it is worth considering exactly what is meant by this term. As noted by many gastroenterologists, a large proportion of patients attending their clinics have no detectable organic cause for their complaints. Among these it is easy to recognise, with experience, a number of symptom patterns which are individually distinct and which have different natural histories and

217

TABLE 12.1. Patients referred
to a gastroenterology clinic in Bristol[a]

Definite organic diagnosis	980
Definite non-organic diagnosis	888
Undiagnosed gastroenterological disease	75
Non-gastroenterological	57
	2000

[a] After Harvey et al., 1983.

responses to therapy, despite the absence of organic disease. Tables 12.1 and 12.2 show the diagnoses of patients newly referred by general practitioners to a gastroenterology clinic in Bristol over approximately a 5-year period (Harvey et al., 1983). About 45% had disturbances of gastrointestinal function* which were not due to organic disease states (Table 12.2). It is extraordinary that so little is understood of the mechanism of production of symptoms in these patients, especially as functional conditions are so common. Because these conditions seem to differ in a number of important respects, and because the possible role of diet in their aetiology and/or treatment varies from one to another, the different clinical types will be described briefly.

A.   "Classical" irritable bowel syndrome

In this type, abdominal pain, usually but not exclusively in the lower abdomen, appears to originate in powerful contractions of colonic smooth muscle. The pain is usually dull and prolonged, with more severe bouts associated with diarrhoea which then relieves the pain. Over a period of time, often a few days, the motions become firmer and less frequent. Abdominal distension, gurgling and rumbling, with the appearance of mucus in the stools, are common at this time. The pain continues or worsens with a further bout of loose frequent motions, and the cycle starts again. Superimposed on this pattern, various external factors may aggravate the pain, notably emotional upsets, certain foods and premenstrual tension. On examination, useful indications that the pain is colonic in origin are tenderness over the descending and sigmoid colon and reproduction of typical pain by puffing air into the colon at sigmoidoscopy. Spastic colon is a term used frequently for this syndrome.

B.   Painless diarrhoea

The only symptom is the passage of frequent loose stools with urgency, often shortly after waking in the morning, and sometimes after meals. Anxiety is frequently an aggravating factor. Because the story is less distinctive than

---

* Throughout this chapter, the term "functional disorder" is used to mean a disorder of function rather than structure, as opposed to a disorder that is psychological in origin.

TABLE 12.2. Non-organic diagnoses made in 2000 outpatients[a]

A	"Classical" irritable bowel syndrome	449
B	Painless diarrhoea	107
C	"Endoscopy-negative dyspepsia"	77
D	Predominant depression with abdominal pain	80
E	Painless constipation	39
F	Habit disorders (aerophagy, rumination, etc.)	34
G	Predominant anxiety with gut symptoms	24
H	"Mad and incurable" pains (5 Munchausen)	15
I	Eating problems (anorexia, food intolerance, carotenaemia)	10
J	Miscellaneous[b]	73

[a] After Harvey et al., 1983.

[b] Acid in the head, vomiting due to pregnancy, nausea, burbulence, wind, halitosis, lonely, unsure why referred, feeling fine.

that of "classical" irritable bowel syndrome and there are no characteristic clinical findings, care should be taken to exclude organic disease—thyrotoxicosis, lactose intolerance and giardiasis in particular.

C. Endoscopy-negative dyspepsia, X-ray-negative dyspepsia

The chief symptom is upper abdominal pain, usually epigastric but sometimes radiating retrosternally, to the right or left hypochondrium or to the back. Belching, fullness, nausea, retching and worsening of symptoms soon after food, alcohol or stress are common. Relief of symptoms with antacids may suggest acid-peptic disease (peptic ulcer or oesophagitis) but upper gastrointestinal tract endoscopy and radiology are normal. The pain is unrelated to bowel action, and there are usually no colonic symptoms.

D. Depression with abdominal pain

In these patients, abdominal pain is associated with symptoms of depression, e.g. weepiness, early waking, feeling "drained", constant nausea. The pain is unlike that of spastic colon or functional dyspepsia in that it tends to be constant and unaffected by eating, distension, bowel action or anything else.

E. Constipation

This is the infrequent, difficult passage of firm motions without abdominal pain, episodes of diarrhoea or evidence of organic disease.

F. Habit disorders

Usually longstanding and somewhat intractable, the most common are air swallowing, rumination (voluntary regurgitation of swallowed food) and functional vomiting.

G. Anxiety with gut symptoms

An anxiety state is usually recognised as such by the patients, and is associated with "butterflies in the stomach", sensations of a lump in the throat (globus), panic and sometimes other somatic manifestations of anxiety such as trembling, overbreathing or tachycardia.

H. "Mad and incurable"

These patients are bizarre people with bizarre complaints, a heterogenous and uncommon type of problem, including patients who are malingerers, some with Munchausen syndrome and those with strange delusions (e.g. "acid in the testicles").

I. Eating problems

On the borderline between functional and organic, this group of patients included several with abdominal symptoms due to excessive coffee or alcohol, or symptoms resulting from strange diets (e.g. carotenaemia), but without organic disease.

J. Miscellaneous

These are patients with usually minor problems, but include depressed patients complaining of unpleasant tastes or smells, halitosis, constant nausea, wind or similar symptoms, but without any disturbance of bowel habit or any abdominal pain.

These brief descriptions are only intended to demonstrate the constitution of the groups of patients with symptoms not due to organic disease which were encountered in this series of 2000 new outpatients. Clinicians will recognise the descriptions, but will also know that in many patients there is overlap in symptoms between the groups. As can be seen from Table 12.2 and the foregoing definitions, groups D and F–K consist largely of patients whose main problem is psychological. Many will respond to appropriate treatment with psychotherapy or anxiolytic or antidepressant drugs, but it seems improbable that their diet is the primary cause of their symptoms, or that dietary manipulation will help them except in a few rare instances, such as coffee intolerance. This leaves groups A, B, C and E, spastic colon, painless diarrhoea, "endoscopy-negative dyspepsia" and painless constipation, a total of 77.1% of those patients without organic disease, or 34.2% of all newly referred outpatients. The first three of these groups are classified together as "irritable bowel syndrome" by some workers, but although there may be overlap of symptoms in some patients, they are considered separately in this chapter.

II. Epidemiology

Although these four disorders of gut function are common in outpatient clinics, little is known of their prevalence in the general population. Thompson and Heaton (1980), in a retrospective survey of several apparently healthy groups of subjects in the United Kingdom, found that 30% of 300 people had abdominal symptoms corresponding to one of these four clinical types, but three-quarters of them had not complained of them to their general practitioners. Very similar findings in a healthy population in Chapel Hill, North Carolina, were recently reported by Drossman and his colleagues (1982). Banks *et al.* (1975) and Morrell (1979) showed in a prospective study of 198 young women that abdominal pain was experienced on 87 occasions over a 1-year period but that this resulted in only 28 consultations. Although other similarly detailed studies are not yet available, abdominal pain without detectable disease is common in many parts of the world, and in doctors from those parts (Fowkes and Ferguson, 1981), and presumably many of the sufferers have a syndrome similar either to the spastic colon or endoscopy-negative dyspepsia as found in the United Kingdom. Thus, in West Africa, Archampong *et al.* (1976) describe the common occurrence of "dyspepsia" without organic disease—"vague abdominal discomfort with heartburn, eructation, flatulence and sometimes diarrhoea". In subjects living in developing countries and on unrefined diets, it is easier to get an idea of the prevalence of diarrhoea or constipation than of abdominal pains. As one might expect, those populations subsisting on unrefined diets have a high incidence of diarrhoea and a low incidence of constipation, however either is defined. In a large prospective survey in South Africa, Walker *et al.* (1982) showed that about 30% of black Africans living in villages passed three or more stools a day, and none fewer than five a week. In contrast, fewer than 1% of white people living in Cape Town passed three or more stools a day, but 11% fewer than five a week and 4% fewer than two a week. The proportion of either group who were unhappy about their bowel habit was not noted, but it seems clear that in the United Kingdom, and possibly also in the United States (Thompson, 1981; Whitehead *et al.*, 1981), those who present themselves for medical help represent only the tip of the iceberg.

III. Pathogenesis of pain

In discussing the pathogenesis of abdominal pain arising from the gastrointestinal tract but in the absence of organic disease, we find a paucity of information which is quite extraordinary considering the size of the problem. Extraordinary, that is, until one reflects that this is also true of most other common pains, whether it is headache, angina pectoris or the pain of a duodenal ulcer. In the gastrointestinal tract, functional pain is most probably

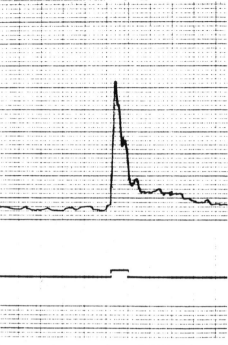

Fig. 12.1. Intracolonic pressure (upper trace) recorded by miniature balloon in the sigmoid colon of a patient experiencing bouts of pain due to colonic spasm. Lower trace shows when patient could feel the pain. The onset of pain is before the greatest rise in intracolonic pressure, which suggests that the muscle contraction itself is responsible (see Harvey and Read, 1973).

produced by forceful contraction of smooth muscle in the wall of the intestine. Figure 12.1 shows a recording of pressure detected by a balloon placed in the sigmoid colon of a patient who was able to detect individual painful contractions of the colon. The pain was felt by the patient before any appreciable rise in intraluminal pressure, and thus must have resulted from the muscular contraction itself rather than from secondary effects such as proximal distension. This same phenomenon can often be observed during labour, when the mother feels the onset of pain before other observers can palpate uterine contraction.

Various studies have shown that in patients with abdominal pain without organic disease, there is abnormally marked or frequent contraction of smooth muscle in the colon (Almy et al., 1949; Chaudhary and Truelove, 1961; Connell et al., 1965; Wangel and Deller, 1965; Harvey and Read, 1973; Sullivan et al., 1978; Burns, 1980). However, as Alvarez (1944) noted when supporting the use of the term "irritable bowel syndrome", "I prefer to say bowel rather than colon because there are reasons for believing that in some of these cases the small bowel and even the stomach share in the irritability". This has been confirmed for the small intestine (Connell *et al.,* 1965; Thompson *et al.,* 1979) and, in addition, abnormalities in the motor function of the oesophagus have also recently been described (Whorwell *et al.,* 1981).

Thus it seems reasonable to suppose that pains referred to different parts of the abdomen, chest or back in patients with irritable bowel syndrome may originate not only in the colon (Ritchie, 1973; Swarbrick *et al.,* 1980) but also in the oesophagus, stomach, small intestine and possibly even the biliary tract.

IV.   Pathogenesis of painless diarrhoea

Contrary to what might be expected, patients with painless diarrhoea show on the average reduced colonic motor activity (Connell, 1962). This decrease in segmenting or static muscular contractions has been described only for the sigmoid colon, which is the easiest part to study, and it is only an average decrease, but it has been suggested as leading to lack of resistance to forward flow (Connell, 1962). In some patients with diarrhoea, there are brief periods of increased motor activity, especially after meals (Waller and Misiewicz, 1972), and it is common experience that diarrhoea with urgency is felt as being associated with a positive effort by the colon to empty itself. It seems probable, therefore, that there are two different mechanisms for diarrhoea due to motor abnormalities (as opposed to secretory diarrhoea). In "low-resistance" diarrhoea, onward flow of ileal effluent is rapid and the few segmenting contractions of the colon do little to slow its progress. In "high-pressure" diarrhoea, sudden rapid propulsion and expulsion of colonic contents is achieved by brief bursts of motor activity, either the brief postprandial events described by Waller and Misiewicz (1972) or the even more impressive though less well documented "mass movements" (Holdstock *et al.,* 1970). One must suppose that functional diarrhoea associated with pain (and therefore by definition falling into the "spastic colon" group) is associated with active colonic contraction. However, despite much work, the pathogenesis of painless diarrhoea remains quite unknown.

Painless diarrhoea without organic disease is quite common in children (Walker-Smith, 1980), and it seems clear that in many adults the tendency to produce loose, frequent motions is lifelong and dates from childhood. There may be a family history of similar complaints. Thus, painless diarrhoea may simply represent one end of a spectrum of bowel behaviour, at the other end of which is a lifelong tendency to constipation and/or abdominal pain, both of which are common in children and often persist into adult life (Apley and Naish, 1958; Apley and Hale, 1973; Christensen and Mortensen, 1975).

V.   Endoscopy-negative dyspepsia

In this condition symptoms suggestive of upper gastrointestinal tract disease predominate. Other terms are ulcer-type dyspepsia, non-ulcer dyspepsia, X-ray-negative dyspepsia, functional dyspepsia and so on. On the continent of Europe, "biliary dyskinesia" is a much more commonly made diagnosis than in the United Kingdom or United States, where such patients would probably be included in this group. The group probably contains at least two types of patient. In most the symptoms clearly arise from the oesophagus, stomach or small bowel, presumably as a result of some disorder of motor function there (Connell et al., 1965; Thompson et al., 1979; Whorwell et al., 1981). However, there are certainly some whose symptoms originate in the colon, but whose pain is felt in the upper abdomen or even the chest (Ritchie, 1973; Swarbrick et al., 1980). The latter patients often respond to the treatment used for ordinary "classical" irritable bowel syndrome (spastic colon), whereas the former usually do not. Reproduction of their typical pain by sigmoidoscopic air insufflation is a very useful diagnostic clue.

VI.   Diet as an aetiological factor in functional gut disorders

It seems improbable that any diet could cause or cure those disorders of gut function which are primarily the result of psychosis, anxiety or depression. However, these (Table 12.2) are relatively infrequent and account for only about one in ten of all patients with functional gut disorders. In an even smaller group, the symptoms can be attributed solely to single obvious dietary items such as alcohol or coffee. Many patients with irritable bowel syndrome, painless diarrhoea or endoscopy-negative dyspepsia find that individual food items, often a wide variety of foods, exacerbate their symptoms. These foods, however, seem to act only as trigger factors rather than as primary causes, as during remissions they have no effect.

A.   Food intolerance

It is surprising that there is still relatively little known about the frequency of food intolerance in functional gut disorders. Lactose intolerance may present with symptoms suggestive of irritable bowel syndrome in both adults (Pena and Truelove, 1972; Ahmed, 1975; Fowkes and Ferguson, 1981) and children (Barr et al., 1979), yet seems relatively uncommon. More children benefit from a lactose-free diet than have objective evidence of lactose intolerance (Dearlove et al., 1983). True food allergy seems to be relatively uncommon if tested for with double-blind food provocation tests. Thus, Bentley et al. (1983) confirmed patients' belief that their symptoms were due to food allergy in only 3 of 27 such cases. These findings disagree with those of Jones *et al.* (1982), who reported a marked beneficial effect of exclusion diets in patients with irritable bowel syndrome, whose symptoms returned when one or more of a wide variety of foods was reintroduced into their diet. Their results were striking and, if confirmed, would completely change current management of the irritable bowel. However, until such confirmation becomes available, it seems more likely that intolerance of specific food items is the result rather than the cause of irritable bowel syndrome in most patients.

B.   Fibre-depleted foods

It is at present impossible to say whether functional gut disorders are more common in those who eat refined fibre-depleted diets, because appropriate population data are not available. It is clearly unsatisfactory to compare symptoms in (say) rural black Africans with white populations, as so many variables other than diet are involved. It would be simple, if tedious, to compare prospectively, by using a health diary (Banks *et al.*, 1975), the bowel symptoms of a supposedly normal Western population living on an unrefined diet with those of a matched group living in the same area on a refined fibre-depleted diet. Until such comparisons become available, the only non-circumstantial evidence that links functional gut disorders with refined diets comes from experience in treating these disorders by dietary means.

VII.   Diet and the treatment of functional gut disorders

It is now very common for patients with either spastic colon syndrome or constipation to be treated with a high-fibre diet or wheat bran, or both. In the United Kingdom, 93 of 100 gastroenterologists reported that they used this treatment for spastic colon syndrome and 84 of 100 used it for painless diarrhoea (Manning and Heaton, 1976). The reason is that the treatment works very effectively in a large proportion of patients. Controlled trials of dietary treatments are for obvious reasons difficult to undertake, but some have been completed. Manning *et al.* (1977) showed that dietary supplementation by bran and/or the substitution of wholemeal bread for white bread resulted in a significant improvement in symptoms of patients with the irritable bowel syndrome, with a decrease in intracolonic pressure. In contrast, Søltoft *et al.* (1976) showed that 30 g of wheat bran baked into biscuits had no detectable effect on transit time, bowel function or symptoms. The need for proper controls in such studies is illustrated by the fact that about 60% of their patients improved when treated with placebo biscuits. Why this dosage of bran should have had no effect is puzzling, but presumably an effect on the stools or transit time is necessary for symptomatic relief to be achieved, and it has been suggested that the type of bran used was inappropriate for this (Weinreich, 1976). Other bulking agents that increase stool water content may also be effective, for example, ispaghula (Ritchie and Truelove, 1979).

Only two other studies of the effects of bran in irritable bowel syndrome have been published to date. Cann *et al.* (1983) in a non-blind, open, 4-week trial of a variable dose of bran (depending on the individual symptomatic response of the patient) found an improvement in about half the patients. However, the improvement was not significantly greater than that seen subsequently with a placebo tablet. As might be expected, those who responded to treatment with bran tended to be those who initially had been constipated. In a crossover study, a daily dose of 30 g coarse wheat bran for 6 weeks was compared with breadcrumbs for a similar period in 18 patients by Arffmann *et al.* (1983). Colonic transit time decreased and faecal weight increased by a mean of 50%, yet there was no reported difference in abdominal pain, distension or "rumbling".

Since the symptoms of uncomplicated diverticular disease are believed to be similar, if not identical, to those of classical irritable bowel syndrome, it is worth considering the results of the three placebo-controlled studies that have been made on the effect of bran on the symptoms of diverticular disease. Brodribb (1977), in a 3-month trial of bran biscuits, found them to be significantly better than placebo. In contrast, Ornstein *et al.* (1981), using similar bran biscuits, found little or no beneficial effect, except on constipation. Weinreich (1982) reported that patients taking coarse bran 24 g/day were relieved of symptoms more often than those on placebo after 3, 6 and 12 months.

The reported trials of bran in the irritable bowel syndrome and diverticular disease differ in many respects, notably in the selection of patients, the form of bran given, its dose, the fibre content of the diet itself and the factors analysed. In addition, there seems to be a placebo effect that can be very marked for almost any form of treatment in irritable bowel syndrome. These problems, and a detailed analysis of all these studies, have been critically reviewed by Heaton (1984).

It seems clear that neither bran nor a high-fibre diet is a panacea for patients with the irritable bowel syndrome who present to the hospital. Nevertheless, there are certainly some who benefit. Further controlled dietary studies are desirable, particularly if they are combined with other measurements of gut function besides faecal weight and colonic transit time, and with selection of patients into more homogeneous, carefully defined groups. At present, the patients most likely to respond to an increased fibre intake seem to be those who have predominantly colonic symptoms, especially with abdominal pain and constipation, who have a short history and who are not unduly anxious or depressed.

References

AHMED, H. F. (1975). *Lancet.* **2**, 319–320.

ALMY, T. P., HINKLE, L. E., JR., BERLE, B. and KERN, F. J. (1949). *Gastroenterology* **12**, 437–450.

ALVAREZ, W. C. (1944). "Nervousness, Indigestion and Pain." Heinemann, London.

APLEY, J. and HALE, B. (1973). *Br. Med. J.* **3**, 7–9.

APLEY, J. and NAISH, J. M. (1958). *Arch. Dis. Child.* **33**, 165–167.

ARCHAMPONG, E. Q., FALAIYE, J. M., KAJUBI, S. J. and PARRY, E. H. O. (1976). *In* "Principles of Medicine in Africa" (E. H. O. Parry, ed.), pp. 407–429. Oxford University Press, Oxford: London and New York.

ARFFMANN, S., ANDERSON, J. R., HEGNHØJ, J., SCHAFFALITZKY DE MUCKADELL, O. B., MORGENSEN, N. B. and KRAG, E. (1983). *Scand. J. Gastroenterol.* **18**, Suppl. 86, 3.

BANKS, M., BERESFORD, S., MORRELL, D., WALLER, J. and WATKINS, C. (1975). *Int. J. Epidemiol.* **4**, 189–195.

BARR, R. G., LEVINE, M. D. and WATKINS, J. B. (1979). *N. Engl. J. Med.* **300**, 1449–1452.

BENTLEY, S. J., PEARSON, D. J. and RIX, K. J. B. (1983). *Lancet* **2**, 295–297.

BRODRIBB, A. J. M. (1977). *Lancet* **1**, 664–666.

BURNS, T. W. (1980). *Arch. Intern. Med.* **140**, 247–251.

CANN, P. A., READ, N. W. and HOLDSWORTH, C. D. (1983). *Gut* **24**, 1135–1140.

CHAUDHARY, N. A. and TRUELOVE, S. C. (1961). *Gastroenterology* **40**, 1–17, 18–26.

CHRISTENSEN, M. F. and MORTENSEN, O. (1975). *Arch. Dis. Child.* **50**, 110–114.

CONNELL, A. M. (1962). *Gut* **3**, 342–348.

CONNELL, A. M., JONES, F. A. and ROWLANDS, E. N. (1965). *Gut* **6**, 105–112.

DEARLOVE, J., DEARLOVE, B., PEARL, K. and PRIMAVESI, R. (1983). *Br. Med. J.* **2**, 1936.

DROSSMAN, D. A., SANDLER, R. S., McKEE, D. C. and LOVITZ, A. J. (1982). *Gastroenterology* **83**, 529–534.

FOWKES, F. G. R. and FERGUSON, A. (1981). *Scott. Med. J.* **26**, 41–44.

HARVEY, R. F. and READ, A. E. (1973). *Lancet* **1**, 1–3.

HARVEY, R. F., SALIH, S. Y. and READ, A. E. (1983). *Lancet* **1**, 632–634.

HEATON, K. W. (1984). *In* "Irritable Bowel Syndrome" (N. W. Read, ed.), pp. 203–218. Academic Press, London.

HOLDSTOCK, D. J., MISIEWICZ, J. J. and SMITH, T. (1970). *Gut* **11**, 91–99.

JONES, V. A., McLOUGHLAN, P., SHORTHOUSE, M., WORKMAN, E. and HUNTER, J. O. (1982). *Lancet* **2**, 1115–1117.

MANNING, A. P. and HEATON, K. W. (1976). *Lancet* **1**, 588.

MANNING, A. P., HEATON, K. W., HARVEY, R. F. and UGLOW, P. (1977). *Lancet* **2**, 417–418.

MORRELL, D. C. (ed.) (1979). "Management of Minor Illness", pp. 107–115. King Edward's Hospital Fund, London.

ORNSTEIN, M. H., LITTLEWOOD, E. R., BAIRD, I. M., FOWLER, J., NORTH, W. R. S. and COX, A. G. (1981). *Br. Med. J.* **282**, 1353–1356.

PENA, A. S. and TRUELOVE, S. C. (1972). *Scand. J. Gastroenterol.* **7**, 433–438.

RITCHIE, J. (1973). *Gut* **14**, 125–132.

RITCHIE, J. A. and TRUELOVE, S. C. (1979). *Br. Med. J.* **1**, 376–378.

SØLTOFT, J., GUDMAND-HOYER, E., KRAG, B., KRISTENSEN, E. and WULFF, H. R. (1976). *Lancet* **1**, 270–272.

SULLIVAN, M. A., COHEN, S. and SNAPE, W. J., JR. (1978). *N. Engl. J. Med.* **298**, 878–883.

SWARBRICK, E. T., HEGARTY, J. E., BAT, L., WILLIAMS, C. B. and DAWSON, A. M. (1980). *Lancet* **2**, 443–446.

THOMPSON, D. G., LAIDLOW, J. M. and WINGATE, D. L. (1979). *Lancet* **2,** 1321–1323.
THOMPSON, W. G. (1981). *Dig. Dis. Sci.* **26,** 281–282.
THOMPSON, W. G. and HEATON, K. W. (1980). *Gastroenterology* **79,** 283–288.
WALKER, A. R. P., WALKER, B. F., BHAMJEE, D., WALKER, E. J. and CONGWANE, J. N. (1982). *S. Afr. Med. J.* **61,** 195–199.
WALKER-SMITH, J. A. (1980). *Arch. Dis. Child.* **55,** 329–330.
WALLER, S. L. and MISIEWICZ, J. J. (1972). *Scand. J. Gastroenterol.* **7,** 93–96.
WANGEL, A. G. and DELLER, D. J. (1965). *Gastroenterology* **48,** 69–84.
WEINREICH, J. (1976). *Lancet* **1,** 860.
WEINREICH, J. (1982). *In* "Colon and Nutrition" (H. Kasper and H. Goebell, eds), pp. 239–249. MTP Press Ltd., Lancaster, England.
WHITEHEAD, W. E., ENGER, B. T. and SCHUSTER, M. M. (1981). *Dig. Dis. Sci.* **26,** 282–283.
WHORWELL, P. J., CLOUTER, C. and SMITH, C. L. (1981). *Br. Med. J.* **282,** 1101–1102.

Chapter 13

Duodenal ulcer

FRANK TOVEY

I. Differences between gastric and duodenal ulcer

In Britain during the nineteenth century duodenal ulcer was uncommon, but gastric ulcer was fairly common and affected mainly young women (Tovey, 1975). Gastric ulcer began to increase in men after 1920, becoming more frequent in men than in women; from 1930 onwards the incidence remained stationary until recent years when it declined and is now highest in men over 50 years of age. Duodenal ulcer began to increase at the beginning of this century, and has always been more frequent in men than in women. It became classifiable as a separate disease by the Registrar General in 1921. Its incidence increased until about 1955; since then it has steadily declined in men, but has remained almost stationary in women (Langman, 1982).

In most parts of the world, the incidence of duodenal ulcer is greater than that of gastric ulcer. There are a few areas where gastric ulcer predominates—the eastern highlands of Papua New Guinea, parts of Japan and in high altitudes in Peru. In western Europe, a high incidence has been reported in France and in two groups of islands inhabited by fishermen in northern Norway. So far no consistent explanation, either geographical or dietary, has been found for these differences.

229

Dietary Fibre, Fibre-Depleted Foods
and Disease

Increasingly, duodenal and gastric ulcers are recognised as two distinct but related diseases. The incidence of these two diseases differs with respect to sex, age, social class, occupation, genetic inheritance factors, gastric secretion, blood groups and secretor status; there are also variations in incidence in terms of history and geography. In Britain it would be difficult to correlate the rise, and even more the fall, of gastric ulcer incidence with the rise in the consumption of sugar and refined flour during the past century. Similarly, no relationship with dietary fibre can be found in other areas of the world where there is a high incidence of gastric ulcer. The discussion, therefore, is now limited to duodenal ulcer, although at times it is interesting to compare its incidence with that of gastric ulcer.

In vast developing countries like India, Bangladesh and in the majority of countries in Africa, it is impossible to obtain exact figures of disease incidence. In determining the distribution of a given disease the picture has to be built up by assessing reports from a variety of sources, such as the opinions of experienced workers, necropsy records, the opinions or figures of radiologists, hospital admission and operation registers. More weight must be given to actual figures when available than to clinical impressions, bearing in mind the fallacies of selection in all hospital figures. However, when information from several sources in a certain area points consistently to a high incidence, and in another area with equal facilities to a low incidence, this can be regarded as significant. By illustration, in 1973 a rural hospital of 700 beds at Kumudini, near Dacca, Bangladesh, was observing 70 positive barium meals and performing 30 operations a week for duodenal ulcer, whereas a similar-sized hospital of 600 beds at Ludhiana in the Punjab, Pakistan, recorded only about 20 cases a year. Likewise, in a 76-bed hospital at Buye, Burundi, Africa, in the Nile-Zaire watershed, over 400 operations for peptic ulcer were performed in a period of less than 3 years by a doctor often working single-handed, whereas in somewhat larger hospitals at Haydom and Mvumi in the adjoining country of Tanzania, duodenal ulcer was seldom seen.

Because of the difficulty in obtaining exact information, areas will be described as having a high incidence when duodenal ulcer has constituted a major problem, and a low incidence when it was not commonly encountered. When figures can be related to adult hospital admissions, an incidence of above 10 cases of duodenal ulcer per 1000 admissions will be regarded as high, 1–10 as moderate, and below 1 as low.

II.   Duodenal ulcer

A.   In Western countries

In Britain, the prevalence rate of duodenal ulcer has been stated to be approximately 4% in men and 1.5% in women, with a male annual incidence rate of approximately 0.15% (Coggon *et al.,* 1981; Wormsley, 1978). The incidence rate in men has steadily declined since 1955 so that the sex ratio, men to women, has fallen from 4.5:1 in 1938 to 1.9:1 in 1970. Duodenal ulcer has remained more common in the north of England and Scotland than in the southern part of England (Langman, 1979). In the 1950s, there was a lower incidence in rural agricultural communities than in urban populations, but this difference had largely disappeared by the late 1960s due to a falling incidence in the urban male population. In the 1930s, duodenal ulcer was predominantly a disease of the moderately affluent, but now, like gastric ulcer, it mainly affects the poor.

The ratio of duodenal ulcer to gastric ulcer has also changed. In the 1950s, it was between 3:1 and 4:1, but has decreased to between 2:1 and 3:1 at the present time. The peak age for duodenal ulceration is in the fifth decade.

The most common complication is haemorrhage, and it has been estimated that 25% of duodenal ulcers bleed at some time. Perforation is less common and its incidence, variously estimated at between 3 and 13%, is falling. Although moderate obstruction may be found in 3 to 4% of hospital cases, severe pyloric obstruction has become almost a rarity.

The same pattern is found in most of northern and western Europe (except France) and in the United States. However, records suggest that in the 1930s duodenal ulcer was uncommon in the Negro population of North America, but since 1940 the prevalence rate has been comparable to that of the white population.

B. In India and Bangladesh

Fig. 13.1 shows the distribution of duodenal ulcer in rural areas of India, northern Pakistan and Bangladesh (Tovey, 1979). There are marked dietary differences between the main areas of relatively high and low incidence. In the low incidence areas of northern Pakistan and north India (Punjab, Rajasthan and parts of Madhya Pradesh, and Uttar Pradesh), the staple food is unrefined wheat, eaten as chapatis. In many of these areas, particularly the Punjab, the diet of unrefined wheat is supplemented by considerably more milk or milk products, pulses and green vegetables than are taken in the regions of high incidence.

In almost all of the high-incidence areas of southern India, Bihar, West Bengal, and Bangladesh the staple diet consists of refined polished rice. This is supplemented in some areas, especially Kerala, by variable amounts of manioc (cassava or tapioca). In southern India, there is a large relatively drier belt of high incidence running horizontally eastwards across Maharashtra and northern Karnataka into Andhra Pradesh (Fig. 13.1,A) wherein the staple diet is *Sorghum vulgare* with occasional rice. In some drier, but smaller areas, the staple diet is maize and duodenal ulcer is common (Fig. 13.1,B);

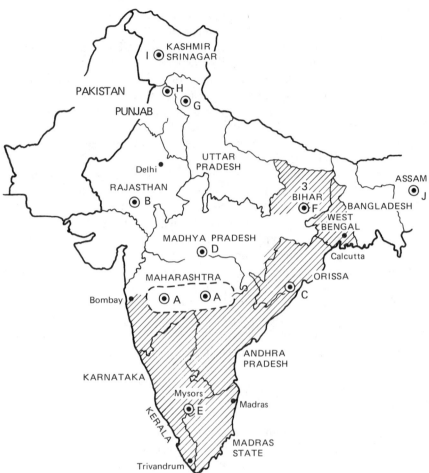

FIG. 13.1 Distribution of duodenal ulcer in rural areas of India and Bangladesh. Areas of high incidence are shaded, those of low incidence are unshaded, special areas of unusual incidence are marked by letters (see text).

such an area is found in the Aravalli Hills surrounded by the low-incidence area of Rajasthan.

In addition there are interesting isolated areas of low incidence with peculiar dietary habits, surrounded by rice-eating areas of high incidence. One such area is found at Udaiyagiri (Fig. 13.1,C) in the eastern Ghats of Orissa where the Kond tribes have a much lower incidence than do the rice-eating Oriyas in the plains. The Kond diet is seasonal, made up of a grass-like cereal called kahari or querry, the pulses Bengal gram and horse gram, mango seeds, jungle plants and roots, and mahula flowers. Another area of low incidence is that inhabited by the Gond tribes around Padhar (Fig. 13.1,D) in southern Madhya Pradesh. They use the millets sava (*Echinochola free-mantacea*) and kutki (*Faricum millare*) cooked into chapatis. A third area of low incidence is found south of Mysore (Fig. 13.1,E) where, for most of the year, the staple diet is the millet ragi (*Eleucine coracana*). A low incidence is also reported in the drier hilly areas of Bihar (Fig. 13.1,E) where more millets and pulses are grown.

There are also isolated islands of rice production with high incidence surrounded by areas of low incidence where the diet is unrefined wheat or millets. Such areas occur around Simla and in the Kangra Hills (Fig. 13.1,G), in Hoshiarpur (Fig. 13.1,H), around Srinagar in Kashmir (Fig. 13.1,I) and in the plains of Assam (Fig. 13.1,J).

Duodenal ulcers in these rural areas show certain characteristics that differ markedly from those met in Western countries. The most common complication is pyloric stenosis, often occurring early in the disease and in as many as 24% or more of hospital cases in some areas. There is often a considerable amount of inflammatory reaction or fibrosis around the ulcer. Haemorrhage and perforation are uncommon. There is a marked male predominance; the average ratio of male to female is approximately 16:1.

These characteristics disappear in duodenal ulcer patients exposed to an urban environment. The picture in Calcutta and Bombay closely resembles that in Western countries. In Madras, although pyloric stenosis is still the most frequent complication, its incidence is falling and the incidence of haemorrhage and perforation is rising.

Gastric ulcer is relatively uncommon in India and Bangladesh; the ratio of duodenal to gastric ulcer varys from approximately 12 to 19:1. The peak age is the third decade, 20 years younger than in Western countries.

C.   In black populations in sub-Saharan Africa

The areas of high and low incidence are shown in Fig. 13.2. High-incidence areas occur along the West Coast, in the Nile-Zaire watershed, and in parts of northern Tanzania and Ethiopia (Tovey and Tunstall, 1975).

Along the West Coast, the highest incidence is in the Cameroons, Nigeria and Ghana. It is higher in the coastal zone and rain jungle, and lower to the north in the savannah regions. The diet in the high-incidence areas is starchy and often refined. It consists of white rice, white wheat flour and maize, together with yams, cocoyams, plantain and manioc, whereas in the low-incidence areas in the north, whole cereals such as millet and sorghum form the staple diet.

The highest incidence of all seems to be in the Nile-Zaire watershed consisting of Rwanda, Burundi, eastern Zaire around Lake Kivu, in extreme western Tanzania adjacent to Burundi, and in southwestern Uganda. In these areas operations for duodenal ulcer form the major part of all abdominal surgery. The area is very fertile, although overpopulated, and the diet con-

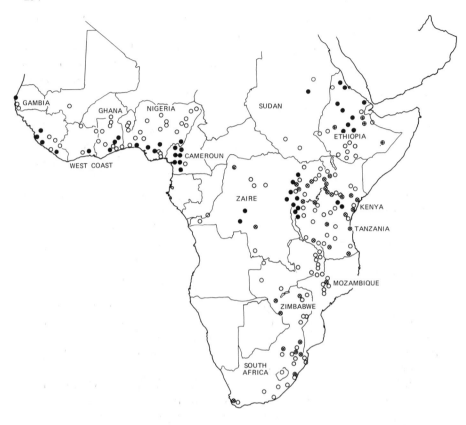

FIG. 13.2. Distribution of duodenal ulcer in black populations of sub-Saharan Africa. Places of high incidence, ●; intermediate incidence, ⊗; low incidence, ○; no data from certain countries wherein there are no incidence signs.

sists largely of unrefined starchy foods such as plantains, maize, sorghum, peas, beans and sweet potatoes according to season. Cassava is eaten in times of food shortage.

A moderate incidence is found on the rainward sides of Mount Kenya where the diet is similar to that in Rwanda. Duodenal ulcer also occurs frequently among the Wachagga living in the rainbelt of Mount Kilimanjaro in northern Tanzania where plantains form the staple food.

In Ethiopa, the incidence is high in the highlands extending from Addis Ababa up to Gondar and Asmara, where the staple food is teff, a small unrefined cereal grain, supplemented by spicy "wot," a stew containing vegetables or meat. It seems to be rare in the lower country areas where maize, millet and wheat are grown and seldom refined.

To the north, in the Sudan, there is a pocket of high incidence northeast of Khartoum where the diet is refined wheat flour, refined maize and dura (a sorghum), and a low incidence in the south where the staple foods are unre- fined dura and a millet called bufra.

The incidence is low in the rural population of northern Uganda, most of Zaire, Tanzania, Zambia, Malawi, Zimbabwe, Lesotho and in Boputhats- wana, Venda, Natal, Transvaal, Transkei, Ciskei and Swaziland in southern Africa. The traditional staple diet in most of the low-incidence areas is unre- fined sorghum and millet, but this has been supplanted in many areas, partic- ularly in South Africa, by maize, mostly unrefined. This is often supple- mented by pumpkin and beans. The picture is not entirely consistent, and there have been isolated reports of high incidence from urban areas of Zaire and Zambia. Duodenal ulcer is rare in the pastoral nomads such as the Masai of Kenya and the Borana of southern Ethiopia whose diet is made up largely of milk, with occasional blood and meat.

Duodenal ulcer, however, is appearing and the incidence is rising in the urban populations of Nairobi, Mombasa, Dar-es-Salaam, Salisbury, Johan- nesburg, Durban and Cape Town, although it is still low compared with the local white population and with those in Western countries.

As in India, the commonest complication in the rural areas of high inci- dence is pyloric stenosis, often occurring early in the course of the disease. Both haemorrhage and perforation are rare. There is a marked male predomi- nance and the ratio of duodenal ulcer to gastric ulcer is high. Where duodenal ulcer is appearing in the urban population, the characteristics resemble those in Western countries.

Duodenal ulcer is common in the Indian population of Durban, South Africa, and follows the Western pattern. It occurs equally in those who originated from the wheat-eating areas of north India and the rice-eating areas of south India; their diets have become modified by a modern urban environment.

D. Other areas in Asia and the Pacific

Duodenal ulcer is rare in the Pacific Islands except for Western Samoa (Mac- Laurin *et al.*, 1979). In the latter area the staple diet is taro, a starchy tuber, whereas elsewhere the diet is varied with several different staple foods. In Malaysia (Alhady and Srinivasan, 1965), duodenal ulcer is rare in the Malay- sians but common in the Indians and Chinese. Duodenal ulcer is common in the Indians in Fiji (Ram, 1975); the ratio of Indians to Fijians with duodenal ulcer is 2:1. In Indonesia (D. P. Burkitt, personal communication, 1976), duodenal ulcer is said to be uncommon in Java, southe. Sumatra and Sul- awesi. In these areas the staple diet is mostly rice and some soya bean cake. The consumption of peppers is one of the highest in the world. Duodenal ulcer is, however, reported in the northern areas of Sumatra and Sulawesi where soya bean cannot be grown.

Duodenal ulcer is widespread both in the rice-eating and wheat-eating areas of China although probably to a lesser degree in the latter. The wheat is refined into a white flour unlike that in north India. Information is being sought about the incidence in the millet-eating areas in the northeast and northwest of China.

III.   Diet and the incidence of duodenal ulcer

A.   Refined and unrefined carbohydrate foods

The rise of duodenal ulcer in Britain during this century until 1955 coincided with the increased consumption of refined sugar but a decreased consumption of white wheat flour. Cleave (1962, 1974) proposed that the prime cause of peptic ulcer (gastric ulcer and duodenal ulcer) was the consumption of refined carbohydrate foods, white wheat flour and sugar. Apart from the dietary changes in Britain, Cleave supported his hypothesis with evidence of the rarity of peptic ulcer in certain underdeveloped countries wherein unrefined carbohydrate foods were eaten, and also with evidence of the disappearance of peptic ulcers in white prisoners of war when compelled to eat unrefined carbohydrate foods.

However, the geographical distribution of duodenal ulcer cannot be related consistently to the consumption of refined carbohydrate foods. Although, broadly speaking, in India duodenal ulcer is uncommon in the unrefined wheat-eating rural areas of the north and common in the refined polished white rice- and manioc-eating areas of the south and east, it is also common in the areas where unrefined sorghum is the staple food. Likewise, in rural Africa although the incidence of duodenal ulcer along the West Coast is high in the southern part where much of the diet is refined staple foods, and the incidence is low in the northern savannah areas where unrefined millet is eaten, which thus supports this hypothesis, elsewhere there is no correlation between the distribution of duodenal ulcer and the consumption of refined carbohydrate foods. For instance, in the highlands of Ethiopia, where the incidence is high, the staple food is the unrefined cereal teff. The diet of the high-incidence areas of Rwanda and Burundi is almost completely unrefined starchy staple foods.

B.   Experimental studies

1.   Buffering effect

Cleave (1962, 1974) suggested that the protective action of unrefined food may be due to its buffer content. Although some unrefined foods (such as brown rice, wheat wholemeal, maize and millet) contain significant quantities of buffer, these foods seem to act as antral stimulants (Tovey, 1974) so that, after a short period of neutralisation, the increased acid output outweighs the buffering effect. The studies from Calcutta of Jalan *et al.* (1979, and personal communication) and S. Nundy from Delhi (personal communication, 1978) showed that the intragastric pH is similar with unrefined wheat diet and with polished refined rice diet despite the different buffer content.

According to Malhotra (1967, 1970), the unrefined wheat diet of north India, taken in the form of chapatis, requires much more mastication than the sloppier rice diet of the south. The increased chewing results in a bigger output of saliva with its content of bicarbonate and mucin, and he showed resultant higher pH levels in the stomach, although Dubey (1981) was unable to reproduce these results. The same situation could apply to the Gond tribes in Madhya Pradesh who also make their millets into tough chapatis. However, the diet in other low-incidence areas, such as those occupied by the Kond tribes in Orissa and the millet (ragi)-eating area in Mysore, is quite sloppy and does not require mastication. In Africa there is no correlation between masticatory diets and the incidence of duodenal ulcer, their diets uniformly requiring minimal mastication.

2.   *Stimulation of acid secretion*

(*a*) *Spices.* The consumption of peppers (capsicum) is high in some areas of high incidence such as south India, Bangladesh, the west coast of Africa and the highlands of Ethiopia, but it is also high in some low-incidence areas such as parts of north India and Indonesia. In addition, in the very high-incidence area of the Nile-Zaire watershed, no peppers are consumed. Peppers recently have been reported as producing a supramaximal acid output (Dubey, 1981; Johnson *et al.*, 1978; Solanke, 1973), particularly in duodenal ulcer subjects, thereby causing an increased DNA turnover and also producing gastritis. There is general agreement that duodenal ulcer patients are relieved of pain if they omit peppers from their diet.

(*b*) *Tea.* It has been shown in India that "black" tea (Dubey, 1981), without milk and sugar, will result in a supramaximal output of acid, more marked in duodenal ulcer patients. The output is reduced if milk and sugar are added. There is, however, no difference in tea consumption between the high- and low-incidence areas of India, and tea is almost absent from the diet of many high- and low-incidence areas of Africa.

3.   *Ulcerogenic factors*

Recent work on animal models for producing experimental peptic ulceration (A.P. Jayaraj, personal communication, 1983) has suggested that some foods may be ulcerogenic, possibly by acting as an irritant on the gastric or duodenal mucosa. For instance, using pylorus ligated rats, it has been shown that adding cassava to a rice diet will increase the rumenal and mucosal ulceration. In addition, although fresh rice bran oil has no effect, stored rice bran oil is markedly ulcerogenic. This is thought to be a result of enzyme action, hydrolysis and autoxidation during storage, and is being investigated further.

4. Protective factors

There is strong evidence that the diet in low-incidence areas of India may contain a protective factor or factors, and that the absence of this may account for the increased duodenal ulceration in high-incidence areas. This concept was supported by Malhotra (1978), who described a group of 50 patients in Bombay who were hospitalised until their ulcers were symptomatically and radiologically healed. After this, one-half continued on their normal rice diet and the other half changed to a Punjabi diet. At the end of 5 years, 21 patients were left in each group. Among those on the Punjabi unrefined wheat diet only 3 (13%) had relapsed in comparison with 17 (81%) of those on their normal rice diet.

More recently from Norway, Rydning et al. (1982) studied two groups of patients following healing of their duodenal ulceration. Over a 6-month period they found 28 (80%) relapses in 35 patients put on a low-fibre diet (median 11 g/day), and 17 (45%) relapses in 38 patients given a high-fibre diet (median 26 g/day).

The work of Cheney (1950a, b, 1952) and of Singh et al. (1962) on animal models of experimental peptic ulceration suggested that certain foods such a whole cream milk, butter, eggs and fresh cabbage contained a substance, or substances protective against ulceration. The possibility of such protective factors (Jayaraj et al., 1980) being present in the diet of low-incidence areas in India was supported by experiments on pylorus ligated rats. Rats pre-fed for 2 weeks on diets from low-incidence areas developed significantly fewer rumenal ulcers after pyloric ligation than rats fed on diets from high-incidence areas. The protective action was found in various items of food from the diets of low-incidence areas. Unrefined wheat and unrefined rice, certain pulses (black gram, green gram, horse gram), some millets (sava, kutki, ragi), soya bean, ladies' fingers (ochra), cabbage, spinach and whole cream milk were protective to varying degrees. Refined wheat, refined white polished rice, refined maize, Sorghum vulgare, sugar, bananas, amaranthus, brinjal, pumpkin, potato, peanut oil, some pulses (Bengal gram, turdhal) and skimmed milk were non-protective. The protective factor was shown to be a liposoluble substance. Horse gram (Dolichus biflorus) was a particularly potent source of this protective factor.

An ether extract of horse gram is active in very small amounts, whether given orally or parenterally. In addition to pylorus ligated rats, it has been shown to be protective against intraperitoneal histamine-induced gastric ulcers in guinea-pigs and both cysteamine-induced duodenal ulcers and alcohol-induced gastric ulcers in rats. Fractionation experiments are currently in progress to identify the active substance. It is not related to carbenoxolone and does not have any steroid-like effects. The evidence suggests that while it does not have any effect on acid or pepsin secretion, it does increase mucosal resistance to ulceration.

The evidence from Africa at present is confusing and, although it is possible that there may be a protective factor or factors in the millets of the low-incidence areas, such as in the savannah areas of West Africa, in Tanzania and the lowlands of Ethiopia, no consistent differences in diet have been found elsewhere between the areas of high and low incidence.

It seems possible that the high intake of soya bean in Java may account for the low incidence there, and that the high intake of taro, which resembles cassava, may be responsible for the high incidence in Western Samoa.

Wheat bran is highly protective, in contrast to wheat germ which is not protective, and it is possible that the diminishing consumption of wholemeal and lightly refined flour in Britain towards the end of the last century may partly account for the rising incidence of duodenal ulcer from that time. The increasing consumption of fresh vegetables, milk, butter and eggs, which have accompanied the increasing affluence, particularly in the south of England, together with the increasing interest in a high-fibre diet, may also account for the falling incidence in this region in recent years.

IV. Conclusions

An important factor in peptic ulceration is the combination of acid and pepsin secretion in association with a decrease in mucosal resistance. Treatment by reduction of acid and pepsin by H_2 antagonists results in the healing of 70 to 80% of ulcers, but the relapse rate is high, probably because of persisting reduced mucosal resistance. The present historical and geographical evidence suggests the possibility that variations in mucosal resistance may be related to diet and that this may account for differences in incidence. If the protective factors in this diet of low-incidence areas can be identified, this could prove a valuable supplement to the present treatment of peptic ulcers.

References

ALHADY, S. M. A. and SRINIVASAN, G. (1965). *Proc. Asian Congr. Gastroenterol., 2nd, 1965,* Vol. 2, pp. 427–428.
CHENEY, G. (1950a). *J. Am. Diet. Assoc.* **26,** 668–672.
CHENEY, G. (1950b). *Stanford Med. Bull.* **8,** 144–161.
CHENEY, G. (1952). *Calif. Med.* **77,** 248–252.

CLEAVE, T. L. (1962). "Peptic Ulcer." John Wright, Bristol.

CLEAVE, T. L. (1974). "The Saccharine Disease", pp. 138–174. John Wright, Bristol.

COGGON, D., LAMBERT, P. and LANGMAN, M. J. S. (1981). *Lancet* **1,** 1302–1304.

DUBEY, P. (1981). "The Effect of Indian Diets on Some Aspects of Gastroduodenal Function in Health and Disease." Ph.D. Thesis, All India Institute of Medical Science, New Delhi.

JALAN, K. N., MAHALANABIS, D., MAITRA, T. D. and AGARWAL, S. K. (1979). *Gut* **20,** 389–393.

JAYARAJ, A. P., TOVEY, F. I. and CLARK, C. G. (1980). *Gut* **21,** 1068–1076.

JOHNSON, L. P., GIMSA, B., ZENABE, H. L., WONDEMU, M. and WORKU, S. (1978). *Ethiop. Med. J.* **16,** 111–113.

LANGMAN, M. J. S. (1979). "The Epidemiology of Chronic Digestive Disease", pp. 9–39. Edward Arnold, London.

LANGMAN, M. J. S. (1982). *Br. Med. J.* **284,** 1063–1064.

MacLAURIN, B. P., WARDILL, T. E. M. and PAAIUASO, S. T. (1979). *N. Z. Med. J.* **89,** 341–344, 376–378.

MALHOTRA, S. L. (1967). *Gut* **8,** 548–555.

MALHOTRA, S. L. (1970). *Am. J. Dig. Dis.* **15,** 489–496.

MALHOTRA, S. L. (1978). *Postgrad. Med. J.* **54,** 6–9.

RAM, P. (1975). *Fiji Med. J.* **3,** 148–153.

RYDNING, A., BERSTAD, A., AACLLAND, E. and ØDEGAARD, B. (1982). *Lancet* **2,** 736–738, 878, 980.

SINGH, G. B., ZAIDI, S. H. and BAJPAL, R. P. (1962). *Indian J. Med. Res.* **50,** 741–749.

SOLANKE, T. F. (1973). *J. Sci. Res.* **15,** 385–390.

TOVEY, F. I. (1974). *Postgrad. Med. J.* **50,** 683–688.

TOVEY, F. I. (1975). *In* "Refined Carbohydrate Foods and Disease: Some Implications of Dietary Fibre" (D. P. Burkitt and H. C. Trowell, eds), pp. 279–309. Academic Press, New York and London.

TOVEY, F. I. (1979). *Gut* **20,** 239–247.

TOVEY, F. I. and TUNSTALL, M. (1975) *Gut* **16,** 564–576.

WORMSLEY, K. G. (1978). *In* "Duodenal Ulcer", pp. 2–4. Eden Press, Canada and England.

Chapter 14

Hiatal hernia and gastro-oesophageal reflux

ISIDOR SEGAL

Hiatal hernia and gastro-oesophageal reflux are controversial entities with regard to nomenclature, aetiology and treatment. One definitive aspect in a sea of uncertainty, however, is the epidemiology of hiatal hernia. In this chapter, pertinent aspects appertaining to classification, epidemiology and the various hypotheses as to the aetiology will be considered.

I. Classification and nomenclature

A. Hiatal hernia

Three types are observed—sliding, para-oesophageal and combined. In the sliding type, the anatomic junction of the stomach and oesophagus lies above the hiatus of the diaphragm. The normal relationship between the oesopha-

Dietary Fibre, Fibre-Depleted Foods
and Disease

gus and the fundus of the stomach is lost. Para-oesophageal hernia is characterised by the oesophagogastric junction remaining in the normal position,
while the fundus and greater curvature roll upward above the diaphragm to
form the hernia. In the combined type, the oesophagogastric junction is
above the diaphragm, but the fundus and greater curvature have extended
upward to a higher level. Sliding hiatal hernia is by far the most common of
the three types and discussion is limited to this condition. In fact, sliding
hiatal hernia is the most common abnormality found on radiological examination of the upper gastrointestinal tract, whether the subjects are symptomatic
or not (Postlethwait, 1979).

B.   Gastro-oesophageal reflux

This is defined as a dysfunction of the distal oesophagus which causes frequent regurgitation of stomach contents into the oesophagus (Herbst, 1981).
Depending on the techniques used, gastro-oesophageal reflux with and without hernia may be revealed with almost equal frequency. Thus, neither a
hiatal hernia nor gastro-oesophageal reflux need be necessarily of clinical
significance.

II.   Epidemiology

A.   Western countries

In 1926, the incidence of hiatal hernia was reported as 2 to 3% of all upper
gastrointestinal tract examinations. By 1950, however, the figure had risen to
15%, and since then has increased to 24% (Hafter, 1974). The diversity in
reported incidence may be due to different radiological techniques and diagnostic criteria, but there is no doubt that hiatal hernia is a common condition
in westernised populations. The most prevalent age distribution is between
40 and 70 years, with a peak in the disease in the sixth decade (Postlethwait,
1979).

B.   Africa

In contrast to Western countries, hiatal hernia and gastro-oesophageal reflux
are uncommon in developing countries, and are not even referred to in
standard texts (Russell and Bremner, 1981). Patients of all ethnic groups in
Johannesburg with gastro-oesophageal reflux are referred to the oesophageal
motility unit of the Johannesburg Hospital. During the past 10 years, only 47
black patients with hiatal hernia and reflux were referred to this unit. This is
in contrast to more than 800 whites in whom the diagnosis was confirmed
(Russell and Bremner, 1981).

   Studies at Baragwanath Hospital, which serves a population of over $1\frac{1}{2}$
million urbanised blacks living in Soweto, adjacent to Johannesburg, further

reflect the rarity of this disease. Thus in 1973, in a series of 250 consecutive barium meal examinations carried out on patients aged 30 years or over at this hospital, only seven patients with hiatal hernia were diagnosed, i.e. 2.8%; this represents 0.03% of the total black adult admissions (Segal et al., 1980). A further study was performed in 1977 to 1978; 1092 consecutive black patients aged 20 years and older were subjected to barium meal examinations because of gastrointestinal symptoms. The diagnosis of hiatal hernia was elicited in 46 patients, i.e. 3.3%, which represents 0.07% of the total black adult hospital admissions (Segal et al., 1980). Moreover, reports available from rural areas in South Africa further reflect the rarity of this condition. This low incidence rate in urban, and especially in the rural, black population is in marked contrast to the frequency of the disease in South African whites, who have a reported incidence of 22% (Segal et al., 1980). Confirmatory evidence that the disease is uncommon in blacks is that complications are rare. In this context it is of significance to note that Russell and Bremner (1981) detected only two oesophageal strictures in their series, and in the past 6 years only two peptic strictures have been detected by the gastrointestinal unit at Baragwanath Hospital.

Studies from other developing countries of Africa also reflect the low prevalence of hiatal hernia and gastro-oesophageal reflux. In Kenya, Whitaker (1966) detected only one case of hiatal hernia and one case of oesophageal reflux in 1314 barium meal examinations. In Nigeria, Bassey et al. (1977), in a prospective study, reported four cases of hiatal hernia and 23 patients with gastro-oesophageal reflux in 1030 upper gastrointestinal tract investigations. In Tanzania, the rarity of hiatal hernia was emphasised by Grech (1965). He found only one case in over 733 barium studies. Moore (1967) found a higher incidence in Uganda—some 25 cases in 786 radiological investigations—but noted that almost all were small.

C.   Asia

The rarity of the disease in Africans is paralleled by the situation in Asia. Kim (1964) found 14 cases in 1000 consecutive radiological investigations carried out at Seoul, South Korea, and emphasised that all were minimal hiatal hernias. In Calcutta, India, Bannerjee observed eight cases in 7 years in a department doing between 300 and 400 upper gastrointestinal tract investigations annually. Similar low incidences were reported in Delhi, northeast India and Iraq (Burkitt, 1975). There can be no doubt, therefore, that there is a marked difference in the prevalence of hiatal hernia between the westernised nations and the developing countries of Africa and Asia.

D.   Age distribution

It has been suggested that the different age distributions in Western and Third World countries might account for the differences in the observed age-related disease patterns. Most urban blacks in South Africa are young—50% are under 15 years. However, in a study of diverticular disease at Barag-wanath Hospital, which is an age-related disease commonly associated with hiatal hernia, the proportion of patients over 60 years of age who had barium enemas was relatively large, yet diverticula were uncommon (Segal and Walker, 1982). Moreover, the mean age of patients with diverticular disease was 62.2 years, which is similar to that of a local series of white patients, and consistent with the age at which diverticular disease is found in Western populations. Further, the proportion of the population over the age of 50 in Western countries is about two and one-half times that in India or Africa, but the disease incidence differs in the region of 50-fold or more. Additional evidence, which supports environmental rather than genetic factors in the aetiology, is that white and black Americans both are similarly affected by the disease (Burkitt, 1981).

III.   Postulated aetiology

A.   Hiatal hernia

Orthodox postulates about the aetiology of the disease include: (1) muscular degeneration with increasing age; (2) increased intra-abdominal pressure as a result of pregnancy, obesity, large ovarian cysts; and (3) an increase of fatty tissue in the hiatus with decreased elasticity of the crus, consequent from obesity (Rains and Ritchie, 1981). These factors can at best only partially explain the contrasting situations found in Africa, Asia and westernised coun-tries. Burkitt (1975) considered that the basic predisposing factor is a de-crease in consumption of high-fibre foods, consequent of westernisation of the diet. The associated ramifications of this diet on the physiology of the gastrointestinal tract are well documented and include the influence of fibre on stool volume, water content and transit time (Walker, 1947; Walker and Walker, 1969; Walker et al., 1970). Burkitt (1975) has consequently postu-lated that abdominal straining during efforts to evacuate hard faeces will increase intra-abdominal pressure, thereby forcing the gastro-oesophageal junction upward into the thoracic cavity and producing, or exaggerating, the herniation through the diaphragmatic hiatus. Straining presumably effects a Valsalva manoeuvre. This theory is substantiated by the work of Light and Routledge (1965), who measured pressures in the sigmoid colon; these reflect intra-abdominal pressures and found that the pressures increased with lifting but were highest during the Valsalva manoeuvre. The manner of defecating may also be important. Thus, Fedail et al. (1979) measured intra-abdominal and intra-thoracic pressures and the gradient between them during defeca-tion. They also compared pressures in the sitting position with those in the squatting position. Their study showed that the intra-abdominal pressures always considerably exceeded the intra-thoracic pressures when straining maximally to defecate. They suggested that if this pressure gradient across the diaphragm occurs often and for prolonged periods, the stomach might gradually be pushed up into the chest.

Squatting for defecation, compared with sitting on a raised toilet seat, was more protective, since the pressure gradient was less, but the difference was not statistically significant. It should be noted that most people in developing countries adopt the traditional squatting position for defecation. In addition, with the passing of soft bulky stools, no straining is present. This contrasts with Western populations who use the less advantageous sitting position, and in whom straining is necessitated because of hard faeces (Burkitt, 1981).

Considering these facts, it seems reasonable, therefore, to conclude that Burkitt's hypothesis does indeed play a role in the causation of hiatal hernia.

Obesity may be another factor. This causes an increased bulk of intra-abdominal contents. In addition, an accumulation of fat in the retroperi-toneal portion of the oesophago-gastric region may be the entering wedge that predisposes to the hernia. It is noteworthy that in the Baragwanath Hospital study the black patients with hiatal hernia were characterised by a high incidence of obesity (Segal et al., 1980). This is one of the features that invariably accompanies urbanisation and westernisation in Third World populations.

B.   Gastro-oesophageal reflux

Although the lower oesophageal sphincter is an important and perhaps the only anti-reflux mechanism, its role in preventing gastro-oesophageal reflux is controversial. Cohen and Harris (1971) consider that "a hiatus hernia apparently has no effect on gastro-oesophageal sphincter competence". Others, however, emphasise that the lower oesophageal sphincter functions best in its normal anatomic position (Postlethwait, 1979; Singh, 1980), and that hiatal hernia is the most common abnormality leading to reflux (Postlethwait, 1979).

The only normal physiologic challenge to the lower oesophageal sphincter is intra-gastric pressure resulting from contraction of the stomach wall against outflow resistance (Edwards, 1981). While the lower oesophageal sphincter may be able to oppose normal increases in intra-gastric pressures, large abnormal increases are opposed by other mechanisms, such as the "flutter valve" mechanism of the abdominal oesophagus (Clark and Cuschieri, 1980), and the narrowing of the hiatus as the diaphragm contracts (Edwards, 1981). This "hiatal mechanism" therefore protects the lower oesophageal sphincter from a challenge that it is not inherently built to withstand. However, abnormal factors that may indeed render the lower oesophageal sphincter susceptible to abnormal pressures are herniation of the spincter and the size and shape of the hiatus (Edwards, 1981). It would seem most probable, therefore, that there is in fact an intimate relationship between the lower oesophageal sphincter and the hiatal mechanism. The role of hiatal hernia in the mechanism of such symptoms should consequently not be ignored.

Other factors that cause a decrease in lower oesophageal sphincter pressure, and which may, therefore, contribute to symptomatology are fat, tobacco smoking (Reed, 1980), and alcoholic consumption (Lipschutz, 1976). From a global perspective on human nitrition, it would appear that a high intake of fat and a low intake of vegetable fibre go hand in hand (Almy, 1981). As far as alcohol is concerned, it may be noteworthy that traditional African brews are low in alcohol content.

C. Association with other diseases

Cholelithiasis, diverticular disease and hiatal hernia are found in association not only in individual patients, but also on a geographical distribution (Burkitt and Walker, 1976). The association of the three diseases is known as "Saint's Triad" (Muller, 1948). These diseases have their highest frequency in Western countries and are infrequent in regions such as rural Africa. Diverticular disease and cholelithiasis are uncommon in South African blacks. All three diseases affect both white and black Americans equally.

It is of significance that recent studies have shown that patients with gallstones have an increased risk of developing hiatal hernia and vice versa (Baldwin, 1978). It has further been shown that patients with hiatal hernia have more lithogenic bile than patients without this defect, and that they are more likely than others to suffer from gallstones (Capron et al., 1978). These associations inevitably suggest some common causative basis for these diseases. Burkitt (1975) has postulated that the common factor that links hiatal hernia with diverticular disease and gallstones is a low-fibre diet.

IV. Summary

1. There is a marked disparity in the prevalence of hiatal hernia between westernised countries and those of Africa and Asia. For instance, in Baragwanath Hospital, Johannesburg, over a thousand black patients having gastro-intestinal symptoms were examined by a barium meal, but only 3.3% were diagnosed as having hiatal hernia.

2. People of developing countries defecate more frequently, have shorter transit times and void a greater weight of soft faeces daily.

3. The major changes that occur in developing countries during the westernisation of diets are the increases in calories and the doubling or more of intakes of sugar and fat. The consumption of cereal foods drops, and moreover they are almost wholly refined in character—in other words, a low-fibre

diet. A decrease in intake of cereal fibre results in a considerable decrease in the diet's bulk-forming capacity (Walker and Burkitt, 1976).

4. Intra-abdominal pressures exceed intra-thoracic pressures when straining to defecate. If this pressure gradient across the diaphragm occurs often and for prolonged periods, the gastro-oesophageal junction might be forced upward into the thoracic cavity, thereby producing or exaggerating, the herniation through the diaphragmatic hiatus.

5. People in developing countries adopt the traditional squatting posture for defecation. This is more protective to the diaphragmatic hiatus than sitting on a raised toilet seat, as in the custom in the West.

6. Certain factors that are part of the usual Western lifestyle directly affect the lower oesophageal sphincter, i.e. dietary fat, smoking and alcohol.

The association of three major Western diseases—hiatal hernia, cholelithiasis and diverticular disease, suggest a common causative factor. It is suggested that a low-fibre diet may be this common factor. Burkitt (1975) suggested that a low-fibre diet produced hard faeces and increased straining at stool. This, as well as the additional factors mentioned previously, are probably the reasons why hiatal hernia and gastro-oesophageal reflux occur commonly in westernised nations but are uncommon in the developing nations.

References

ALMY, T. P. (1981). *Am. J. Clin. Nutr.* **34,** 432–433.

BALDWIN, J. A. (1978). *Lancet* **2,** 992.

BASSEY, O. E., EYO, E. E. and AKINHANMI, G. A. (1977). *Thorax* **32,** 356–359.

BURKITT, D. P. (1975). *In* "Refined Carbohydrate Foods and Disease: Some Implications of Dietary Fibre" (D. P. Burkitt and H. C. Trowell, eds), pp. 161–169. Academic Press, London.

BURKITT, D. P. (1981). *Am. J. Clin. Nutr.* **34,** 428–431.

BURKITT, D. P. and WALKER, A. R. P. (1976). *S. Afr. Med. J.* **50,** 2136–2138.

CAPRON, J. P., PAYENNEVILLE, H., DUMONT, M., DUPAS, J. L. and LORRIAUX, A. (1978). *Lancet* **2,** 329–331.

CLARK, K. and CUSCHIERI, A. (1980). *Br. J. Surg.* **67,** 559–603.

COHEN, S. and HARRIS, L. D. (1971). *N. Engl. J. Med.* **284,** 1053–1056.

EDWARDS, D. A. W. (1981). *J. Clin. Gastroenterol.* **3,** 109–113.

FEDAIL, S. S., HARVEY, R. F. and BURNS-COX, C. J. (1979). *Br. Med. J.* **1,** 91.

GRECH, P. (1965). *East Afr. Med. J.* **42,** 106–116.

HAFTER, E. (1974). *In* "Diseases of the Oesophagus" (G. Van Trappen and J. Hellemans, eds), pp. 741–782. Springer-Verlag, Berlin.

HERBST, J. J. (1981). *J. Pediatr.* **98**(6), 859–870.

KIM, E. O. (1964). *N. Engl. J. Med.* **271,** 764–768.

LIGHT, H. G. and ROUTLEDGE, J. A. (1965). *Arch. Surg.* (*Chicago*) **90,** 115–117.

LIPSCHUTZ, W. H. (1976). *In* "Recent Advances in Gastroenterology" (I. A. D. Bouchier, ed.), pp. 1–26. Churchill-Livingstone, Edinburgh.

MOORE, E. W. (1967). *East Afr. Med. J.* **44,** 513–517.

MULLER, C. J. B. (1948). *S. Afr. Med. J.* **22,** 376–382.

POSTLETHWAIT, R. W. (1979). *In* "Surgery of the Oesophagus" (R. W. Postlethwait, ed), pp. 196–255. Appleton-Century-Crofts, New York.

RAINS, A. J. H. and RITCHIE, H. D. (1981). *In* "Bailey and Love's Short Practice of Surgery" (A. J. H. Rains and H. D. Ritchie, eds), 18th edition, pp. 789–809. Lewis, London.

REED, P. I. (1980). *Practitioner* **224,** 357–363.

RUSSELL, R. D. and BREMNER, C. G. (1981). *S. Afr. J. Surg.* **19,** 189–190.

SEGAL, I. and WALKER, A. R. P. (1982). *Digestion* **24,** 1, 42–46.

SEGAL, I., SOLOMON, A., OU TIM, L., RABIN, M., and WALKER, A. R. P. (1980). *S. Afr. Med. J.* **58,** 404–405.

SINGH, S. V. (1980). *Scand. J. Thor. Cardiovasc. Surg.* **14,** 311–315.

WALKER, A. R. P. (1947). *S. Afr. Med. J.* **21,** 590–596.

WALKER, A. R. P. and BURKITT, D. P. (1976). *Semin. Oncol.* **3,** 341–350.

WALKER, A. R. P. AND WALKER, B. F. (1969). *Br. Med. J.* **3,** 238.

WALKER, A. R. P., WALKER, B. F. and RICHARDSON, D. B. C. (1970). *Br. Med. J.* **3,** 48–49.

WHITAKER, L. R. (1966). *East Afr. Med. J.* **43,** 336–340.

Chapter 15

Obesity: the interaction of environment and genetic predisposition

PHILIP JAMES

I. Environment and individual susceptibility

Obesity is one of the least understood public health problems of affluent societies. The glib assumption that the condition develops because of either gluttony or lethargy is unwarranted since formal studies of obese subjects rarely show that they eat more or do less than their lean counterparts. Yet several societies, e.g. China, have very few obese individuals with little evidence of a scarcity of food, whilst Western countries characteristically have a population in whom excess weight is an extraordinarily prevalent condition.

249

It is therefore important to understand the environmental basis for obesity and the reason why particular individuals in Western societies are affected.

II.   Prevalence of overweight and obesity

Measurements in 1980 of the adult population in Britain show that the problem of excess weight and obesity is extremely common and affects all age groups. About 15% of 16- to 19-year-old boys are overweight; this proportion, which increases with age until including 40% of men in the fourth and fifth decades of life, have a weight in excess of the low-risk optimal range shown in Table 15.1. The statistics in this table, based on the original Metropolitan Life Insurance statistics, were endorsed by an expert group from the United States (Bray, 1979) and the Royal College of Physicians of London. The table no longer specifies a weight for each frame size since frame sizes were never defined in the original data. For simplicity one can consider anybody with weight in excess of the "acceptable" values to be overweight; a 20% increase above the limit signifies the presence of obesity. Although recently there has been a tendency to consider these figures as too rigid a limit on appropriate weights, the latest American actuarial analyses (Society of Actuaries, 1979) confirm their validity since the risk from overweight, particularly in men before the age of 40, increases progressively in proportion to the excess weight carried. The risks relate particularly to cardiovascular disease and are largely accounted for by the increases in plasma lipids and blood pressure which occur as weight is gained. A detailed analysis of epidemiological data provides reasons for maintaining these body weight values and is presented in the Obesity Report from the Royal College of Physicians of London (1983).

Some of the relationships between weight and mortality have been confused by the assessment of risk in groups where smokers and non-smokers are included in a single category. Recent studies from the American Cancer Society (Fig. 15.1) show that smokers at whatever weight have a much higher mortality rate and suggest that stopping smoking is beneficial, even if a considerable gain in weight occurs thereafter. In practical terms, therefore, giving up smoking is the first priority in an overweight smoking adult.

Despite the widespread emphasis on slimness and the prevalence of dieting, women do not have a low prevalence rate of excess weight; about 12% of 16- to 19-year-old adolescent girls are still overweight in Britain; 20% of 20-year-olds also weigh more than the acceptable values listed in Table 15.1 and 35% are overweight in their forties. In addition to these large percentages, there are more women than men with obesity; 4% of 16- to 19-year-old women are classified as obese and this figure increases to 16% in the 60- to 65-year-old group.

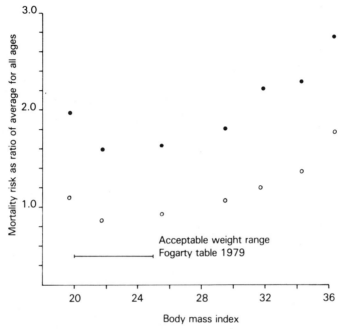

FIG. 15.1. Mortality, weight and smoking. An analysis of the mortality rate of women either smoking over 20 cigarettes per day (●) or for those who never smoked (○) based on recalculated data from the American Cancer Society Study (Lew and Garfinkel, 1979). (From Royal College of Physicians Report, "Obesity", 1978, with permission.)

III.   Secular changes in adiposity, exercise and diet

The problem of excess weight becomes more frequent as a society becomes more affluent. The estimated average body fat of adults has risen over the last 40 years in Britain with a smaller increase within the last 20 years when standards of living have risen sharply.

In Western societies, there has been a striking change in work and leisure activities in the last 30 years, with a marked reduction in working hours and the arrival of television-watching as the principal leisure time activity of the population. There has also been a compensatory fall in food intake, which may reflect a physiological controlled reduction in hunger and not simply the response of individuals who are determined to stay slim. The downward trend in food consumption is seen even in 5-year-old schoolchildren (Whitehead *et al.*, 1981) who now spend an average of 4 h a day watching television. Both boys and girls are affected; adolescents in Glasgow, for example, showed a reduction in food intake of 7 to 11% between 1964 and 1971 when there were marked changes in leisure time activities (Durnin *et al.*, 1974).

TABLE 15.1. Acceptable body weight, overweight and obesity in men and women

Height (m)	Men (weight in kg)				Women (weight in kg)			
	Acceptable average	Acceptable weight range	Overweight	Obese	Acceptable average	Acceptable weight range	Overweight	Obese
1.45					46.0	42–53	58	64
1.48					46.5	42–54	59	65
1.50					47.0	43–55	61	66
1.52					48.5	44–57	63	68
1.54					49.5	44–58	64	70
1.56					50.4	45–58	64	70
1.58	55.8	51–64	70	77	51.3	46–59	65	71
1.60	57.6	52–65	72	78	52.6	48–61	67	73
1.62	58.6	53–66	73	79	54.0	49–62	68	74
1.64	59.6	54–67	74	80	55.4	50–64	70	77
1.66	60.6	55–69	76	83	56.8	51–65	72	78
1.68	61.7	56–71	78	85	58.1	52–66	73	79
1.70	63.5	58–73	80	88	60.0	53–67	74	80
1.72	65.0	59–74	81	89	61.3	55–69	76	83
1.74	66.5	60–75	83	90	62.6	56–70	77	84
1.76	68.0	62–77	85	92	64.0	58–72	79	86
1.78	69.4	64–79	87	95	65.3	59–74	81	89
1.80	71.0	65–80	88	96				
1.82	72.6	66–82	90	98				
1.84	74.2	67–84	92	101				
1.86	75.8	69–86	95	103				
1.88	77.6	71–88	97	106				
1.90	79.3	73–90	99	108				
1.92	81.0	75–93	102	112				

Despite this fall, the body fat of boys remained the same and that of girls actually rose.

The fall in energy intake in Britain has been accompanied by major shifts in the proportions of nutrients contributing to energy intakes. Since the war, less starch has been consumed but sugar and fat intakes have remained the same in absolute terms and therefore come to represent a higher proportion of the energy in the diet. Cereal fibre intakes have fallen as bread consumption has dropped, and foods are now being sold in different forms; fewer people, for example, are buying potatoes as such but they are eating equivalent amounts in the processed form of crisps, chips and other potato products.

Given these behavioural changes, of which many medical practitioners are aware, one may then question why some individuals seem particularly susceptible to weight gain. There is little evidence to suggest that the overweight individual is eating a diet which is particularly abnormal, e.g. excessively high in sugar and fat. Formal studies of energy turnover show that obese individuals eat the same types of food in equivalent amounts as lean subjects and that their general level of activity is comparable. If, therefore, one wishes to invoke a difference in the type of food eaten or an abnormality in the control of energy intake or in physical activity as the cause of obesity, then very subtle differences must be present to elude the scrutiny of investigators. It is more likely that the obese individual has a peculiar susceptibility to weight gain in the unfavourable environment of an affluent society. On this basis, one has to consider whether specific dietary and exercise patterns are particularly linked to individual susceptibility to weight gain before one can explain why some children and adults become overweight and why there has been a change in the prevalence of obesity in Britain. Figure 15.2 shows some of the factors (a high-fat and energy-dense diet but reduced exercise) that affect the population distributions, using migrant Japanese as an example. In Japan they are much thinner than when living in the United States yet have similar genetic stock; the genetic variability within the population in part explains the distribution of weights within the population.

IV. Genetic susceptibility

It has long been known that some individuals require less energy than others to sustain the same body size and equivalent rates of physical exertion (James, 1983). It would therefore seem logical to consider individuals with small energy needs as particularly susceptible to weight gain and obesity. This has been confirmed by the finding that children of obese parents with a recognised increased risk of obesity eat on the average 20% less than children of normal weight families. Even in adults it is possible to show a clear relationship between the energy needs of a mother and her adult daughter

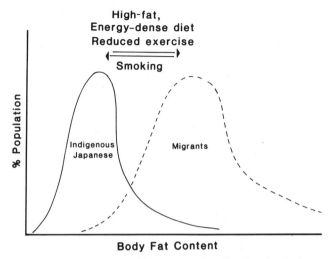

FIG. 15.2. The influence of environmental factors on the adiposity of a single race. The Japanese are chosen since there are extensive studies on migrants living in Hawaii and California. Within each population group there is a range of adiposity which relates not only to the personal habits of the individual but also to his genetic predisposition for leanness or adiposity.

(James, 1982). These findings suggest that the well-known familial aggregation of obesity does depend on different energy needs of families and that this is genetically determined. Twin studies in Britain confirm that weight gain is under strong genetic as well as environmental influences (Brook *et al.*, 1975).

A.   Subnormal metabolic response to dietary fat

Recently studies have begun to unravel the basis for this metabolic susceptibility to obesity. It has now been shown that obese, and even formerly obese adults from obese families, have a subnormal metabolic response to a mixed meal, the obese showing only half the increase in metabolism seen in lean individuals (Shetty *et al.*, 1981). When each of the principal components of the meal is tested separately, then surprisingly there are no differences between lean and obese subjects in their response to starch or protein; however, there is a much smaller increase in metabolism in obese patients when the effect of dietary fat is tested. The metabolic response to adding fat to the diet of obese patients is astonishingly small: if they are provided with an extra 1000 kcal of fat per day in their food then very accurate total 24-h measurements in whole-body calorimeters show that only about 40 (4%) of the 1000 extra kcal are dissipated as heat; the rest are conserved and presumably deposited in white adipose tissue. Thin volunteers on the average metabolise about 150 (15%) of the extra kcal when tested after 5 days on the diet. However, when thin American prisoners were fed a high-fat diet for prolonged periods of time, then after a month of very modest weight gains, body weights steadied and, despite eating twice their normal energy intakes, the subjects failed to gain any more weight (Sims, 1976).

B.   Metabolic response in markedly obese subjects

When markedly obese subjects are compared with normal weight subjects few differences are observed in the immediate metabolic response to carbohydrate, fat or protein intake. However, subjects with this extreme form of obesity have a system for appetite control which is substantially disturbed and hyperphagia is common. It is then likely that the "forced feeding" has led these very obese subjects to adapt to the high inflow of food by increasing their sub-normal metabolic response to normal levels (Nair et al., 1983). With pronounced hyperphagia, one would have expected a supranormal response to food if thermogenesis were adapting normally in these very obese subjects.

C.   Brown adipose tissue in rodents

Adding fat to the diet is a particularly good method of displaying the differences in susceptibility to weight gain; this technique has been widely used for inducing obesity in some strains of animals. Increasing the fat content of the diet is also particularly effective in producing huge increases in body fat in genetically susceptible rodents such as the ob/ob mouse and the Zucker rat. These animal models of obesity have as a key feature a sub-normal activity of their brown adipose tissue which consumes fatty acids as its primary fuel. This tissue is very important in maintaining the body temperature of small animals and newborn babies. Activity of this tissue can be stimulated by infusing noradrenaline, which immediately triggers the combustion of fatty acids in a unique system within the mitochondria, which bypasses the normal mechanism for oxidative phosphorylation.

D.   Brown adipose tissue in man

If this infusion technique with noradrenaline is applied to adult humans, then each individual shows an immediate response with a sharp increase in metabolic rate. Moderately obese or formerly obese adults from fat families, however, have a sub-normal response. In this they mimic the response of genetically obese animals where noradrenaline also produces a subnormal increase in the metabolism of brown adipose tissue. If, therefore, one attempts to link the evidence on the proposed relationships between dietary fat, brown adipose tissue and obesity then one hypothesis (Fig. 15.3) involves the inflow of dietary fat by chylomicra from the gut to adipose tissue. The flow to adipose tissue rather than to muscle is determined by the fluctuating activity of the

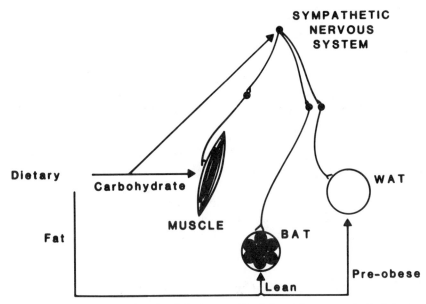

FIG. 15.3. Potential integration of carbohydrate- and fat-induced thermogenesis. Carbohydrate after ingestion is distributed to a wide range of tissues, e.g. muscle, once it has passed the liver. Experiments suggest it activates the sympathetic system which in turn affects white adipose tissue (WAT) and residual brown adipose tissue (BAT). The thyroid (not shown) also responds to this inflow and modulates cellular activity as well as the sympathetic nervous system. Dietary fat is readily deposited in WAT but can also be oxidised for heat dissipation in activated BAT. The hypothesis is that constitutionally lean individuals have more active BAT than the obese.

enzyme lipoprotein lipase in the different organs. If there is active brown adipose tissue (BAT) within the adipose organ, then fatty acid combustion and an increase in metabolism occurs. If triglyceride does not enter brown adipose tissue and induce a surge in metabolism then the triglyceride is deposited at little cost in white adipose tissue (WAT), to remain there as a store of energy. The noradrenaline studies suggest that familial obese and pre-obese individuals have less brown adipose tissue; they therefore show the minimal response to feeding fat expected and dissipate only the small amounts of energy needed for the cost of transporting dietary triglyceride from the lumen of the intestine to the white adipocytes.

From this scheme we can begin to understand how a pre-obese individual with a low energy requirement would, if encouraged to take a normal amount of Western food rich in fat, readily put on weight. As his weight increases, so would the supporting protein-rich tissues in adipose tissue and muscle. As the protein mass increases, so will the metabolic rate increase until eventually the person has increased his metabolic output to match his new intake. On this basis one then explains the paradoxical finding of an obese patient having a high basal metabolic rate with its associated large lean body mass despite having a metabolic pre-disposition to obesity. The corollary of this is that as the obese patient slims he loses the excess protein as well as the excess fat and therefore reduces his metabolic rate, thereby reducing his ability to metabolise food. Dietary adjustments to reduce energy intakes must therefore be permanent if weight is not to be regained.

E. A more complicated picture

1. Increased energy intakes in obesity

The overall picture presented so far seems straightforward but unfortunately data are accumulating which point to a somewhat more complicated picture. Not only are abnormalities of heat production (thermogenesis) difficult to document in very obese individuals, for reasons that have been suggested, but it is becoming apparent that even moderately obese subjects may be ingesting slightly more energy than lean individuals despite the co-existence of demonstrable thermogenic abnormalities and their own conviction that they consume substantially less food than normal. Formal tests of energy expenditure, e.g. by keeping moderate or markedly obese patients in a whole body calorimeter for 24 h on a controlled intake of food, show that they have a slightly elevated 24-h energy expenditure, implying that they usually eat slightly more than normal if they take a normal amount of exercise.

2. Transition from pre-obese child to obese adult

How, on this basis, a pre-obese child converts from having an energy requirement which is 20% less than normal to an obese adult, who still displays metabolic abnormalities but has an energy requirement for stabilising his excess weight which is 5% above normal, is obscure. Some alteration in appetite control seems to have occurred, but why obese adults do not regulate their intake at the sub-normal level appropriate to a normal body weight with a lower energy requirement is uncertain. This concept of a physiological control of appetite is more likely than simply considering obese patients to be unduly emotional and overeating for "psychological reasons". Although psychological drives can lead to the use of food for emotional satisfaction, this explanation is too readily accepted as a general determinant of weight gain.

V.   Environment

A. Energy-dense diets, more sugar and fats, less fibre

Although few of us are aware of it, there is a physiological regulation of appetite which usually manages, in both obese and lean individuals, to adjust food intake to within about 15% of the amount of energy that is expended.

The adjustment by unknown mechanisms is slow and takes several days to come into effect. When lean and obese subjects are unwittingly offered a less energy-dense diet, both groups show a compensatory increase in the weight of food consumed. However, the adjustment in energy intake is imperfect, so a persistent small decrement in energy stores will ensue until energy expenditure falls by metabolic adaptation, or simply as a consequence of a falling body weight, to a level equivalent to the new intake of energy. A diet that has a low energy density contains not only less sugar and fat but it is also usually rich in dietary fibre with its associated water; the bulkier diet may limit any tendency to overeat since satiety from gastric distention and other potential gut-based stimuli may occur. This aspect of the use of fibre-rich foods in promoting satiety has been described in a recent report of the Royal College of Physicians of London (1980).

B.   Implications for diets of affluent communities

These concepts, developing from studies on appetite regulation, have important implications for the dietary practices of affluent communities. A complex interaction between several dietary factors seems to be involved in the surprising frequency with which adults in Europe and North America become obese and helps to explain both the prevalence of this condition and why some individuals seem unduly susceptible to weight gain. The recent physiological studies on appetite control and the calorimetry work on thermogenic responses to overfeeding suggest that a reasonably accurate control of energy intake occurs in man but that the last 15% adjustment depends on the range and flexibility of thermogenesis, which need not be marked to help in maintaining energy balance. Small and subtle differences in energy expenditure will, if persistent, accumulate and explain the gain in weight in susceptible individuals.

VI.   Management of overweight patients

A.   High-risk groups

A doctor may decide that if 4 in 10 of all patients walking into his surgery are likely to be overweight, he can either consider being overwhelmed by managing everybody individually or devise alternative methods for coping with the large numbers, e.g. by the use of retrained nurses or health visitors, or even a dietitian. He may ignore this approach to all the overweights and concentrate his efforts on trying to identify the high-risk groups for treatment. Given the increasing recognition that an effective programme of preventive medicine requires that a patient's blood pressure be taken routinely if he has not been seen within a year, then it would seem a reasonable policy to weigh all new patients at a practitioner's surgery and then relate the value to an individual's height. An overweight patient who is also smoking or mildly hypertensive should benefit from dietary advice, providing the advice is appropriate (see below). Similarly, those overweight individuals with a family history of coronary artery disease should have their plasma cholesterol and triglyceride concentrations measured, the blood sample being taken in a fasting state. Overweight hyperlipidaemic patients need dietetic management, whereas overweight subjects without this problem are at a lower risk.

The link between increases in plasma lipids and blood pressure and a gain in weight is important because it suggests a method for communicating with and managing overweight men who traditionally regard the development of a middle-aged paunch as a normal feature of ageing and one that is not disfiguring. Men do not normally present to physicians for treatment of their obesity unless their condition is extreme, there being a 1:6 ratio of men to women in those attending special obesity clinics in hospitals. However, men respond well to advice to lose weight provided it is linked by the physician to their other physical problems (Garrow, 1981).

B. The aim: slow persistent weight loss

It is important to recognise that every 5 kg of excess weight represents about 40,000 kcal of excess energy stored. To lose 1000 kcal per day on a rigid dietary scheme is a substantial target more readily achieved by tall, young active men than short, older, sedentary women. Even a rapid rate of weight loss of up to 1 kg per week requires 5 weeks to effect the loss of 40,000 kcal and a weight loss at half this rate would not be surprising once the initial loss of water at the onset of dieting had passed. An appropriate weight loss of 0.5 kg adipose tissue per week is frequently obscured by small fluctuations in water balance, and weighing more than fortnightly can be very misleading. Patients need to be told that a 10-kg weight loss will take 3 months to achieve.

C. Key features of the reducing diet

The key features of the dieting scheme are readily understood if the underlying problem is remembered. A high-fat reducing diet can now be seen as not only medically harmful in view of its effect on blood lipids, but potentially less effective metabolically than a high-protein or high-carbohydrate diet. The advantages of the old-fashioned low-carbohydrate diet were that patients readily accepted the injunction not to eat bread and potatoes, and saw a rapid weight loss as glycogen levels fell in muscle and liver and sodium and water diuresis ensued. As ketonaemia developed the patients felt less hungry and thereby reduced their overall energy intake. They came to regard the constipation of dieting as a small price to pay for a slimmer figure and fortunately did not know that their hyperlipidaemia remained untreated or was exacerbated. This short-term view of dietary management, geared simply to slimming and not to other aspects of health, was encouraged by dietitians and doctors who failed to recognise the need for a permanent change in eating habits and the desirability of a substantial reduction in fat intake. It could even be argued that the medical profession has amplified the morbidity problems of obese patients by advocating diets that induce the very complications which the obese patient seeks to avoid by slimming!

1.   *Changing the diet of the whole family*

Given the familial predisposition to obesity, a doctor could be charged with failing to tackle the problem properly if he suggests simply a change in diet for the obese individual only; a change of the whole family's diet is essential, not only to aid the patient's adherence to a new regimen but also to prevent the development of obesity in other members of the family. The problem really is that many dietitians as well as doctors have an inappropriate diet themselves and remain ignorant of how to assess the dietary pattern of their patients. Questioning patients about their previous diet is often a waste of time and a detailed record of each item eaten and drunk for 2 to 4 weeks *while weight is maintained* is often invaluable in highlighting problems. Additional questions about household purchases help; for example, housewives will declaim their tenacity at dieting, their knowledge of cooking and pride in feeding the family well while readily admitting to sugar purchases of over 1 kg (2.2 lb) per month per person, the use of cooking oil in excess of 1 litre (1.8 pint) per year for the family and combined purchases of butter, margarine or lard in excess of 250 g (8.9 oz) per fortnight per person. Their food record then reveals the plentiful use of fried foods and the consumption of salami, pork pies, Cornish pasties, sausage rolls, crisps and peanuts—items that might well be considered as requiring labelling with a government health warning! Doctors, patients and many dietitians still consider beef, pork and lamb to be necessary protein-rich items in the diet, when evidence suggests that protein deficiency in the community is the least of our nutritional problems; these meats are best consumed in limited quantities and replacing them with the low-fat meats such as chicken and turkey would be advisable. Other simple dietary goals, such as the liberal use of potatoes (providing only 80 kcal per 100 g) and the consumption of three to five thick rounds of wholemeal bread per day to give 250–500 kcal, would help to limit pangs of hunger while providing a substantial proportion of the body's protein, mineral and vitamin needs. The doctor only needs to provide himself with a simple calorie counting book to rid himself of the prejudices that bedevil good dietary practice. In this way the physician ends up regarding fried bacon and eggs for breakfast as a curious mediaeval custom appropriate to societies involved in hard physical activity, now to be replaced by sugar-free cereal and bread as the principal ingredients. Similarly, rice-based dishes from Spain, China and

India are increasingly familiar to the public and, as long as they are not subtly adulterated by the addition of fat, provide a much more varied and interesting diet than the extraordinarily unimaginative menus which are evident when one simply asks a cross-section of the British or American public to record what they eat.

2. *Specific advice for an obese patient*

An obese patient needs specific advice. Diet sheets based on the low-carbohydrate principle should now be discarded and replaced by a low-fat and low-sugar system. Reducing calorie intakes below 1000 kcal is rarely needed except in handicapped or very arthritic patients. Additional advice is readily obtainable in Britain in the booklet *Diet Revolution,* distributed by W. H. Smith, and the bi-monthly *Slimming Magazine* is an additional source of reliable and useful dietary advice. Gimmicky diets should be avoided and exercise encouraged on a regular basis. Adjusting the regimen to suit the individual's own needs in relation to working conditions, food preference and cooking skills requires only a few minutes. Encouragement to continue the process of changing dietary habits can be linked to the development of self-help groups in the clinic or health centre and there is not necessarily any need to consider medical counselling on a weekly or fortnightly basis.

3. *Preventing obesity in susceptible families*

Preventive measures depend not only on dealing with the single patient, but also on recognising the opportunities for preventing weight gain. During pregnancy mothers are anxious to learn what is best for their children. Yet we continue to be complacent in our use of antenatal and children's clinics, considering them mainly as a place to identify high-risk groups for conditions such as toxaemia of pregnancy or childhood deafness, rather than seeing the opportunity to develop a preventive approach to modern diseases. These diseases have a strong environmental component, compounded in susceptible families by their genetic predisposition to obesity, hypertension, heart disease and diabetes. As the metabolic basis of these conditions is unravelled, we may be able to develop more sophisticated tests for genetic predisposition, but in the meantime the familial aggregation of the diseases should highlight the need for advice on changing diets to provide food that is rich in starch and fibre and low in sugar and fat. The general practitioner is in the unique position of knowing the families with these problems; the young adults in these families are often aware of their own increased risk and seem very amenable to advice.

Current evidence suggests that the present approach is an appropriate way of limiting the risk in those who are metabolically prone to obesity. The approach has advantages in terms of general health as well as slimming so that if attempts to slim are only moderately successful, the modest dietary changes will at least contribute to, rather than detract from, the patient's well-being.

References

BRAY, G. A. (ed.) (1979). "Proceedings of the 2nd Fogarty International Centre Conference on Obesity", No. 79. U.S. Department of Health, Education and Welfare, Washington, D.C.

BROOK, C. G. D., HUNTLEY, R. M. C. and SLACK, J. (1975). *Br. Med. J.* **2**, 719–721.

DURNIN, J. V. G. A., LONERGAN, M. E., GOOD, J. and EWAN, A. (1974). *Br. J. Nutr.* **32**, 169–179.

GARROW, J. S. (1981). "Treat Obesity Seriously." Churchill-Livingstone, London.

JAMES, W. P. T. (1982). *In* "Nutrition and Health: A Perspective" (M. R. Turner, ed.), pp. 123–134. M.T.P. Press Ltd., Lancaster.

JAMES, W. P. T. (1983). *Lancet* **2**, 386–389.

LEW, E. A. and GARFINKEL, L. (1979). *J. Chronic Dis.* **32**, 563–576.

NAIR, K. S., HALLIDAY, D. and GARROW, J. S. (1983). *Clin. Sci.* **65**, 307–312.

Royal College of Physicians of London (1980). "Report on Medical Aspects of Dietary Fibre." Pitman Medical, London.

Royal College of Physicians of London (1983). *J. R. Coll. Physicians London* **17**, 5–65.

SHETTY, P. S., JUNG, R. T., JAMES, W. P. T., BARRAND, M. A. and CALLINGHAM, B. A. (1981). *Clin. Sci.* **60**, 519–525.

SIMS, E. A. H. (1976). *Clin. Endocrinol. Metab.* **5**, 377–395.

Society of Actuaries (1979). "Build Study." Association of Life Insurance Medical Directories of America.

WHITEHEAD, R. G., PAUL, A. A. and COLE, T. J. (1981). *J. Hum. Nutr.* **35**, 339–348.

Chapter 16

Diabetes mellitus: some aspects of aetiology and management of non-insulin-dependent diabetes

JIM MANN

On a broad street of a certain peaceful New England village there once stood three houses side by side, as commodious and attractive as any in the town. Into these three houses moved in succession four women and three men—heads of families—and of this number all but one subsequently succumbed to diabetes. The remaining member of the group died of cancer of the stomach at the age of 77 years. Although six of seven persons dwelling in these adjoining houses died from a single cause, no one spoke of an epidemic. Contrast the activities of the local and state boards of health if these deaths had occurred from scarlet fever, typhoid fever or tuberculosis. Consider the measures that would have been adopted to discover the sources of the outbreak and to prevent a recurrence. Because the disease was diabetes and because deaths occurred over a considerable interval of time, the fatalities passed unnoticed

(Joslin, 1921).

263

Dietary Fibre, Fibre-Depleted Foods
and Disease

I. Introduction

This decription by Joslin of diabetes as an epidemic disease represented the begining of a serious scientific attempt to explore the aetiology of the disease. The condition had of course been described some 2000 years previously in India but little research had been undertaken. Thomas Willis (1679) implicated dietary excess as a major factor: "Diabetes was so rare among the ancients that many famous physicians made no mention of it and Galen knew of only two sick of it. But in our age given to good fellowship and gushing down chiefly of unalloyed wine, we meet with examples and instances enough, I may say daily, of this disease".

A fascinating interpretation of mortality statistics for New York City during the years 1866–1923 was published by Emerson and Larimore (1924). During this time there was a fall in overall death rate but a steady and impressive rise in diabetes death rates, which are most striking in the over-45 age group. Interestingly, in the earlier period there was little difference between sexes, but by the end of the period there was a striking preponderance among females. The authors discussed at length factors other than an increasing frequency of the disease which might explain the increasing rates, but reasonably concluded that, at least to an appreciable extent, the increase must be real. Interestingly, at that time diabetes took precedence over all other jointly reported causes of death (except diphtheria, pulmonary tuberculosis and typhoid fever) so under-recording was less likely. An attempt is made to explain the rates in terms of race (Jewish origins), affluence, lack of physical activity and, in particular, changes in food habits in the United States (most notably the greater abundance of all foods). The authors interpreted their rather crude data with caution. The extent to which their tentative conclusions have been substantiated by subsequent study will be discussed later, but the data served to illustrate well the emergence of diabetes as a disease capable of reaching epidemic proportions and suggested the probable importance of environmental factors in the aetiology.

This chapter attempts to examine the data that suggest that various dietary and other environmental factors are involved in the aetiology of diabetes. The dietary management of diabetes is also discussed since some of the data are in fact relevant to a discussion concerning aetiology. Particular attention is given to non-insulin-dependent diabetes mellitus (NIDDM) or type 2 diabetes since, in almost all societies, this is the most common type of diabetes and the form that has been the most clearly established as a Western disease. Indeed, insulin-dependent diabetes mellitus (IDDM) or type 1 diabetes almost certainly has a different aetiology: it is strongly associated with certain HLA antigens, autoimmunity and possibly also with viral infections. There is no evidence that nutritional factors are involved in the aetiology and this type of diabetes is therefore not discussed further, unless specifically mentioned.

II. Methodological problems in establishing aetiological factors

Several techniques have been used to look for an association between diabetes and various nutritional and environmental factors. One of the most widely used techniques has been the examination of mortality statistics (either trends over time in one population, or rates in various countries or communities) in relation to food consumption figures. Such studies may provide clues for further research but underestimate the prevalence of diabetes. Data on food intakes also are often unreliable and short term; the best data are derived from monitored wartime rations such as occurred in Britain during World War II (p. 269). In 1938 the Registrar General of England and Wales altered the regulations that had reported deaths in diabetics. Previously diabetes took precedence over almost all other diseases, but after this year mortality figures reported deaths due to diabetes rather than deaths in diabetics dying from some other disease. Correction factors were published which showed that the reduction in the figures was not large, and this allowed long-term trends to be studied more accurately.

A better approach is the survey technique. Here, frequency of diabetes is actually measured in randomly selected populations, usually by means of some form of glucose tolerance test, and information concerning prevalence is correlated with food intake in the sample. The problems here are costliness of the exercise, differing criteria for the diagnosis of diabetes and difficulty in actually measuring food intake. The most precise method is one where all food eaten for 1 week is weighed and recorded. This is usually supervised by a dietician and samples are often collected for chemical analysis. This method is not usually practical for large epidemiological surveys and is subject to several biases, the most important being the fact that the week chosen may not be a representative one and that the methodology may actually influence eating habits. A compromise approach is to use detailed questionnaires based on dietary recall. Most of the questionnaires used are based on the method originally described by Burke (1947). It is possible to develop simplified questionnaires when one is principally interested in obtaining information concerning only one factor. Such a questionnaire has been developed to assess intake of total dietary fibre (Gear et al., 1981).

Comparisons of food intake of newly diagnosed diabetics with people of the same age and sex who have not developed the disease (case control studies) are subjected to many biases. Recall of diet before the onset of diabetes may be strongly and selectively influenced by the fact that the condition has just developed. The observer who is usually aware of who is a case and who is a control may also be biased. One of the most convincing within-population epidemiological approaches is the prospective or cohort study. Here, dietary information is collected from disease-free individuals who are then followed for 5 to 10 years, or even longer, and the development of diabetes may then be related to measurements made at the onset of the study. This is clearly a lengthy and costly procedure, but the approach is free from most of the biases applicable to other types of investigation and consequently findings in such studies are almost always far more reliable than those from any other approach. The methods by which dietary data are obtained in case–control and cohort studies are the same as for the surveys described above.

A major difficulty in interpreting associations between dietary factors and diabetes is that dietary variables are interrelated. When more than one positive or negative association emerges, it may prove to be virtually impossible to determine whether the association is primary or merely secondary.

III.   Evidence for a nutritional aetiology

A.   Sucrose

The suggestion that a high intake of sucrose might be causally related to diabetes existed in the very early literature. Indian physicians described sweet and sticky urine nearly 2000 years ago and Willis in 1679 described diabetic urine as tasting "wonderfully sweet, as if combined with honey or sugar" (Singer and Underwood, 1962). Whether or not sugar consumption does increase the risk of diabetes has a major controversy for at least the past 100 years; West (1978) has listed some of the scientific publications that argue for and against this theory (Table 16.1; West, 1978, p. 249). He concluded that the evidence from all sources appeared to exclude sugar consumption as a dominant and universal aetiological agent.

The hypothesis that sugar has an aetiological role in the development of diabetes has been based on several assumptions. Sucrose is said to present a challenge to the β-cells of the pancreas which is more immediate and produces higher blood glucose levels than other carbohydrates. Nevertheless, studies where sucrose has been compared on an equimolar basis with glucose or starch have reported a lesser rise in blood glucose and insulin. This is due to the fructose component of sucrose; this has little effect on blood glucose and no direct effect on insulin secretion (Thompson et al., 1978; Bohannon et al., 1977).

The most frequently quoted argument in favour of the sugar hypothesis is the striking positive correlation between sugar consumption in various countries and prevalence of diabetes. Yudkin (1964) has reported a correlation coefficient (r) of 0.73 (p <0.001) when examining the relationship between pre-war sugar intake and mortality due to diabetes some 20 years later in 22 countries. The problems associated with this approach have been described earlier. In addition, the findings of such strong positive correlations depend upon the populations selected for study. West (1978) has drawn attention to the discrepancies which exist and the consequent change in correlation coeffi-

TABLE 16.1. Some of the major publications that argue for and against a role of excessive sucrose intake in the aetiology of diabetes[a]

Yes or probably		No or probably not	
Greisinger (1859)	Cohen (1961)	Brigham (1868)	Mills (1930)
Cantani (late 19th century)	Campbell (1963)	Naunyn (1898)	Himsworth (1935–1936)
Mitra (1903)	Gelfand (1963)	Von Noorden (1900)	Walker (1966)
Havelock Charles et al. (1907)	Alpert (1964)	Sandwith (1907)	Tsai (1970)
Wilcox (1908)	Yudkin (1964)	Saundby (1908)	Baird (1972)
LeGoff (1911)	Ziegler (1967)	Benedict (1909)	Stare (1973)
Morse (1913)	Tsuji (1970)	Lemann (1911)	Truswell (1973)
Harris (1950)	Schaefer (1971)	Allen (1913)	Keen (1974)
Del Greco (1953)	Edginton (1972)	Joslin (1917)	Bierman (1975)
Cleave (1956)	Pfeiffer (1973)	Emerson (1924)	Medalie (1975)
	Wales (1976)	Dutt (1928)	Walker (1977)

[a] From West, 1978, p. 249.

cient when countries other than those considered by Yudkin are included. For example, sugar intake is greater in Costa Rica than Malaya and yet diabetes rates are about the same.

In some countries diabetes mortality rates have paralleled sugar intake with notable falls during the period of rationing during the two World Wars. The failure to show a similar immediate association in other countries has been explained by the need for a 20-year incubation period in communities not previously exposed to a high sugar intake. The "rule of 20 years" was first postulated by Campbell (1960) in the case of the urbanised Zulu in Natal, South Africa, and has also been used to explain the emergence of diabetes in Yemenite immigrants to Israel (Cohen *et al.*, 1961). All the criticisms of demographic associations are equally applicable to these considerations. Once again there is conflicting evidence: in Fiji, diabetes rates have increased despite low levels of sugar intake (Hawley and Jansen, 1971), and in Taiwan changes in diabetes rates do not relate at all to sugar intake (Tsai, 1971). Studies of sugar cane cutters have produced conflicting results; some researchers have suggested increased diabetes rates amongst labourers who consume vast amounts of refined sugar as well as the raw sugar cane, but others have found no increase in rates (Cleave, 1974). However, on the whole, this labour is carried out by young men, often migrants, working for a relatively short period each year. Dietary influence could well be modified by the huge energy expenditure associated with this work. Poor migrants often tend to increase sugar intake in a new westernized environment. Many other factors also change so that it is impossible to relate any one dietary factor to change in diabetes incidence.

Within-population studies provide no confirmation: case–control studies suggest that diabetics do not habitually consume more sugar than non-diabetic controls (Baird, 1972). Such studies are, of course, subject to various biases already discussed. Cohort studies such as that carried out in Israel in which diet histories were taken from 10,000 healthy men, then followed for 10 years for the subsequent development of diabetes, showed no relation between sugar intake and subsequent risk of diabetes (Medalie *et al.*, 1975). No association has been found between intake of sugar and glucose intolerance (Keen *et al.*, 1979). Carbohydrate tolerance has actually been shown to improve when both non-diabetics and well-controlled diabetics were changed from a low-carbohydrate diet to an equicalorie diet high in simple sugars including dextrose (Brunzell *et al.*, 1974).

B.   Dietary fibre and starchy foods

There is more evidence for, and less against, the hypothesis that dietary fibre and the starchy foods are important nutritional factors in the aetiology and treatment of diabetes (NIDDM) than for the sugar hypothesis. The principal protagonist of this hypothesis has been Trowell (1974, 1975, 1978, 1981) whose conclusions are based on several approaches. First, there were his personal observations in East Africa with corroboration from others in Africa and from the historical literature. During 6 years as a physician in Kenya (from 1929 to 1935), he had not treated a single case of glycosuria, whereas diabetes, usually seen in association with obesity, is now commonplace throughout East Africa. There are few data available concerning glucose and insulin levels in primitive people, but African bushmen, who still follow their traditional hunter-gatherer lifestyle, have low blood glucose and also reduced insulin response to a glucose load. Rural Africans who, 30 years ago were still following a fairly traditional lifestyle of peasant cultivators of crops, were reported as having fasting blood glucose ranging from 40 to 70 mg/100 ml (Trowell, 1960). Even those living in the cities of southern Africa had lower insulin levels in response to glucose loads than comparable groups of whites. Black African students in Zimbabwe, whose diet was semi-westernised, had glucose levels and insulin responses which were intermediate between those of African cleaners, whose diet contained large amounts of only lightly refined high-fibre corn meal, and those seen in white students. These differences are likely to be associated with some aspect of dietary change that accompanies westernisation of the food and lifestyle. The traditional African diet of southern and eastern Africa still tends to contain very large amounts of lightly processed maize meal or millet meal which are high in dietary fibre; they also are low-fat diets. The differences described (low fasting blood glucose and insulin levels and a low incidence of diabetes, type 2, and of obesity) accompany the consumption of this primitive-type diet and tend to parallel intake of dietary fibre. Trowell (1981) also draws support from the emergence of diabetes in India as a common disease about 2000 years ago with the production of white rice, low in dietary fibre. Diabetes was a rare disease in the ancient empires of Rome and Greece and only became common, together with obesity, in British upper classes in the eighteenth century.

Second, Trowell was impressed by the work of Himsworth (1935a, b) who, in the 1930s, showed that carbohydrate tolerance in healthy adults was improved by increasing the proportion of carbohydrates in the diet. Himsworth's conclusions that a low-carbohydrate, high-fat diet might increase the risk of diabetes was supported by a case–control study of newly diagnosed diabetics (Himsworth and Marshall, 1935) and by various demographic associations which demonstrated a strong correlation between such diets and high rates of diabetes. The most impressive of these geographic observations appeared to be the decrease in diabetes death rates in those cities most affected by food shortages during World War I (1914–1918), i.e. Berlin and London, and the absence of changed death rates in cities like New York and Tokyo where food supplies were unaffected by war. The argument was supported by the unchanging diabetic mortality rates in rural Prussia where food supplies had been unaffected. Himsworth quoted several nutritional reports that suggested that the principal dietary changes in these war-affected cities had been an increase in carbohydrate and a decrease in fat. He conceded that reduction in total energy intake also occurred, but considered that this was unlikely to be the major dietary factor, since this did not occur to a great extent in the United Kingdom, where death rates also fell.

Third, Himsworth (1949) subsequently reported declining English diabetes death rates had occurred also during the World War II (1939–1945) and he ascribed this to decreasing fat consumption. Trowell (1974), however, re-examined these data and extended the period of survey until 1970. (Fig. 16.1). He used the recently published official diabetes mortality indices. These had remained virtually stationary in both sexes from 1933 until 1941, the third year of the war, although fat supplies per head had fallen 14% and sugar had fallen 25% for at least 2 years. Strict food controls and the monitoring of all supplies were imposed in 1939; they were vital to ensure the health of a nation that was at war and which imported much food. They were even continued after the war during the years of food shortages until 1954. Special attention was paid to the energy supplies so essential for the war effort; these remained approximately at pre-war levels throughout all these years.

In 1942, however, serious shortages of imported cereals necessitated the introduction of the high-extraction, high-fibre National flour to replace completely the low-extraction, low-fibre white flour. National flour remained mandatory for everyone until 1953; then it was replaced by the white flour. Diabetes mortality rates started falling in 1942 and continued falling regular-

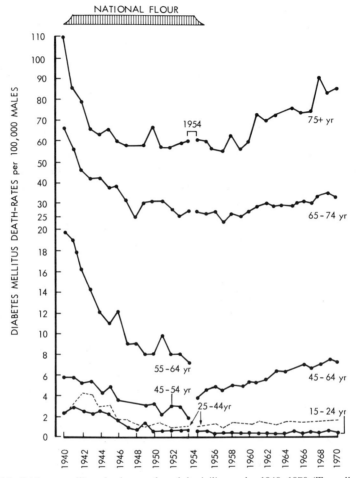

FIG. 16.1. Diabetes mellitus death rates for adult civilian males 1940–1970 (Trowell, 1974).

ly almost every year until about 1954 to 1955, by 55% in men and 54% in women; subsequently they rose again (Fig. 16.1). This coincided closely with the years of the National flour, which was frequently analysed and reported for its fibre content—about three to four times that of the white flour. In addition, flour and bread supplies rose about 20% during many of the years of the National flour. This led to the formulation of the dietary fibre hypothesis of the aetiology of diabetes (type 2), i.e. fibre-depleted starchy foods are a risk factor and fibre-rich starchy foods are a protective factor (Trowell, 1974, 1975, 1978).

This hypothesis, founded on diabetes mortality rates, receives partial sup-

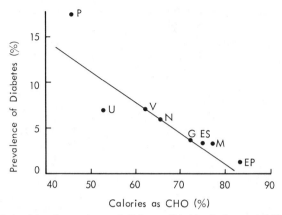

FIG. 16.2. Relationship of prevalence of diabetes (2-h blood glucose >149 mg/100 ml) and percentage of calories as carbohydrate in eight populations. Data were limited to subjects more than 34 years of age. Populations designated by their initials (left to right) are Pennsylvania, Uruguay, Venezuela, Nicaragua, Guatemala, El Salvador, Malaya and East Pakistan (West, 1972).

port by the careful surveys of West (1974a,b). In selected populations he reported a strong inverse association of diabetes prevalence and the percentage of calories derived from carbohydrate (starch and sugar). Further examination of his data, which did not report the fibre content of the carbohydrate foods, would have demonstrated that the highest prevalence occurred in affluent Pennsylvania (P) where low-fibre white flour would have contributed nearly 30% of the calories, while the lowest prevalence occurred in impoverished East Pakistan (EP) where wheat wholemeal, leguminous seeds and vegetables would have contributed nearly 70% of the calories. Other countries stand in order of their affluence and westernization of the diet, U (Uruguay) and V (Venezuela) before G (Guatemala), ES (El Salvador) and M (Malaya) (Fig. 16.2).

Some might cite contrary evidence, such as the high prevalence of diabetes in Mabuig islanders, living to the north of Australia, but there were no details of their diet; it was noted, however, that they were obese and indolent (Tulloch, 1962), neither of which occur in a poor peasant community. Eskimos formerly ate no fibre and rarely suffered from diabetes. This supports and does not contradict the dietary fibre hypothesis which regards fibre-depleted starch foods as the main diabetogenic factor in Western diets. The high incidence of diabetes among Japanese Sumo wrestlers, who are very obese and consume much carbohydrate (Kuzuya et al., 1975), does not contradict the dietary fibre hypothesis. These well-to-do sportsmen presumably eat much low-fibre white rice and have a high consumption of fat and a high energy intake, which fattens them up for combat.

Although dietary fibre intake has not been related to diabetes incidence in cohort studies, investigations in which diabetic patients have been fed high-fibre, high-carbohydrate diets provide strong corroborative evidence. This is discussed later.

C.   Fat

As has already been indicated, a high fat intake is almost invariably associated with a low intake of starch, usually refined and low in fibre. Himsworth (1935a, b), on the basis of his case–control study and geographic correlations, suggested that an excessive intake of dietary fat might be an important risk factor in diabetes. There has been little supporting evidence for this hypothesis until recently. As discussed later, obesity is certainly a major factor in the production of diabetes. Recent research has suggested that a high intake of fat may be a major factor in Western communities in producing overweight susceptible phenotypes (James, 1983 and p. 254–257).

D.   Excessive energy intake

Excessive energy intake is another potential aetiological dietary factor. Much of the geographical data used to support the association between high energy intake and diabetes are identical to those which have been used to implicate other dietary factors such as high intakes of fat or sugar or refined low-fibre starch. For example, the data relating to wartime rationing and diabetes mortality have sometimes been used to implicate a protective effect of calorie reduction in generally over-nourished societies, as have the data from Emerson and Larimore (1924). The highest incidence of diabetes in the world occurs in wealthy Nauru islanders who live on a mineral-rich island in the Pacific Ocean; 42% of men and women over 20 years of age have been classified as diabetic after a glucose tolerance test; energy intakes were estimated to be double those of most Caucasian people (Zimmet, 1979).

Within-population studies should, in theory at least, prove more reliable. Using the case-control approach, Baird (1972) found that before the onset of their disease diabetics ate more than non-diabetic siblings did. There was no difference in the various proximate food constituents, they merely ate more of everything. Medalie et al., (1975), in their prospective study of 10,000 Israeli men, were able to find no association between energy intake (and indeed any other aspect of the diet history) and subsequent development of diabetes. Keen et al., (1979) actually demonstrated a negative correlation between total food energy intake and various indices of glucose tolerance (Keen et al., 1979). These apparently conflicting data may be due to the fact that diet-history methodology is insufficiently sensitive to detect differences in total energy intake. However, data relating energy intake to obesity (discussed below) may explain some of the findings. There is no firm evidence

TABLE 16.2. Distribution of body weights in Joslin's series of 1000 patients and in "controls" insured with the New England Life Insurance Company[a]

	Below standard weight (%)			Average zone (%)	Above standard weight (%)					
	>20	20–11	10–6	+5 → −5	6–10	11–20	21–30	31–40	41–50	>50
Diabetics	0.5	5.0	5.2	15.9	10.6	18.6	16.9	12.1	6.7	8.5
New England Life Insurance Company Control Data	1.3	18.0	17.8	43.3	6.9	8.1	3.0	0.8	0.2	0.1

[a] Table adapted from data given in the publication; Joslin, 1921.

for incriminating energy excess alone, at least in the absence of obesity, as a predisposing factor.

IV. Obesity

The first unequivocal declaration concerning the role of obesity in the aetiology of NIDDM in modern literature was made by Joslin (1921) on the basis of a series of over 1000 consecutive cases. His conclusions were based principally on a comparison of the distribution of weight of diabetics with that of generally healthy people in the general population, admittedly derived from Life Insurance Company statistics, but the differences were striking (Table 16.2). On the basis of these data and the calculation that those 6–20% above average weight are from 6 to 12 times as liable to diabetes as their counterparts in the corresponding group below average weight, he concluded that obesity was far more important in determining the frequency of diabetes than other factors previously thought to be important, such as a predisposition among Jews, affluence and heredity. These factors, including heredity, might, he considered, be explained by unusual exposure to an environment that encourages obesity.

He recognised the difference between the milder forms of diabetes seen in obese people and that seen in those who were not obese, the latter usually developing the disease at a younger age. He described the latter as probably representing a "purer, simpler and more dangerous group of diabetics", but occurring far less frequently. He was acutely aware of the epidemic proportions of diabetes, declaring that a "physician should consider it as important to prevent his patients acquiring diabetes as he feels it incumbent on himself to vaccinate them against smallpox".

Early data from Life Insurance Company statistics showed that in obese people diabetes risk was greater than that of any other disease (Metropolitan Life Insurance Company, 1937). Some more recent statistics are shown in

TABLE 16.3. Principal causes of death
among men and women rated for overweight.
Numbers in brackets are not significantly different from 100.
(Standard insurance rate = 100% death rate)[a]

	Standard death rate (%)	
Cause of death	Men	Women
Diabetes mellitus	383	372
Cirrhosis of the liver	249	(147)
Appendicitis	223	195
Biliary calculi	206	284
Cardiovascular–renal diseases	149	177
Accidents	(111)	135
Pneumonia	(102)	(129)
Leukaemia and Hodgkins disease	(100)	(110)
Cancer	(97)	(100)
Suicide	(78)	(73)
Peptic ulcers	67	—
Tuberculosis	21	35

[a] From Mann, 1976.

Table 16.3. Numerous sets of epidemiological data have been quoted in support of the association between obesity and diabetes. For example, Slome et al. (1960) showed in Durban, Natal, that migration of Zulus from rural to urban communities was associated with a marked increase of obesity. This change coincided with a marked increase in diabetes prevalence. Vinke et al. (1959) have suggested that the female preponderance in the prevalence of NIDDM may be primarily due to the greater frequency of obesity in women. They found that rates of IDDM were similar in the sexes at all ages, but NIDDM was much more common in women than in men in proportion to the degree of overweight. Jackson (1978) found rates of diabetes in Natal Indians which ranged from 1.9% in very lean individuals to 17.8% in those who were markedly obese. A particularly interesting study was that of West and Kalbfleisch (1971) who showed an immensely strong correlation between rates of NIDDM and mean percent of standard weight (Fig. 16.3). Their studies included many different ethnic groups and it is especially noteworthy that racial differences were found to be insignificant when adjusting for obesity. Further evidence for the importance of obesity came from the study of certain populations who recently became affluent and had little excercise, e.g. the Pima Indians and Nauruans (Bennett et al., 1976; King et al., 1983).

Of course, in all these studies it is conceivable that factors other than obesity might explain the differences. It should be remembered that even the carefully conducted studies of West and Kalbfleisch (1971) were carried out

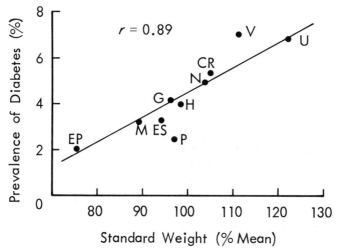

FIG. 16.3. Relationship of average fatness and prevalence of diabetes among populations of 10 countries (East Pakistan, Malaya, El Salvador, Guatemala, Panama, Honduras, Nicaragua, Costa Rica, Venezuela and Uruguay). Data applied to only those over 29 years of age (West and Kalbfleisch, 1971).

in populations possibly selected because of frequency or rarity of diabetes and one cannot assume that the correlation would have been similar had other populations been included.

For this reason, the findings from prospective studies within a population are particularly important. Figure 16.4 shows the data from a study in Oslo in which 3751 men aged 40–49 years at the start were followed for the development of diabetes during 10 years (Westlund and Nicolaysen, 1972). In those less than 10% of standard weight, diabetes was not seen in the follow-up period. Amongst those with gross obesity (45% or more overweight), more than 12% developed diabetes during the relatively short follow-up period. There was a generally steady gradient between the extremes, but at 25 to 35% overweight the curve became steeper. Other prospective studies (Medalie *et al.*, 1975) have confirmed this association. It is worth stressing that no other nutritional variable has ever been prospectively shown within a population to be related to the subsequent development of diabetes. It is just conceivable that this association might be a secondary rather than a primary one, but the consistent gradient of increasing risk with increasing obesity makes this unlikely unless the true association is with some factor still to be clarified which is very strongly associated with obesity.

There are some reports wherein an association has not been demonstrated between obesity and diabetes. Usually failure to demonstrate an association can be fairly easily explained. First, Tulloch (1962) found that a substantial proportion of newly diagnosed patients in Jamaica were not obese at the time

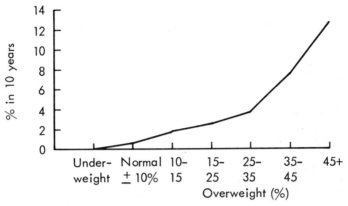

FIG. 16.4. Incidence of diabetes in 3737 Norwegian men (aged 40–49 years at the outset) followed prospectively for 10 years (Westlund and Nicolaysen, 1972).

of presentation. However, the majority of these had been obese earlier and presumably the weight loss was a consequence of the illness, a phenomenon recognised by Joslin (1921). Second, obesity of short duration is not associated with diabetes, something that was first noted by Watson (1939). Thirdly, the widely used body mass index (weight/height^2) is probably appropriate for use in most populations, but may be misleading when used for comparative purposes in some racial groups (Bassett and Schroffner, 1970; Fredman, 1972). Finally, prevalence studies in older people may not show an association between diabetes and obesity since many of the obese diabetics may have already died.

V. Ethnic groups and genetic factors

A. Ethnic groups

There are other studies where failure to find an association between diabetes and obesity is less easily explained. Jackson and his colleagues (1970; Jackson, 1978) have studied the frequency of diabetes in five ethnic groups living in South Africa. Although there appears to be an association with obesity within some of these groups, the association is not always strong. For example, the prevalence of diabetes among non-obese Africans is 1.6%, rising to only 2.3 among the obese. Furthermore, in this country obesity clearly does not explain the different frequencies in the different ethnic groups. The two most obese groups (White and Bantu) had the lowest frequency of diabetes. A similar situation seems to prevail in some Pacific Islands: For example, in rural New Caledonia, the prevalence of diabetes is higher in part-Polynesians than in comparable age groups of Melanesians—males 6.6% versus 0.5%, females 6.3% versus 3.5%, respectively. Degree of obesity appeared similar in the two ethnic groups and while it is not possible to exclude some qualitative aspects of diet or other differences in environmental factors (e.g. physical activity), it seems most likely that differences here are largely genetically determined (Zimmet et al., 1982). There are several examples amongst other populations (both indigenous and migrant) where obesity appears to play a less important role.

B. Genetic factors

The association between obesity and diabetes frequency seems to be very consistent in traditional westernised populations. Within these populations there is in addition strong evidence for genetic factors even though the precise mode of inheritance is uncertain. The findings from certain twin studies suggest a strong genetic factor in some European populations, at least in type 2 (NIDDM) diabetes. Two other studies also provide strong confirmation of an interaction between genetic and environmental factors.

Kobberling (1971) studied 392 randomly chosen outpatient NIDDM persons with an age at onset of 25 years or more and interviewed them about their family history. Information was then obtained about body weight before the onset of the disease, and the ideal body weight also was calculated. The percentage overweight was then multiplied by the interval in years between the onset of overweight and the onset of diabetes. Using this product, diabetics were allocated to one of three groups. In the most overweight (group III), the expected frequency of diabetes in the siblings was significantly lower than either group I or group II (Fig. 16.5).

Thus, the frequency of diabetes among the siblings falls with increasing overweight of the diabetic probands. This suggests that there is a stronger genetic influence in the development of NIDDM in the lean than in those who are obese. However, when patients with IDDM were studied in the same way, no relationship was found between overweight and family history of diabetes. This suggests that the interaction between obesity and diabetes is limited to NIDDM.

Kobberling's findings were supported by data from a study performed in Edinburgh by Baird (1973). The cases consisted of all new diabetics aged 45–65 years diagnosed over a 2-year period in a defined geographical area, and their non-diabetic brothers and sisters. Non-diabetic brothers and sisters of controls, matched with the diabetics for age, sex, social class and obesity, were also studied. All siblings were tested for diabetes; 10% of the siblings of diabetics were found to be diabetic compared with 3.8% of the siblings of controls (Table 16.4). When obesity of the propositi was considered, it was found that 15% of the siblings of non-diabetic patients were diabetic, compared with 7.3% of the siblings of obese diabetic patients, while there was no

J. MANN

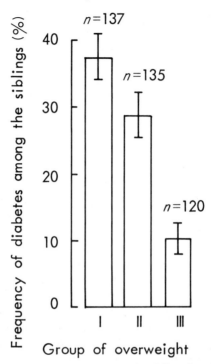

FIG. 16.5. Expected frequency of diabetes among the siblings in relation to the degree of overweight. Probands: adult-onset diabetes with oral or diet therapy in three groups of different overweight; n = number of probands (Kobberling, 1971).

difference in the rates of diabetes between siblings of obese and non-obese controls (4.1% and 3.4%, respectively). The differences were enhanced when obesity in the siblings was also considered (Table 16.5). The rate of diabetes in the obese siblings of non-obese diabetics was as high as 30%, compared with 10% in the obese siblings of obese diabetics.

Assuming that obesity is particularly important in the aetiology of NID-DM at least in some countries, failure to find a consistent association with energy intake is surprising. One simple explanation is that obese individuals

TABLE 16.4. Rates of diabetes in the siblings
of 238 diabetics and matched controls,
grouped by obesity[a]

	Obese	Non-obese	Total
Diabetic (%)	7.3	15.0	10.0
Control (%)	4.1	3.4	3.8

[a] From Baird, 1973.

TABLE 16.5. Rates of diabetes
in the obese and non-obese siblings
of 238 obese and non-obese diabetics[a]

	Diabetics	
	Obese	Non-obese
Siblings		
Obese (%)	10	30
Non-obese (%)	5	6
Total (%)	7.3	15

[a] From Baird, 1973.

either intentionally or unintentionally underestimate their energy intake, or that they are already reducing energy intake to reduce obesity. Another is the fact, previously mentioned, that energy intake is so difficult to assess accurately. However, the survey of three normal populations by Keen *et al.* (1979) previously referred to, provides a third intriguing possibility. Dietary histories were obtained for 3454 subjects for whom a fasting blood sugar (1005), a blood glucose 2 hours after a carbohydrate load (2449), or a full glucose tolerance test (220—a subset of one of the populations) were also available. Blood sugar concentrations and indices of glucose tolerance correlated positively with the degree of adiposity but were negatively correlated with total food energy intake and its component nutrients (total carbohydrate, sucrose and fat). This inverse association was accounted for by an impressive inverse correlation between food energy intake and adiposity, a relationship present in both sexes and all three populations studied. Thus, obesity and increased risk of diabetes are both associated with a lower total energy expenditure. The data do not prove that a "low-energy throughput state" is a cause of obesity; indeed it could be a consequence of it, or both might be manifestations of an individual's setting in a range of energy utilisation. This study, however, provides strong support for the suggestion that adiposity is a major determinant of diabetes and glucose intolerance and that the relationship between food consumption and diabetes and obesity is far more complex.

VI.   Dietary management

A.   Weight reduction

In view of the strong association between obesity and diabetes, it is hardly surprising that raised levels of blood glucose respond to weight reduction in overweight diabetic patients. Failure to show an association between energy intake and diabetes is of course quite irrelevant to the importance of this therapeutic aspect in the overweight diabetic individual. Energy restriction for such diabetics is probably the only uncontroversial dietary recommendation. The value of changing individual nutrients is less clear. A reduction in sucrose, other simple sugars, refined carbohydrate and indeed total carbohydrate, have until recently been the cornerstone of diabetic dietary advice throughout the Western world. However, in even the most well-conducted studies claiming to show a benefit of restricting these foods, the improvement has only been seen in patients who have lost weight (Perkins *et al.*, 1977). The value of restricting sucrose and other simple sugars lies principally in the fact that these are energy-dense food sources and restricting them, as well as fat intake, may aid weight reduction. On the other hand, it seems that increasing fibre-rich starch carbohydrate in the diet improves diabetic control in a way that is independent of energy balance.

B. *Dietary fibre and starch foods*

The idea that low-fat diets high in fibre and lightly processed starch foods may be beneficial to diabetics is certainly not new. On the basis of the epidemiological evidence (described previously), anecdotal case reports and inadequately controlled trials, a few individuals have claimed that such diets are preferable to the more widely used low-carbohydrate diets (Mann, 1980). It was Anderson's group (Anderson and Ward, 1978) in Lexington, Kentucky (U.S.A.) who demonstrated how striking were the effects of such a diet, described as the high-carbohydrate, high-fibre (HCF) diet (Fig. 16.6). Twelve lean diabetic men were treated with a control diet (low-carbohydrate, low-fibre) for a few days, then changed to an isocaloric HCF (high-carbohydrate, 70% energy, high-fibre 65 g/day) diet. Diabetics treated with oral hypoglycaemic agents or low doses of insulin were able to reduce, or in some cases eliminate, their drug therapy and diabetic control was greatly improved. The improvement was sustained on a maintenance 60% carbohydrate diet with 51 g/day dietary fibre. It is important to stress that although many of the patients studied were taking insulin, the great majority were not insulin dependent, as defined by WHO, and these findings should not, therefore, be extrapolated to true type 1 or ketosis-prone patients (IDDM).

We have studied patients with non-insulin-dependent diabetes (on diet alone or diet plus oral therapy) as well as ketosis-prone insulin-dependent patients (R. W. Simpson *et al.*, 1979 a,b; H. C. R. Simpson *et al.*, 1981). In these controlled studies, the carbohydrate has usually provided about 60% total energy, and the fibre content, derived from readily available whole cereal products and vegetables, has ranged from 50 to 90 g/day. In both groups of patients we have observed an improvement when such diets have been compared with traditional low-carbohydrate, high-fat diets (Fig. 16.7).

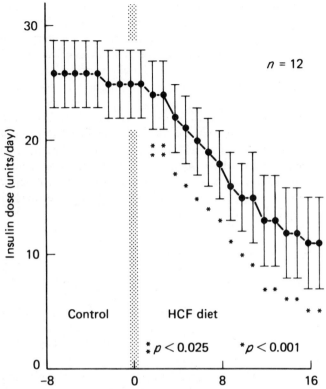

FIG. 16.6. Insulin requirements of diabetic men on low doses of insulin given a control diet, followed by a high-carbohydrate (70% energy), high-fibre (65 g/day dietary fibre) diet. Similar findings were observed in patients taking oral agents (Anderson and Ward, 1978).

These changes occurred without changes in body weight. Similar results have now been reported in diabetic children living in Oxford, England (Kinmoth *et al.*, 1982) and numerous other groups have confirmed the observations in adult diabetics.

It is of interest that diets high in fibre-rich cereals and tuberous vegetables tend to result in an improvement in basal (fasting and pre-prandial) blood glucoses. Post-prandial levels seem to improve only if fibre from leguminous sources (e.g. various types of dried beans) forms part of the diet. The effects are most striking with gel-forming fibres, guar and pectin (Jenkins *et al.*, 1976), but as these substances do not occur in significant amounts in the diets of most populations, they are not discussed in detail here. Our results and those of other groups have in general not been as impressive as those reported by Anderson and Ward (1978). There are several possible reasons for this. First, they have not been quite so high in total high-fibre carbohydrate as those of Anderson and colleagues and this might be essential in order to

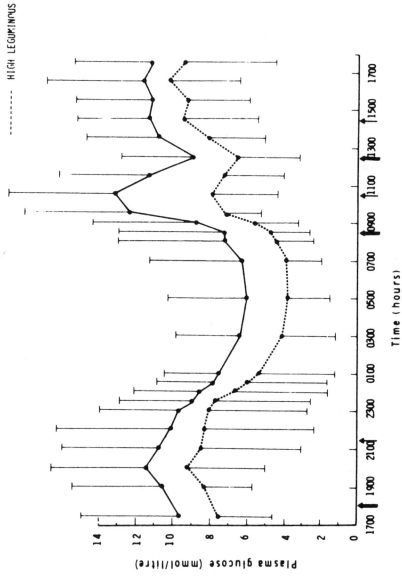

Fig. 16.7. Twenty-four hour blood glucose profiles of patients taking a "low-carbohydrate" diabetic diet (upper line) or a diet containing 60% carbohydrate energy and high in dietary fibre, particularly from leguminous sources (lower dotted line) (Simpson *et al.*, 1981).

TABLE 16.6. Total plasma cholesterol and lipoprotein cholesterol sub-fractions of NIDDM patients on high- and low-fibre diets (HF and LF)[a]

Cholesterol (mmol/litre)	HF	LF	p
Total	4.12 ± 1.00	4.81 ± 0.90	<0.01
LDL	2.62 ± 0.83	3.23 ± 0.90	<0.01
VLDL	0.52 ± 0.26	0.43 ± 0.29	NS
HDL	1.06 ± 0.21	1.18 ± 0.25	NS
HDL/LDL (%)	44.7 ± 17.3	40.1 ± 15.6	<0.05
Total triglycerides (mmol/litre)	1.31 ± 0.43	1.84 ± 0.41	NS

[a] From Simpson et al., 1981.

observe the regression phenomenon described by them. Second, it is conceivable that their diets were, at least during the induction phase, associated with some energy reduction even though appreciable weight changes did not occur. It is well recognised that diabetic patients show a decrease in blood glucose levels with energy restriction even before weight has started to fall. HCF diets rapidly produce satiety and may well be associated with reduced energy intake.

Most studies that have examined diets of this kind have observed favourable changes in blood lipids, a decrease in LDL cholesterol, an increase of HDL/LDL cholesterol ratio and often a reduction in triglycerides (Table 16.6) (Simpson et al., 1981). We have in addition observed a reduction of several coagulation factors (Table 16.7) in diabetics. These have been shown in prospective studies of non-diabetics to be important predictors of subsequent ischaemic heart disease (IHD) (Simpson et al., 1982). These changes in the hypercoagulable state associated with diabetes together with the change in blood lipids provide an additional reason for recommendation of such diets to diabetics whose risk of developing IHD is greatly increased.

TABLE 16.7. Mean values of clotting factors in non-insulin-dependent diabetics after high-fibre and low-fibre diets for 6 weeks. Results pooled for each period[a,b]

	Factor VIIc (%)	Factor VIIIc (%)	Factor VIIIAg (%)	Factor Xc (%)	Fibrinogen (g/litre)
High fibre	92.7	87.4	40.3	82.7	3.56
Low fibre	115.4	82.3	48.9	95.3	3.57
Change	−22.7[c]	5.1	−8.6	−12.6[c]	−0.01
SE of change	6.21	3.26	2.42	3.56	0.12

[a] From Simpson et al., 1982.

[b] Clotting factor values expressed as percentage of one standard; not directly comparable with values in other reports on Northwick Park Heart Study based on other standards.

[c] $p < 0.01$.

The precise mechanisms by which these effects are produced are not yet clear. Insulin secretion is not increased. Monocyte insulin binding is increased on the diets described (Ward et al., 1982). Gel-forming fibres delay gastric emptying and result in delayed, though not impaired, absorption. Unprocessed and lightly processed carbohydrates are surrounded by fibre and available carbohydrate is released more slowly. Apart from the obvious consequences of slower glucose absorption, no major hormonal changes have been demonstrated to account for the differences between high-carbohydrate, high-fibre diets and low-carbohydrate diets. It is still uncertain whether the beneficial effects are due entirely to dietary fibre or whether more digestible carbohydrate itself might confer some additional benefit. There is certainly some evidence to suggest that digestible carbohydrate may influence, at least to some extent, basal blood glucose levels (Simpson et al., 1982). Furthermore, it has been clearly shown in studies using the gel-forming fibre guar, that the beneficial effect of a high-fibre diet is only apparent when guar is given as part of a high-carbohydrate diet.

C. Practical considerations

Advice concerning a reduction of fat and increase in fibre-rich carbohydrate have recently been incorporated into the official dietary recommendations of the British Diabetic Association (Nutrition Subcommittee of the British Diabetic Association's Medical Advisory Committee, 1982). It is not yet clear precisely how low fat intake should be and how much fibre should be included. Most of the research studies using common foods have given at least 50 g/day dietary fibre, a level of intake which is 10 g higher than amongst British vegetarians and one which we found to be acceptable to many of our well-motivated patients in the long term. Indeed, an intake of even 40 g/day involves a major change in the present Western eating habits. Further investigations concerning the effects of this level of fibre and starch intakes are needed, More information is also required concerning the different effects of various high-fibre foods. Recent research from Jenkins and colleagues (1983) showed that glycaemic response to carbohydrate-containing foods varies greatly; it is not related simply to total dietary fibre content.

Diet manuals describing how to translate some of this advice into practice are now available (Mann and the Oxford Dietetic Group, 1982; British Diabetic Association, 1982).

VII.   Conclusions

There would seem to be no doubt that, although genetic factors play a role in the aetiology of NIDDM, the frequency of this disease in most populations is primarily determined by obesity. Undetermined environmental and nutritional factors probably also operate. Obesity seems to be the most important factor but as yet it is impossible to exclude non-nutritional factors, such as lack of physical activity frequently associated with obesity. Obesity and genetic factors appear to interact and in a susceptible individual the development of obesity is associated with a very high risk (West, 1978a).

The evidence that excesses or deficiencies of individual digested and absorbed dietary factors are directly involved in the aetiology of NIDDM is inconclusive. There is, however, strong circumstantial evidence that diets containing much highly processed, fibre-depleted starch foods are associated with an increased risk of developing diabetes.

Studies showing that diabetic control is improved by diets that contain much lightly processed, full-fibre starchy foods provide confirmatory evidence and leave no doubt about the importance of dietary fibre and starch foods in the management of NIDDM and IDDM.

IDDM is less common in some countries where NIDDM is also infrequent, such as much of rural Africa, but there is little evidence to incriminate any particular dietary or other environmental factor.

The importance of obesity rather than energy excess suggests that public health measures aimed at reducing the frequency of diabetes in high-risk populations should emphasise weight reduction.

References

ANDERSON, J. W. and WARD, K. (1978). *Diabetes Care* 1, 77–82.

BAIRD, J. D. (1972). *Acta Diabetol. Lat.* **9**,(Suppl.), 621–637.

BAIRD, J. D. (1973). *Publ—R. Coll. Physicians Edinburgh* **42**, 83–99.

BASSETT, D. R. and SCHROFFNER, W. G. (1970). *Arch. Intern. Med.* **125**, 476–487.

BENNETT, P. H., RUSFORTH, W. B., MILLER, M. and LE COMPTE, P. M. (1976). *Recent Prog. Horm. Res.* **32**, 333–376.

BOHANNON, N. V., KARAM, J. H., LORENZI, M., GERICH, J. E., MATIN, S. B. and FORSHAM, P. H. (1977). *Diabetologia* **13**, 503–508.

British Diabetic Association (1982). "Better Cookery for Diabetics," London.

BRUNZELL, J. D., LERNER, R. L. and PORTE, D. (1974). *Diabetes* **23**, 138–142.

BURKE, B. S. (1947). *J. Am. Diet. Assoc.* **23**, 1041–1046.

CAMPBELL, G. D. (1960). *S. Afr. Med. J.* **34**, 332.

CLEAVE, T. L. (1974). "The Saccharine Disease". Wright, Bristol.

COHEN, A. M., BAYLY, S. and POZNANSKY, R. (1961). *Lancet* **2**, 1399–1401.

EMERSON, H. and LARIMORE, L. D. (1924). *Arch. Intern. Med.* **34**, 585–630.

FREDMAN, H. (1972). *S. Afr. Med. J.* **46**, 1836–1837.

GEAR, J. S. S., BRODRIBB, A. J. M., WARE, A. C. and MANN, J. I. (1981). *Br. J. Nutr.* **45**, 77–82.

HAWLEY, T. G. and JANSEN, A. A. J. (1971). *N.Z. Med. J.* **24**, 9–21.

HIMSWORTH, H. P. (1935a). *Clin. Sci.* **2**, 67–94.

HIMSWORTH, H. P. (1935b). *Clin. Sci.* **2**, 117–148.

HIMSWORTH, H. P. and MARSHALL, E. M. (1935). *Clin. Sci.* **2**, 95–115.

HIMSWORTH, H. P. (1949). *Lancet*, **1**, 465–472.

JACKSON, W. P. U. (1978). *Adv. Metab. Dis.* **9**, 111–145.

JACKSON, W. P. U., VINIK, A. I., JOFFE, B. I., SACKS, A. and EDELSTEIN, I. (1970). *S. Afr. Med. J.* **44**, 1283–1287.

JAMES, W. P. T. (1983). *Lancet* **2**, 386–389.

JENKINS, D. J. A., GOFF, D. V., LEEDS, A. R., ALBERTI, K. G. M. M., WOLEVER, T. M. S., GASSULL, M. A. and HOCKADAY, T. D. R. (1976). *Lancet* **2**, 172–174.

JENKINS, D. J. A., WOLEVER, T. M. S., JENKINS, A. L., THORNE, M. J., LEE, R., KALMUSKY, J., REICHERT, R. and WONG, G. S. (1983). *Diabetologia* **24**, No.4, 257–264.

JOSLIN, E. P. (1921). *JAMA, J. Am. Med. Assoc.***76**, 79–84.

KEEN, H., THOMAS, B. J., JARRETT, R. J. and FULLER, J. H. (1979). *Br. Med. J.* **1**, 655–658.

KING, H., BALKAN, B. and ZIMMETT, P. (1983). *Am. J. Edidemiol.* **117**, 659–666.

KINMONTH, A-L., ANGUS, R. M., JENKINS, P. A., SMITH, M. A. and BAUM, J. D. (1982). *Arch. Dis. Child.* **57**, No.3, 187–194.

KOBBERLING, J. (1971). *Diabetologia* **7**, 46–49.

KUZUYA, T., IRIE, M. and NIKI, Y. (1975). *In* "Diabetes Mellitus in Asia" (S. Baba, Y. Goto and I. Fukui, eds), Proc. 2nd Symp., Kyoto, pp. 137–143. Excerpta Medica, Amsterdam.

MANN, J. I. (1976). *In* "Nutrition in the Community" (S. McLaren, ed.), pp. 101–116. Wiley, New York.

MANN, J. I. (1980). *Diabetologia* **18**, 89–95.

MANN, J. I. and the OXFORD DIETETIC GROUP (1982). "The Diabetics' Diet Book." Martin Dunitz, London.

MEDALI, J. H., PAPIER, C. M., GOLDBOURT, U. and HERMAN, J. B. (1975). *Arch. Intern. Med.* **135**, 811–818.

Metropolitan Life Insurance Company (1937). "Girth and Death." *Stat. Bull. Metropolitan Life Ins. Co.* **18**, 2–5.

Nutrition Sub-Committee of the British Diabetic Association's Medical Advisory Committee (1982). Dietary recommendations for the 1980's - A policy statement by the British Diabetic Association *Hum. Nutr.: Appl. Nutr.* **36a**, 378–386.

PERKINS, J. R., WEST, T. E. T., SONKSEN, P. H., LOWY, C. and ILES, C. (1977). *Diabetologia* **13**, 607–614.

SIMPSON, H. C. R., SIMPSON, R. W., LOUSLEY, S., CARTER, R. D., GEEKIE, M., HOCKADAY, T. D. R. and MANN, J. I. (1981). *Lancet* **1**, 1–5.

SIMPSON, H. C. R., MANN, J. I., CHAKRABARTI, R., IMESON, J. D., STIRLING, Y., TOZER, M., WOOLF, L. and MEADE, T. W. (1982). *Br. Med. J.* **284**, 1608.

SIMPSON, R. W., MANN, J. I., EATON, J., MOORE, R. A., CARTER, R. D. and HOCKADAY, T. D. R. (1979a). *Br. Med. J.* **,1** 1753–1756.

SIMPSON, R. W., MANN, J. I., EATON, J., CARTER, R. D. and HOCKADAY, T. D. R. (1979b). *Br. Med. J.* **2**, 523–525.

SINGER, C. and UNDERWOOD, E. A. (1962). "A Short History of Medicine", 2nd edition, p. 544. Oxford University Press (Clarendon), London.

SLOME, C., GAMPEL, B., ABRAMSON, J. H. and SCOTCH, N. (1960). *S. Afr. Med. J.* **34**, 505–509.

THOMPSON, R. G., HAYFORD, J. T., and DANNEY, M. M. (1978). *Diabetes* **27**, 1020–1026.

TROWELL, H. C. (1960). "Non-Infective Disease in Africa", pp. 303–310. Edward Arnold, London.

TROWELL, H. C. (1974). *Lancet* **2**, 998–1004.

TROWELL, H. C. (1975). *Diabetes* **24**, 762–765.

TROWELL, H. C. (1978). *Am. J. Clin. Nutr.* **31**, 553–557.

TROWELL, H. C. (1981). *In* "Western Diseases: Their Emergence and Prevention" (H. C. Trowell and D. P. Burkitt, eds), pp. 22–26. Edward Arnold, London.

TSAI, S. H. (1971). *In* "Diabetes Mellitus in Asia" (S. Tsuji and M. Wadar, eds), p. 104. *Excerpta Medica*, Amsterdam.

TULLOCH, J. A. (1962). "Diabetes Mellitus in the Tropics", p. 73. Churchill-Livingstone, Edinburgh.

VINKE, B., NAGELSMIT, W. F., VAN BUCHEN, F. S. P. and SMID, L. J. (1959). *Diabetes* **8**, 100–104.

WARD, G. M., SIMPSON, R. W., SIMPSON, H. C. R., NAYLOR, B. A., MAHN, J. I. and TURNER, R. C. (1982). *Eur. J. Clin. Invest.* **12**, 93–96.

WATSON, B. A. (1939). *Endocrinology (Baltimore)* **25**, 845–852.

WEST, K. M. (1972). *Acta Diabetol. Lat.* **9** (Suppl 1), 405–428.

WEST, K. M. (1974a). *In* "Is the Risk of Becoming Diabetic Affected by Sugar Consumption?" (S. Hillibrand, ed.), Proc. 8th Symp. Int. Sugar Res. Found. pp. 33–43. International Sugar Research Foundation, Bethesda, Maryland.

WEST, K. M. (1974b). *Diabetes* **23**, 841–855.

WEST, K. M. (1978). "Epidemiology of Diabetes and its Vascular Lesions", pp. 231–248. Elsevier, Amsterdam.

WEST, K. M. and KALBFLEISCH, J. M. (1971). *Diabetes* **20**, 99–108.

WESTLUND, K. and NICOLAYSEN, R. (1972). *Scand. J. Lab. Clin. Invest.* **30**, (Suppl. 127), 3–24.

WILLIS, T. (1679). "Of the Diabetes of Pissing Evil", Chapter 3. Dring, Harper and Leight, London.

YUDKIN, J. (1964). *Lancet* **2**, 4–5.

ZIMMET, P. (1979). *Diabetes Care* **2**, 144–153.

ZIMMET, P., CANTELOUBE, D., GENELLE, B., LE GONIDEC, G., COUZIGOU, P., PEGHINI, M., CHARPIN, M., BENNETT, P., KUBERSKI, T., KLEIBER, N. and TAYLOR, R. (1982). *Diabetologia* **23**, 393–398.

Chapter 17

Gallstones

KENNETH HEATON

I.   Fibre-depleted food hypothesis

The hypothesis that the main cause of human gallstones is the consumption of fibre-depleted foods, especially those containing much carbohydrate and formerly called refined carbohydrate, was developed in the early 1970s (Heaton, 1972, 1973a, 1975) at a time of rapid expansion of knowledge about the biochemistry of bile. Inevitably, some aspects of the hypothesis have been proved to be wrong but, overall, it still seems reasonable and no better one has been put forward.

The origin of the hypothesis was the joining of two very different streams of thought, a biochemical and an epidemiological one. Biochemically, there was growing evidence that a major risk factor for the production of bile supersaturated with cholesterol, and hence for cholesterol-rich gallstones, was a small bile acid pool (implying a lack of detergent to keep cholesterol in solution). The small bile acid pool was considered most likely due to a defect in the synthesis of bile acids. The hypothesis coupled this popular theory with two well-established facts from animal research: (1) semi-synthetic diets rich in fibre-depleted carbohydrate suppress the liver synthesis of bile acids

289

Dietary Fibre, Fibre-Depleted Foods
and Disease

and lead to shrinkage of the bile acid pool (Portman and Murphy, 1958; Hellström *et al.*, 1962; Gustafsson and Norman, 1969; Redinger, *et al.*, 1973); and (2) similar diets had been used, often but not always, with added fat and cholesterol, to induce cholesterol-rich gallstones in a variety of rodents (Dam and Christensen, 1952; Hikasa *et al.*, 1969; Tepperman *et al.*, 1964; Brenneman *et al.*, 1972; Borgman and Haselden, 1968) and also in a primate, the squirrel monkey (Osuga and Portman, 1971).

Hence, it was proposed that, in susceptible humans, consumption of fibre-depleted food leads to impaired bile acid synthesis and shrinkage of the bile acid pool and thus to a relative excess of cholesterol in the gallbladder. The mechanism was speculated to be excessive absorption from the colon of a toxic bacterial metabolite of bile acids, lithocholic acid. Lithocholic acid was known to be a powerful suppressor of bile acid synthesis (and of other hepatic functions) and its physicochemical properties were such as would cause it to bind to food residues.

The epidemiological stream of thought began with the author's introduction to Cleave's hypothesis (Cleave *et al.*, 1969). Cleave postulated that cholecystitis was one of a range of diseases (collectively called the Saccharine disease) which modern man had brought upon himself by his technological skill in refining carbohydrate, i.e. in separating sugars and starches from the fibrous matrix or wrapping in which they were formed. The author was impressed by Cleave's arguments, which blamed obesity and diabetes on refined carbohydrate and was intrigued by his claims that gallstones were closely associated with these two diseases and that all three were rare in primitive communities. These claims were tested and, broadly, vindicated in a thorough review of published work on the epidemiology of gallstones (Heaton, 1973a), though the evidence was patchy. The fact that Cleave held to the discredited view of gallstones as secondary to cholecystitis was unimportant and, in fact, he later accepted the modern view of gallstones as a metabolic disease (Cleave, 1974).

Thus, the unifying hypothesis proposed in the early 1970s is shown in Fig. 17.1.

The remainder of this chapter traces the development of knowledge and ideas relevant to this hypothesis and indicates how it has been modified. The term *fibre-depleted foods* is used in place of refined carbohydrates, as explained in Chapter 2.

II.   Fibre-depleted foods and surplus energy intake

The idea that the eater of fibre-depleted foods unwittingly inflates his energy intake was proposed by Cleave (Cleave and Campbell, 1966) and developed by Heaton with more emphasis on the satiating properties of dietary fibre, especially in its intact, chewy form (Heaton, 1973b, 1980). The satiating

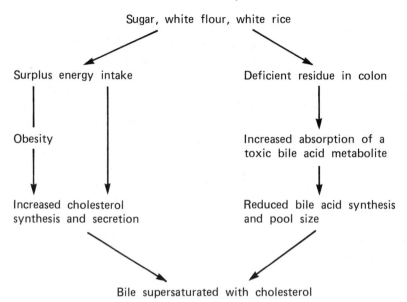

FIG. 17.1. The unifying hypothesis proposed in the early 1970s.

effect of the fibre in fruit has been demonstrated using apples (Haber *et al.,* 1977), oranges and grapes (Bolton *et al.,* 1981). The cereal fibre in whole-meal bread was shown to have a satiating effect in one study (Grimes and Gordon, 1978) but not in another (Bryson *et al.,* 1980). More importantly, it was found that when fibre-depleted foods were eaten in normally consumed amounts over a 6-week period, energy intake was 28% higher than when fibre-depleted foods were excluded but unrefined foods were allowed ad libitum (Heaton *et al.,* 1983). The extra energy provided by the fibre-depleted foods was almost entirely attributable to the sugar in the diet.

III. Energy intake of gallstone patients and gallstone-prone populations

In 1957, 1963 and 1967, Sarles' group in Marseilles carried out three surveys of the eating habits of gallstone patients and of matched healthy controls. All three studies showed the gallstone patients to have a higher intake of energy (Sarles *et al.,* 1970). In 1978, a fourth survey by the same group failed to show a significant difference, though a similar trend was apparent (Sarles *et al.,* 1978b). Similarly, in Melbourne, Wheeler *et al.* (1970) found no difference in energy intake but the controls were hospital patients. In Edmonton, Smith and Gee (1979) actually found, by 48-h dietary recall, that 76 female gallstone patients claimed to take in less energy than controls. This could be related to the fact that the patients were interviewed quite soon after cholecystectomy, but most denied altering their food habits. Intake of fibre (estimated as crude fibre) was low, but so too were intakes of protein and fat.

Asymptomatic people unaware that they have gallstones are presumably the best ones to study, and Williams and Johnston (1980) identified 20 such people in a small town in Nova Scotia by doing a cholecystographic survey. There were no differences in dietary intake between them and stone-free controls except that their energy intake varied less from day to day. The same workers made a parallel observation in 46 Indian women who provided bile samples and dietary records; there was a weak but significant inverse correlation between the cholesterol content of bile and the range of calorie intakes over 4 days (Williams et al., 1981). The authors could not explain why a lack of variation in energy intake should predispose to gallstones. In the 13 Indian women who had gallstones, there was stated to be a correlation between cholesterol concentration in bile and the daily intake of carbohydrate. Unfortunately, no data were given and the type of carbohydrate was not specified, but these Indians are known to be large consumers of refined carbohydrate (Johnston et al., 1977).

Is there a correlation between liability to gallstones and energy intake on a national level? Sarles and his colleagues (1978a) sought to answer this question by comparing the autopsy prevalence of gallstones with food intake data for France, Portugal, Sweden, India, Japan, Uganda and South Africa. There was a good correlation up to an intake of 3000 kcal/day, but not thereafter.

Case–control studies have inherent limitations. When a whole population is exposed to a pathogenic agent, the decisive factor in expression of disease may be susceptibility to the agent rather than level of exposure to the agent. Obese people do not consume more energy than the rest of the population— in some studies they consume less (Keen et al., 1979). Nevertheless, it is undeniable that obesity is due to people consuming more energy than they need. Perhaps the same is true of people with cholesterol-rich gallstones. The data are consistent with this possibility.

IV.   Energy intake and bile composition

Does energy intake affect the cholesterol saturation of bile independently of its effect on body fatness? Sarles et al. (1968) found a correlation between the cholesterol concentration of T-tube bile and the average energy intake of 13 patients with gallstones in experiments lasting 3–37 days, but the studies were performed in an unphysiological setting. Werner et al. (1984) found no difference in the cholesterol saturation of bile nor in the secretion rate of cholesterol in 12 gallstone patients after 6 weeks on a high-sucrose diet and after 6 weeks on a low-sucrose diet although energy intake was 370 kcal (1.55 MJ) higher on the high-sugar diet. Bennion and Grundy (1975) fed a very high-energy diet to two slim men for one month; their weight rose but only by 3 kg. One man responded to excessive energy intake with increased cholesterol secretion, the other did not. Obviously, more data are needed but it seems unlikely that, in the short term, small changes in energy intake have any important effect on bile composition.

V.   Body fatness as a risk factor

The age-old clinical impression that gallstone patients tend to be fat has been confirmed by numerous surveys, in both living and autopsied subjects. Obesity predisposes to gallstones because it leads to increased secretion of cholesterol into bile (Bennion and Grundy, 1975; Shaffer and Small, 1977). There is a significant correlation between the cholesterol saturation of gallbladder bile and indices of body fatness throughout the whole range of body weight (Bennion et al., 1978; Duane and Hanson, 1978; Haber and Heaton, 1979) and fat people have supersaturated bile even if their plasma lipids are normal (Angelin et al., 1981).

The increased biliary secretion of cholesterol in obesity is probably due to increased hepatic synthesis of cholesterol. Certainly, total body synthesis of cholesterol is increased in proportion to body fatness (Miettinen, 1971; Nestel et al., 1973; Leijd, 1980) and it has recently been found that there is increased activity of the rate-limiting enzyme in cholesterol biosynthesis, HMGCoA reductase, in the livers of obese patients (Angelin et al., 1981).

However, obesity does not explain all cholesterol-rich gallstones. In the first place, by no means are all gallstone patients obese and a few are really slim. Second, obese people do not necessarily have supersaturated bile. Certainly, in Western countries almost all obese people have supersaturated bile. However, in a study of bile from obese, middle-aged African women from rural Zimbabwe it was found that bile was unsaturated in 9 out of 10 women (Heaton et al., 1977). Similarly, bile was usually unsaturated in obese Polynesian women on a remote Tongan island (Stace et al., 1981). These findings agree with the well-documented rarity of gallstones in rural Third World communities (Burkitt and Tunstall, 1975), despite the commonness of obesity in middle-aged women in many such communities. This discrepancy is unexplained but it may be relevant that fibre intake is very high in Tonga and rural Zimbabwe. Fat intake is low, but the level of fat intake seems not to affect bile saturation (Sarles et al., 1970).

VI.   Other clinical associations

After obesity, the best documented association of gallstones is *hypertriglyceridaemia*. Gallstone patients have higher fasting serum triglyceride levels than controls (Bell *et al.*, 1973; Kadziolka *et al.*, 1977) even if they are matched for body fatness. Conversely, people with fasting hypertriglyceridaemia have a high prevalence of gallstones (Ahlberg *et al.*, 1979) and their bile is usually supersaturated with cholesterol (Ahlberg *et al.*, 1980). Even within the normal range of plasma triglycerides, there is a relationship between the plasma triglyceride concentration and the cholesterol saturation of bile (Thornton *et al.*, 1981). It is well known that the plasma triglyceride concentration varies with the intake of carbohydrate, unless it is fibre-rich. In some people plasma triglyceride is very sensitive to the intake of sucrose (Reiser *et al.*, 1978).

Whether *coronary heart disease* and gallstones are significantly associated with each other is still a moot point, but on balance the evidence is in favour (Heaton, 1973a) and is strongest in middle-aged women. In a California survey of 16,000 women under 55 years, myocardial infarction was reported in 26. Of these, 9 gave a history of gallbladder disease, which was 6.6 times higher than the expected number (Petitti *et al.*, 1979). The link between the two diseases could be a low plasma concentration of high-density lipoprotein. Californian women with a low HDL cholesterol level were more likely to report having had gallstones (Petitti *et al.*, 1981) while in Bristol women an inverse correlation was found between plasma HDL cholesterol and bile cholesterol saturation (Thornton *et al.*, 1981). These findings are consistent with the accepted role of HDL as a carrier of cholesterol from the tissues to the liver for excretion. In a discordant and puzzling paper, Barker *et al.* (1979) reported that in nine British towns, there was in men an inverse correlation between gallstones prevalence and mortality from ischaemic heart disease. Perhaps men and women behave differently in this respect.

An association with *diabetes* is well documented from autopsy studies (Heaton, 1973a) but it is not clear whether it is diabetes itself or the often associated obesity which increases the risk of gallstones. In a study where the non-diabetic controls were carefully matched for body fatness as well as for age and sex, there was no difference between them and the diabetics in the cholesterol saturation of bile (Haber and Heaton, 1979). In another study, bile was just as supersaturated in non-obese as in obese type 2 diabetics (Ponz de Leon *et al.*, 1978). However, both studies agreed that type 1 (insulin-dependent) diabetics have unsaturated bile.

The well-known Saint's triad of gallstones, hiatal hernia and diverticular disease is unsupported by statistical evidence. However, patients with *hiatal hernia* have twice the expected prevalence of gallstones and their gallbladder bile is unexpectedly rich in cholesterol (Capron *et al.*, 1978). Since there is no obvious mechanism whereby hiatal hernia could cause gallstones, or vice versa, these findings suggest that there is a common factor in the aetiology or pathogenesis of the two diseases. It has been proposed that hiatal herniation results from straining at stool (Burkitt and James, 1973) and such straining does cause an appropriate pressure gradient between abdomen and thorax (Fedail *et al.*, 1979). However, a connection between constipation and gallstones, though possible, is highly speculative.

An association between gallstones and *diverticular disease of the colon* has been reported by Capron *et al.* (1981). Of 102 patients with diverticular disease, 45% had gallstones on oral cholecystography, compared with 22% of closely matched controls. However, in an autopsy series there was no association between the two diseases (Eide and Stalsberg, 1979). A link with diverticular disease would, of course, suggest that a low-residue diet is a causative factor for gallstones.

Recently, a link with *cancer* has been reported. Lowenfels (1981) compared the age-adjusted autopsy prevalence of gallstones with the age-adjusted mortality from cancer in 15 countries and found a significant correlation, especially with uterine cancer ($r = 0.92$) and large bowel cancer ($r = 0.73$ in women, 0.63 in men). Even more strikingly, Lowenfels *et al.* (1982) found that Swedish women who had died of cancer under the age of 50 had 2.2 times the expected prevalence of gallstones, and the relative risk rose to 3.3 for the "diet-related cancers" (gut, breast and reproductive organs). A plausible but unproven explanation for these findings is that obesity predisposes to these cancers as well as to gallstones.

VII.   Small bile acid pool as a risk factor

It is generally accepted that in the non-obese gallstone patient the circulating bile acid pool is reduced from its normal mean of 3 g to 1.5/2.0 g and that the consequent lack of detergent to keep cholesterol in solution contributes to the supersaturation of bile in the gallbladder. However, the origin of the small pool is uncertain and no evidence has yet been put forward to support the hypothesis that it has a dietary origin. On the contrary, the theory has gained ground that the size of the bile acid pool depends on how often it circulates in 24 h, on the basis that the level of feedback inhibition of bile acid synthesis and thus the pool size is determined by the bile acid concentration in portal blood returning to the liver (Low-Beer and Pomare, 1973). The chief delaying factor in the enterohepatic circulation is the storage of bile in the gallbladder. Hence, the frequency of bile acid circulation depends chiefly on the rate and completeness of gallbladder emptying. Duane and Hanson (1978) found that, in normal men, there is a significant correlation between the gallbladder emptying time and the size of the bile acid pool and Maudgal *et al.* (1980) showed that, in patients with presumed cholesterol gallstones, the gallbladder empties faster in response to a test meal than in matched controls. It is unclear why the gallbladder should empty faster because it contains gallstones and it seems more likely that rapid emptying came first. Is rapid emptying an abnormality or just a variant of normal and, if it is an abnormality, is it congenital or acquired? No answer can be given to these questions at the present time.

The same difficulties of interpretation apply to the finding that the bile acid pool size correlates with the small bowel transit time (Duane and Hanson, 1978). Nevertheless, the idea that faster small bowell transit can speed up the enterohepatic circulation and so contribute to a smaller bile acid pool is logical and it is supported by experimental evidence. When small bowel transit was speeded up by feeding the unabsorbed carbohydrate sorbitol, there was a fall in the bile acid pool and a slight rise in the cholesterol saturation of bile (Duane, 1978), whereas when small bowel transit was slowed down by administering the anticholinergic drug propantheline bromide, there was a rise in the bile acid pool (Duane and Bond, 1980).

There are several difficulties in accepting the concept that recycling time determines bile acid pool size and that this in turn determines the cholesterol saturation of bile. First, it is controversial whether the size of the bile acid pool is, indeed, a determinant of cholesterol saturation (Valdivieso et al., 1979). Second, when the pool was expanded by propantheline treatment, there was no fall in saturation (Duane and Bond, 1980). Third, the small bile acid pool of gallstone patients tends to contain excessive amounts of the secondary bile acid, deoxycholate (Pomare and Heaton, 1973a), whereas the small pool associated with rapid small bowel transit contains subnormal amounts of deoxycholate (Duane and Hanson, 1978; Duane, 1978). Fourth, when the overnight storage of bile in the gallbladder was measured, no difference was found between gallstone patients and controls (van Berge Henegouwen and Hofmann, 1978). Finally, the difference in gallbladder emptying rates between gallstone patients and controls is small compared to the difference in bile acid pool size.

When to the above uncertainties is added the fact that, to date, no dietary manipulation has succeeded in altering the size of the bile acid pool in man, one is driven to suspect that further studies of the bile acid pool size are unlikely to throw light on the aetiology of human gallstones.

However, the composition of the bile acid pool is certainly important in determining the cholesterol saturation of bile and this can be altered by dietary fibre.

VIII.   Deoxycholic acid, bile cholesterol saturation and dietary fibre

The original hypothesis that lack of dietary fibre could lead to over-absorption of lithocholic acid and hence to shrinkage of the bile acid pool has been discarded. While the hypothesis has not been tested directly, evidence has accumulated to exonerate lithocholic acid from having toxic effects in man.

On the other hand, there is now much evidence that the proportion of deoxycholic acid in the bile acid pool is an important factor that determines the cholesterol saturation of bile, probably by an effect on cholesterol secretion. Deoxycholic acid is a secondary bile acid, formed in the colon by bacterial dehydroxylation of the primary bile acid cholic acid (lithocholic acid is the equivalent bacterial metabolite of chenodeoxycholic acid). About 30 to 50% of deoxycholic acid is absorbed and, after conjugation with glycine or taurine, it is secreted into bile and recirculated alongside the primary bile acids. The normal composition of the bile acid pool is about 45% cholic acid, 35% chenodeoxycholic acid and 20% deoxycholic acid.

The deoxycholic acid pool can be *expanded* within physiological limits either by feeding small amounts (100–150 mg daily) of deoxycholic acid itself or, in some people, by feeding its precursor, cholic acid. When these manoeuvres have been done in normal people and in gallstone patients, respectively, their bile has become more saturated with cholesterol (Low-Beer and Pomare, 1975; Carulli *et al.*, 1981). In the gallstone patients, the cholesterol saturation index rose from 1.07 to 1.42 despite an increase in the total bile acid pool from 2.6 to 4.1 g (Carulli *et al.*, 1981). Feeding large amounts (750 mg or more daily) of deoxycholic acid does not have this effect (LaRusso *et al.*, 1977; Ahlberg *et al.*, 1977; Carulli *et al.*, 1980), possibly because in high concentration deoxycholic acid is toxic to the small bowel mucosa and impairs cholesterol absorption.

The deoxycholic acid pool can be *contracted* by several manoeuvres—by administering antibacterial drugs, by giving lactulose and by feeding bran (Table 17.1). Metronidazole and ampicillin act presumably by reducing the number of anaerobic bacteria in the colon capable of dehydroxylating cholic acid. Lactulose is thought to act by reducing the pH of the colonic contents,

TABLE 17.1. Methods and effects of reducing biliary deoxycholate

Agents	Subjects	Deoxycholic acid % of biliary bile acids		Cholesterol saturation index of "gallbladder bile"		Reference
		Control	Agent	Control	Agent	
Metronidazole	Normal men	24.0	6.6	1.00	0.83	Low-Beer and Nutter (1978)
Ampicillin	Gallstone patients	24.0	5.4	1.25	0.95	Carulli *et al.* (1981)
Lactulose	Overweight women	28.4	15.6	1.40	1.19	Thornton and Heaton (1981)
Wheat bran	Gallstone patients	27.1	13.8	1.49	1.29	Pomare and Heaton (1973b); Pomare *et al.* (1976)
	Gallstone patients	32.0	22.9	1.39	0.72	McDougall *et al.* (1977)
	Normal women	25.6	19.2	1.36	0.94	Watts *et al.* (1978)
	Normal young men	22.7	16.5	0.56	0.62	Wicks *et al.* (1978)

which inhibits the bacterial enzyme 7α-dehydroxylase. The mode of action of bran is uncertain. It could act by reducing colonic pH since a proportion of bran is metabolised to acids, the volatile fatty acids, and bran has been shown to lower the caecal pH in rats (Jacobs and Lupton, 1982). Alternatively, it could bind deoxycholic acid and thus prevent its absorption from the colon. A binding mechanism is rendered less likely by the fact that, in man, bran takes several weeks to show an effect on bile (Wicks *et al.*, 1978).

Every manoeuvre which reduces biliary deoxycholate also reduces the cholesterol saturation of bile-rich fluid aspirated from the duodenum after cholecystokinin injection; this fluid closely approximates to gallbladder bile in its lipid composition (Table 17.1). This presumably suggests a common mode of action. One possibility is that deoxycholic acid, whose detergent properties are superior to those of any other bile acid, leaches out excessive amounts of cholesterol from the liver cell membrane that lines the bile canaliculus. Another possibility is that deoxycholic acid stimulates the synthesis of cholesterol in the liver cell. This is less likely since feeding deoxycholic acid tends to lower both the serum cholesterol concentration and, when it has been measured, the liver cell activity of HMGCoA reductase (Carulli *et al.*, 1980). A third possibility is that deoxycholic acid selectively suppresses the synthesis of chenodeoxycholic acid and reduces its circulating pool. This selective suppressive effect has been shown in only four subjects (Pomare and Low-Beer, 1975), and could not be duplicated with supra-physiological doses (LaRusso *et al.*, 1977), but it is an attractive idea because of the well-known ability of chenodeoxycholic acid to suppress cholesterol secretion and render bile less saturated (Northfield *et al.*, 1975). It is also attractive because in most studies with bran, and in the metronidazole and lactulose studies, the fall in biliary deoxycholate was balanced by a rise in biliary chenodeoxycholate. However, this did not happen in the ampicillin study, nor in one bran study (Watts *et al.*, 1978). At present the deleterious effect of deoxycholic acid on bile remains unexplained.

The beneficial effect of bran on the cholesterol saturation of bile has been found in all appropriately designed studies (Fig. 17.2). To show benefit from a natural, physiological material it is presumably necessary that the subjects to be studied are not already normal. On this basis, there is no difficulty in explaining why bran feeding had no effect in two studies in which the subjects were healthy young people—their bile was already unsaturated (Wicks *et al.*, 1978; Huijbregts *et al.*, 1980b). It is, however, anomalous that in one of these studies an initially low level of biliary deoxycholate actually increased (Huijbregts *et al.*, 1980b).

Other anomalous findings are the reports of unsaturated bile in the face of quite high deoxycholate levels in the bile of rural African women eating large amounts of unrefined maize (Heaton *et al.*, 1977) and of very high deoxycholate levels in rural Tongans eating large amounts of fruit and root vegetables

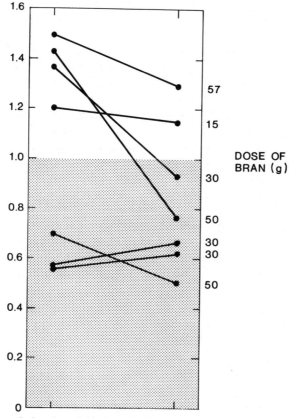

FIG. 17.2. Effect of wheat bran (g/day) on the cholesterol saturation index of bile; mean values
from all published reports (shaded area indicates unsaturated bile).

(Stace *et al.*, 1981), and also of increased dehydroxylation of cholic acid in
Dutch vegetarians (Huijbregts *et al.*, 1980a). Perhaps different kinds of dietary fibre have different effects on bile acid metabolism in the colon. There
is a remarkable lack of studies on sources of fibre other than bran and their
effect on bile acid metabolism and bile composition.

IX. Animal studies

There is no animal model that accurately reproduces the human disease of
cholelithiasis. However, cholesterol-rich gallstones have been induced by
giving artificial diets to hamsters, mice, prairie dogs, rabbits and squirrel
monkeys. Heaton (1975) has pointed out that, although the experimental
diets have varied greatly, they have one feature in common—they are all

semi-synthetic or semi-purified. In practice, this means that their carbohydrate component is always in refined or fibre-depleted form, usually glucose or sucrose, but sometimes cornstarch. An exception to this rule is a gerbil model in which cholesterol stones form on ordinary, unrefined chow, but this is achieved only by adding to the chow such large amounts of cholesterol that the liver becomes stuffed and swollen with it (Bergman and van der Linden, 1971).

The idea that lack of fibre explains the lithogenicity of these diets is supported by two observations. First, in the hamster, the diet loses its lithogenic effect if it is supplemented with bulking agents such as agar and carboxymethyl cellulose, or even if the animal is allowed to eat the straw laid on the floor of its cage (Hikasa et al., 1969). Second, in the rabbit, stones dissolve rapidly if ordinary chow is fed.

There have been few relevant studies of diet-induced gallstones in recent years. Addition of 5% lignin reduces the lithogenic effect of a diet deficient in essential fatty acids in hamsters and when lactulose was added the lithogenic effect disappeared (Rotstein et al., 1981). However, lignin increased faecal bile acids fivefold, whereas in man dietary fibre has little if any effect on faecal bile acids.

X.   Effect of fibre-depleted foods in man

The crucial experiment of comparing bile composition on diets of fibre-depleted and full-fibre foods has recently been reported from Heaton's laboratory (Thornton et al., 1983). Thirteen women with asymptomatic, radiolucent gallstones were studied after 6 weeks on a diet containing frequently consumed amounts of refined sugar and fibre-depleted starch, then subsequently after 6 weeks on a diet devoid of these products but with free access to all lightly processed full-fibre foods. The cholesterol saturation index of bile was 1.50 on the fibre-depleted foods diet and 1.20 on the full-fibre foods. It was lower on the full-fibre foods in all but one subject (who ate immoderately of nuts and gained weight). This clearly indicated that fibre-depleted foods are a risk factor for gallstones. The mechanism is unclear. Bile acid pool size was unchanged so presumably there was a change in cholesterol secretion. Weight fell on the full-fibre foods and rose on the fibre-depleted foods but the changes were too small (1.6 kg) to explain the biliary changes. The difference in energy intake was substantial (480 kcal or 1.92 MJ/day), and this may have been relevant. However, in a subsequent and similarly designed study in which only sucrose, and hence energy, varied, there was no change in bile saturation (Werner et al., 1984). Dietary fibre intake was higher on the full-fibre foods (27 vs. 14 g/day) but there was only a slight fall in biliary deoxycholate.

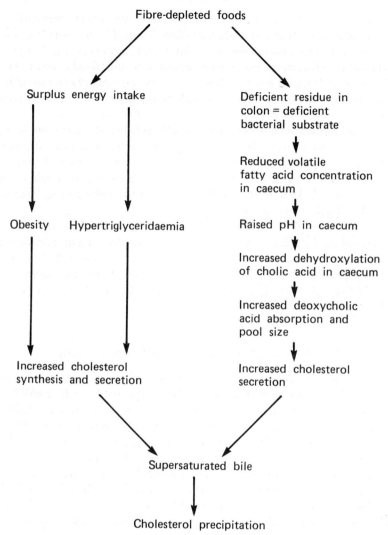

Fibre-depleted foods

Surplus energy intake

Deficient residue in
colon = deficient
bacterial substrate

Reduced volatile
fatty acid concentration
in caecum

Obesity   Hypertriglyceridaemia

Raised pH in caecum

Increased dehydroxylation
of cholic acid in caecum

Increased deoxycholic
acid absorption and
pool size

Increased cholesterol
synthesis and secretion

Increased cholesterol
secretion

Supersaturated bile

Cholesterol precipitation

FIG. 17.3. Suggested working hypothesis of aetiology of gallstones.

XI.   Summary

The refined-carbohydrate hypothesis, now called the fibre-depleted foods
hypothesis for human gallstones, first proposed in 1972, has had to be modified but remains valid. It has not been possible to show that the size of the
bile acid pool varies significantly with changes in the diet. A small pool may
not even be an acquired defect but rather a constitutional trait which confers
susceptibility to a rise in cholesterol secretion by the liver. However, numer-

ous studies point to a raised level of biliary deoxycholate as a risk factor and this can undoubtedly be lowered by feeding bran. Obesity, and possibly a high energy intake without obesity, is the most important risk factor for gallstones, and fibre-depleted sugars are certainly liable to inflate energy intake. In patients with gallstones, avoidance of fibre-depleted carbohydrate foods consistently leads to a fall in the cholesterol saturation of bile. A suggested working hypothesis for the aetiology of gallstones is shown in Fig. 17.3. (For a comprehensive review of diet and gallstones, see Heaton, 1984).

References

AHLBERG, J., ANGELIN, B., EINARSSON, K., HELLSTRÖM, K. and LEIJD, B. (1977). *Clin. Sci. Mol. Med.* **53,** 249–256.

AHLBERG, J., ANGELIN, B., EINARSSON, K., HELLSTRÖM, K. and LEIJD, B. (1979). *Dig. Dis. Sci.* **24,** 459–464.

AHLBERG, J., ANGELIN, B., EINARSSON, K., HELLSTRÖM, K. and LEIJD, B. (1980). *Gastroenterology* **79,** 90–94.

ANGELIN, B., EINARSSON, K., EWERTH, S. and LEIJD, B. (1981). *Scand. J. Gastroenterol.* **16,** 1015–1019.

BARKER, D. J. P. , GARDNER, M. J., POWER, C. and HUTT, M. S. R. (1979). *Br. Med. J.* **2,** 1389–1392.

BELL, G. D., LEWIS, B., PETRIE, A. and DOWLING, R. H. (1973). *Br. Med. J.* **3,** 520–523.

BENNION, L. J. and GRUNDY, S. M. (1975). *J. Clin. Invest.* **56,** 996–1011.

BENNION, L. J., DROBNY, E., KNOWLER, W. C., GINSBERG, R. L., GARNICK, M. B., ADLER, R. D. and DUANE, W. C. (1978). *Metab. Clin. Exp.* **27,** 961–969.

BERGMAN, F. and VAN DER LINDEN, W. (1971). *Acta Pathol. Microbiol. Scand.* **79,** 476–486.

BOLTON, R. P., HEATON, K. W. and BURROUGHS, L. F. (1981). *Am. J. Clin. Nutr.* **34,** 211–217.

BORGMAN, R. F. and HASELDEN, F. H. (1968). *Am. J. Vet. Res.* **29,** 1287–1292.

BRENNEMAN, D. E., CONNOR, W. E., FORKER, E. L. and DENBESTEN, L. (1972). *J. Clin. Invest.* **51,** 1495–1503.

BRYSON, E., DORE, C. and GARROW, J. S. (1980). *J. Hum. Nutr.* **34,** 113–116.

BURKITT, D. P. and JAMES, P. A. (1973). *Lancet* **2,** 128–130.

BURKITT, D. P. and TUNSTALL, M. (1975). *J. Trop. Med. Hyg.* **78,** 140–144.

CAPRON, J-P., PAYENNEVILLE, H., DUMONT, M., DUPAS, J.-L. and LORRIAUX, A. (1978). *Lancet* **2,** 329–331.

CARULLI, N., PONZ DE LEON, M., ZIRONI, F., IORI, R. and LORIA, P. *(1980).* *Gastroenterology* **79,** 637–641.

CARULLI, N., PONZ DE LEON, M., LORIA, P., IORI, R., ROSI, A. and ROMANI, M. (1981). *Gastroenterology* **81,** 539–546.

CAPRON, J. P., PIPERAUD, R., DUPAS, J.-L., DELAMARRE, J. and LORRIAUX, A. (1981). *Dig. Dis. Sci.* **26,** 523–527.

CLEAVE, T. L. (1974). *"The Saccharine Disease".* John Wright, Bristol.

CLEAVE, T. L. and CAMPBELL, G. D. (1966). "Diabetes, Coronary Thrombosis and the Saccharine Disease." John Wright, Bristol.

CLEAVE, T. L., CAMPBELL, G. D. and PAINTER, N. S. (1969). "Diabetes, Coronary Thrombosis and the Saccharine Disease." 2nd edition. John Wright, Bristol.

DAM, H. and CHRISTENSEN, F. (1952). *Acta Pathol. Microbiol. Scand.* **30,** 236–242.

DUANE, W. C. (1978). *J. Lab. Clin. Med.* **91,** 969–978.

DUANE, W. C. and BOND, J. H. (1980). *Gastroenterology* **78**, 226–230.

DUANE, W. C. and HANSON, K. C. (1978). *J. Lab. Clin. Med.* **92**, 858–872.

EIDE, T. J. and STALSBERG, H. (1979). *Gut* **20**, 609–615.

FEDAIL, S. S., HARVEY, R. F. and BURNS-COX, C. J. (1979). *Br. Med. J.* **1**, 91.

GRIMES, D. A. and GORDON, C. (1978). *Lancet* **2**, 106.

GUSTAFSSON, B. E. and NORMAN, A. (1969). *Br. J. Nutr.* **23**, 627–635.

HABER, G. B. and HEATON, K. W. (1979). *Gut* **20**, 518–522.

HABER, G. B., HEATON, K. W., MURPHY, D. and BURROUGHS, L. (1977). *Lancet* **2**, 679–682.

HEATON, K. W. (1972). "Bile Salts in Health and Disease." Churchill-Livingstone, Edinburgh.

HEATON, K. W. (1973a). *Clin. Gastroenterol.* **2**, 67–83.

HEATON, K. W. (1973b). *Lancet* **2**, 1418–1421.

HEATON, K. W. (1975). *In* "Refined Carbohydrate Foods and Disease: Some Implications of Dietary Fibre" (D. P. Burkitt and H. C. Trowell, eds), pp. 173–194. Academic Press, London.

HEATON, K. W. (1980). *In* "Medical Aspects of Dietary Fiber" (G. A. Spiller and R. M. Kay, eds), pp. 223–238. Plenum, New York.

HEATON, K. W. (1984). *Nutr. Abstr. Rev., Rev. Clin. Nutr.* **54**, 549–560.

HEATON, K. W., WICKS, A. C. B. and YEATES, J. (1977). *In* "Bile Acid Metabolism in Health and Disease" (G. Paumgartner and A. Stiehl, eds), pp. 197–202. M.T.P. Press, Lancaster.

HEATON, K. W., EMMETT, P. M., HENRY, C. L., THORNTON, J. R., MANHIRE, A. and HARTOG, M. (1983). *Hum. Nutr. Clin. Nutr.* **37C**, 31–35.

HELLSTRÖM, K., SJÖVALL, J. and WIGAND, G. (1962). *J. Lipid Res.* **3**, 405–412.

HIKASA, Y., MATSUDA, S., NAGASE, M., YOSHINAGA, M., TOBE, T., MARUYAMA, I., SHIODA, R., TANIMURA, H., MURAOKA, R., MUROYA, H. AND TOGÓ, M. (1969). *Arch. Jpn. Chir.* **38**, 107–124.

HUIJBREGTS, A. W. M., VAN SCHAIK, A., VAN BERGE-HENEGOUWEN, G. P. and VAN DER WERF, S. D. J. (1980a). *Eur. J. Clin. Invest.* **10**, 443–449.

HUIJBREGTS, A. W. M., VAN BERGE-HENEGOUWEN, G. P., HECTORS, M. P. C., VAN SCHAIK, A. and VAN DER WERF, S. D. J. (1980b). *Eur. J. Clin. Invest.* **10**, 451–458.

JACOBS, L. R. and LUPTON, J. R. (1982). *J. Nutr.* **112**, 592–594.

JOHNSTON, J. L., WILLIAMS, C. N. and WELDON, K. L. M. (1977). *Can. Med. Assoc. J.* **116**, 1356–1359.

KADZIOLKA, R., NILSSON, S. and SCHERSTÉN, T. (1977). *Scand J. Gastroenterol.* **12**, 353–355.

KEEN, H., THOMAS, B. J., JARRETT, R. J. and FULLER, J. H. (1979). *Br. Med. J.* **1**, 655–658.

LARUSSO, N. F., SZCZEPANIK, P. A., and HOFMANN, A. F. (1977). *Gastroenterology* **72**, 132–140.

LEIJD, B. (1980). *Clin. Sci.* **59**, 203–206.

LOW-BEER, T. S. and NUTTER, S. (1978). Lancet **2**, 1063–1065.

LOW-BEER, T. S. and POMARE, E. W. (1973). *Br. Med. J.* **2**, 338–340.

LOW-BEER, T. S. and POMARE, E. W. (1975). *Br. Med. J.* **1**, 438–440.

LOWENFELS, A. B. (1981). *Gut* **21**, 1090–1092.

LOWENFELS, A. B., DOMELLÖF, L., LINDSTRÖM, C. G., BERGMAN, F., MONK, M. A. and STERNBY, N. H. (1982). *Gastroenterology* **83**, 672–676.

McDOUGALL, R. M., WALKER, K. and THURSTON, O. G. (1977). *Surg. Forum* **28**, 416–418.

MAUDGAL, D. P., KUPFER, R. M., ZENTLER-MUNRO, P. L. and NORTHFIELD, T. C. (1980). *Br. Med. J.* **1**, 141–143.

MIETTINEN, T. A. (1971). *Circulation* **44**, 842–850.

NESTEL, P. J., SCHREIBMAN, P. H. and AHRENS, E. H. (1973). *J. Clin. Invest.* **52**, 2389–2397.

NORTHFIELD, T. C., LaRUSSO, N. F., HOFMANN, A. F. and THISTLE, J. L. (1975). *Gut* **16**, 12–17.

OSUGA, T. and PORTMAN, O. W. (1971). *Proc. Soc. Exp. Biol. Med.* **136**, 722–726.

PETITTI, D. B., WINGERD, J., PELLEGRIN, F. and RAMCHARAN, S. (1979). *JAMA, J. Am. Med. Assoc.* **242**, 1150–1154.

PETITTI, D. B., FRIEDMAN, G. D. and KLATSKY, A. L. (1981). *N. Engl. J. Med.* **304**, 1396–1398.

POMARE, E. W. and HEATON, K. W. (1973a). *Gut* **14**, 885–890.

POMARE, E. W. and HEATON, K. W. (1973b). *Br. Med. J.* **4**, 262–264.

POMARE, E. W. and LOW-BEER, T. S. (1975). *Clin. Sci. Mol. Med.* **48**, 315–321.

POMARE, E. W., HEATON, K. W., LOW-BEER, T. S. and ESPINER, H. J. (1976). *Am. J. Dig. Dis.* **21**, 521–526.

PONZ DE LEON, M., FERENDERES, R. and CARULLI, N. (1978). *Am. J. Dig. Dis.* **23**, 710–716.

PORTMAN, O. W. and MURPHY, P. (1958). *Arch. Biochem. Biophys.* **76**, 367–376.

REDINGER, R. N., HERMANN, A. H. and SMALL, D. M. (1973). *Gastroenterology* **64**, 610–621.

REISER, S., HALLFRISCH, J., MICHAELES, O. E., LAZAR, F. L., MARTIN, R. E. and PRATHER, E. S. (1978). *Am. J. Clin. Nutr.* **32**, 1659–1669.

ROTSTEIN, O. D., KAY, R. M., WAYMAN, M. and STRASBERG, S. M. (1981). *Gastroenterology* **81**, 1098–1103.

SARLES, H., HAUTON, J., LAFONT, H., TEISSIER, N., PLANCHE, N. E. and GÉROLAMI, A. (1968). *Clin. Chim. Acta* **19**, 147–155.

SARLES, H., HAUTON, J., PLANCHE, N. E., LAFONT, H. and GÉROLAMI, A. (1970). *Am. J. Dig. Dis.* **15**, 251–260.

SARLES, H., GÉROLAMI, A. and CROS, R. C. (1978a). *Digestion* **17**, 121–127.

SARLES, H., GÉROLAMI, A. and BORD, A. (1978b). *Digestion* **17**, 128–134.

SHAFFER, E. A. and SMALL, D. M. (1977). *J. Clin. Invest.* **59**, 828–840.

SMITH, D. A., and GEE, M. I. (1979). *Am. J. Clin. Nutr.* **32**, 1519–1526.

STACE, N. H., POMARE, E. W., PETERS, S., THOMAS, L. and FISHER, A. (1981). *Gastroenterology* **80**, 1291.

TEPPERMAN, J., CALDWELL, F. T. and TEPPERMAN, H. M. (1964). *Am. J. Physiol.* **206**, 628–634.

THORNTON, J. R. and HEATON, K. W. (1981). *Br. Med. J.* **282**, 1018–1020.

THORNTON, J. R., HEATON, K. W. and MACFARLANE, D. G. (1981). *Br. Med. J.* **283**, 1352–1354.

THORNTON, J. R., EMMETT, P. M. and HEATON, K. W. (1983). *Gut* **24**, 2–6.

VALDIVIESO, V., PALMA, R., NERVI, F., COVARRUBIAS, C., SEVERIN, C. and ANTEZANA, C. (1979). *Gut* **20**, 997–1000.

VAN BERGE HENEGOUWEN, G. P. and HOFMANN, A. F. (1978). *Gastroenterology* **75**, 879–885.

WATTS, J. McK., JABLONSKI, P. and TOOULI, J. (1978). *Am. J. Surg.* **135**, 321–324.

WERNER, D., EMMETT, P. M. and HEATON, K. W. (1984). *Gut* **25**, 269–274.

WHEELER, M., HILLS, L. L. and LABY, B. (1970). *Gut* **11**, 430–437.

WICKS, A. C. B., YEATES, J. and HEATON, K. W. (1978). *Scand. J. Gastroenterol.* **13**, 289–292.

WILLIAMS, C. N. and JOHNSTON, J. L. (1980). *Can. Med. Assoc. J.* **122**, 664–668.

WILLIAMS, C. N., JOHNSTON, J. L., McCARTHY, S. and FIELD, C. A. (1981). *Dig. Dis. Sci.* **26**, 42–49.

Chapter 18

Lipid metabolism and coronary heart disease

DAVID KRITCHEVSKY

I. Introduction

There is no unequivocal diagnostic indicator of state or severity of coronary disease. A number of risk factors for coronary disease have been identified in man. The major risk factors are elevated blood pressure, cigarette smoking and elevated serum or plasma cholesterol levels (Kannel *et al.*, 1961), but Hopkins and Williams (1981) have identified 246 factors that play a role in the development of coronary heart disease (CHD). Because of its role as a risk factor and because cholesterol feeding can be atherogenic in some animal species, this sterol has been the focus of research in this area. However, elevated triglyceride levels has also been impugned as metabolic contributors to this disease. In the circulating blood the lipids are present in a series of lipid–protein molecules called lipoproteins. The lipoproteins constitute a family of molecules of varying size, composition and function. They may be identified and separated by a number of techniques and are usually classified by density or electrophoretic mobility. The low-density, cholesterol-rich lipoproteins (β-lipoproteins or LDL) were implicated as important factors in

Dietary Fibre, Fibre-Depleted Foods
and Disease

the development of atherosclerosis over 30 years ago (Gofman *et al.*, 1950). At about the same time, Barr *et al.* (1951) recognized that the protein-rich lipoproteins (α-lipoproteins or HDL) might play a protective role, a concept that was dormant until it was revived by Miller and Miller (1975) and has since assumed a central position in discussion of the prevention and treatment of heart disease.

Results of studies of dietary effects on lipid metabolism are discussed in the light of their possible influence on CHD. In man, the only approach is to measure serum lipids or lipoproteins or lipid metabolism. Studies in experimental animals provide a further endpoint in that the influence of diet on aortic and coronary atherosclerosis can be assessed directly.

II. Carbohydrate effects

Little *et al.* (1979) reviewed data relating to carbohydrate influences on lipidaemia in man and concluded that fructose and sucrose are more lipidaemic than glucose or starch. In rabbits fed semi-purified, cholesterol-free diets containing 40% carbohydrate, fructose and sucrose were more cholesterolaemic and atherogenic than starch, glucose or lactose (Kritchevsky *et al.*, 1968, 1973). The addition of cholesterol to a lactose-containing diet renders it very atherogenic for rabbits (Wells and Anderson, 1959). Different carbohydrates have no special influence on lipidaemia in spider monkeys fed a diet high in safflower oil but when the diet contains coconut oil sucrose is more lipidaemic than either starch or glucose (Corey *et al.*, 1974). Lang and Barthel (1972) found that carbohydrate effect is a function of the species of monkey used. They fed ringtail monkeys, rhesus monkeys and stumptailed macaques diets containing 0.5% cholesterol and 66% sucrose or dextrin. There were no differences in the stumptailed macaques. Dextrin was more cholesterolaemic and atherogenic than sucrose in the rhesus monkeys and more atherogenic but not more cholesterolaemic in the ringtailed monkeys. Vervet monkeys were fed semi-purified diets containing fructose, sucrose or glucose for 6 months. Monkeys fed the fructose diet exhibited significantly more aortic sudanophilia and several had atherosclerotic lesions (Kritchevsky *et al.*, 1974a).

Baboons were fed semi-purified diets containing 40% fructose, sucrose, starch or glucose for 1 year (Kritchevsky *et al.*, 1974b). Cholesterol levels were similar in all four groups but compared with controls triglyceride levels were elevated by 65% and 49% in baboons fed fructose and sucrose, respectively, and by 36% in baboons fed the other two carbohydrates. Aortic sudanophilia (%) ranged from 11.2 in the fructose-fed animals to 6.2 in those fed glucose. In a second study (Kritchevsky *et al.*, 1980), a lactose-fed group was added and the diets contained 0.1% cholesterol. There were no striking differences in cholesterol level among the test groups and the baboons fed fructose exhibited the highest triglyceride levels. Baboons fed fructose plus 0.1% cholesterol did not exhibit more severe sudanophilia than when the diet was cholesterol-free, but three of six animals displayed atherosclerotic lesions. Sudanophilia and atherosclerosis were most severe in the baboons fed lactose. In view of the small differences in serum cholesterol and lipoprotein levels, the reason for the differences in atherogenicity must be sought elsewhere, possibly in the level and composition of aortic glycosaminoglycans.

III. Fibre

A. Rats

The influence of dietary fibre on serum lipids in animals and man has been the subject of recent reviews (Kay and Truswell, 1980; Story and Kelley, 1982). Wells and Ershoff (1961) fed rats a basal diet containing 1% cholesterol and observed a modest increase in serum cholesterol levels and a 10-fold increase in the level of liver cholesterol. Addition of 5% pectin to the diet reduced serum cholesterol level from 131 to 106 mg/dl and liver cholesterol from 24.7 to 11.2 mg/g. Guar or locust bean gums or pectin from various sources also reduced liver cholesterol levels (Ershoff and Wells, 1962), as did alfalfa and lignin (Kritchevsky et al., 1975b; Story et al., 1981). Cellulose, agar, pectic and alginic acids actually increased liver cholesterol levels under these experimental conditions (Wells and Ershoff, 1961; Kiriyama et al., 1969; Story et al., 1981).

Chen and Anderson (1979a) fed rats a diet containing 1% cholesterol, 0.2% cholic acid and 10% of cellulose, pectin, guar gum or oat bran. Levels of plasma total cholesterol (mg/dl) and plasma HDL cholesterol (mg/dl) were: cellulose, 133 and 18; pectin, 84 and 26; guar gum, 105 and 31; and oat bran, 113 and 25. In a second study, Chen and Anderson (1979b) compared cellulose, wheat bran and guar gum and found that bran had no effect on plasma total, cholesterol HDL or liver cholesterol; guar decreased plasma and liver cholesterol levels and raised plasma HDL-cholesterol levels significantly.

B. Rabbits

Lambert et al. (1958) found that they could induce atherosclerosis in rabbits by feeding a cholesterol-free diet containing 20% coconut oil for 3 months. Malmros and Wigand (1959) reported that 8% of butter fat, coconut oil or trilaurin were sufficient to render a diet atherogenic for rabbits. Other workers did not find these fats to be atherogenic. Collation of the literature (Kritchevsky, 1964) revealed that addition of hydrogenated cottonseed oil,

TABLE 18.1. Effect of commercial ration components on serum lipids and atherosclerosis in rabbits[a]
(fed for 6 months)

Regimen	No.	Serum lipids (mg/dl ± SEM)		Serum, HDL/LDL cholesterol	Average atherosclerosis[c] (arch + thoracic/2)
		Cholesterol	Triglyceride		
SP[b]	11	207 ± 36	79	0.15	0.85
SP + RF	12	249 ± 41	64	0.24	0.90
RE + HCNO	7	64 ± 9	21	0.24	0.40
CR + HCNO	14	35 ± 2	24	0.37	0.25
CR	6	40 ± 9	23	0.37	0.15

[a] After Kritchevsky and Tepper, 1965, 1968.
[b] Semi-purified diet (SP): 40% sucrose, 25% casein, 14% hydrogenated coconut oil (HCNO), 15% cellulose, 5% salt mix, 1% vitamin mix. SP + RF: SP containing 12% HCNO and 2% of fat extract from commercial ration (RF). RE + HCNO: Residue (RE) from lipid extraction of commercial ration (85%), HCNO (14%). CR + HCNO: Commercial ration (88%) + HCNO (12%). CR: Commercial ration.
[c] Graded on 0–4 scale.

cream or coconut oil (HCNO) to stock diet were neither hyperlipidaemic nor atherogenic, whereas addition of saturated fat to a semi-purified diet rendered it atherogenic. Since the dietary fat was similar in the two types of diet, some other component was assumed to determine the atherogenic response. The most obvious candidate was the dietary fibre.

Most commercial rabbit ration contains about 2 to 4% unsaturated fat (iodine value about 115) and an experiment was designed to determine if this, rather than fibre, was the protective factor in commercial ration. Groups of rabbits were fed one of the following five diets (Table 18.1): (1) Semi-purified diet (SP) containing 14% HCNO and 15% cellulose; (2) SP diet containing 12% HCNO and 2% fat (RF) extracted from the commercial ration (CR); (3) the residue (RE) from lipid extraction of the ration (CR) 85%, 1% vitamin mix and 14% HCNO; (4) CR plus 12% HCNO; and (5) CR alone (Kritchevsky and Tepper, 1965, 1968). It is evident that the addition of 2% of unsaturated fat did not inhibit cholesterolaemia or atherosclerosis but the delipidized ration residue did. The residue was of plant origin and contained carbohydrates and fibre.

Moore (1967) compared the effects of several types of fibre in rabbits fed a semi-purified diet containing either 20% corn oil or 20% butter oil. The fibre was fed as 19% of the diet. In the corn oil study the fibres used were wheat straw, cellulose and cellophane. Serum cholesterol levels (mg/dl) and degree of atherosclerosis (%) were: wheat straw, 23 and 0.7; cellulose, 61 and 1.3; and cellophane, 71 and 5.0. A fourth fibre (cellophane-peat 14:5) was added for the experiment involving butter. Serum cholesterol levels in the four groups were: wheat straw, 114; cellulose, 133; cellophane, 216; and cellophane peat, 141. Degree of atherosclerosis were 13 for the rabbits fed wheat straw; 21 for those fed cellulose; 38 in the cellophane group; and 11 in rabbits ingesting the cellophane-peat mixture.

Cookson *et al.* (1967) fed rabbits calf meal (CM) or a 9:1 mixture of alfalfa and calf meal (ACM) together with 600 mg of cholesterol daily. After 10 weeks the average serum cholesterol level of rabbits fed CM were 1345 ± 212 mg/dl and in those fed ACM the average level was 45 ± 5. In another study, five rabbits were fed ACM for 6 weeks, then CM for 10 weeks, ACM without cholesterol for 6 weeks and ACM for another 10 weeks. Average serum cholesterol levels were 53 ± 8, 1202 ± 330, 68 ± 12, and 80 ± 21, respectively. Howard *et al.* (1967) fed rabbits a semi-purified diet containing beef tallow and cellophane and observed mean plasma cholesterol levels of 275 mg/dl and average atherosclerosis of 1.6 (on a 1–3 scale); dilution of the diet with an equal amount of stock diet inhibited atherosclerosis and reduced plasma cholesterol to 92 mg/dl.

Berenson *et al.* (1975) added 5% pectin to an atherogenic rabbit diet and effected a 33% decrease in serum cholesterol and a 25% fall in β + pre-β-lipoprotein cholesterol. Kritchevsky *et al.* (1977) added 15% wheat straw, cellulose or alfalfa to semi-purified diets whose protein was either casein or soya protein. In both cases, serum cholesterol levels and degree of average atherosclerosis were highest in rabbits fed cellulose and lowest in those fed alfalfa. The ratio of serum α/β-lipoprotein cholesterol was highest in rabbits fed alfalfa.

C. Chicken

Fisher *et al.* (1966) fed chickens diets containing 0.6% cholesterol and 3% cellulose or pectin. Plasma cholesterol levels and incidence and severity of aortic and coronary atherosclerosis were significantly lower in birds fed pectin.

D. Primates

In Vervet monkeys fed atherogenic semi-purified diets containing 15% cellulose, wheat straw or alfalfa for 23 weeks, Kritchevsky *et al.* (1981) found average serum cholesterol levels and ratios of α/β-lipoprotein cholesterol to be: cellulose, 174 and 0.49; wheat straw, 167 and 0.66; and alfalfa, 153 and 0.74. Average sudanophilia (%) was: cellulose 3.8 ± 1.5; wheat straw, 1.5 ± 0.4; and alfalfa 4.1 ± 2.9. Malinow *et al.* (1978) induced atherosclerosis in female cynomologous monkeys by feeding a diet containing butter and cholesterol for 6 months. One group was killed at this time and exhibited a cholesterol level of 701 mg/dl, a ratio of α/β + pre-β-cholesterol of 0.09 and average atherosclerosis of 3.0. A group maintained on a semi-purified diet for 18 months more had a cholesterol level of 287 mg/dl, α/β + pre-β-cholesterol ratio of 0.21 and the severity of atherosclerosis had increased to 3.7. A third

TABLE 18.2. Cholesterol metabolism in rabbits
fed semi-purified or commercial diet for 6 months[a]

	Diet[b]	
	Commercial (5)[c]	Semi-purified (9)
Serum		
^{3}H × 10^5	0.38 ± 0.11	4.03 ± 0.36
^{14}C	ND	2757
Liver (dpm)		
^{3}H × 10^5	1.34 ± 0.44	4.41 ± 0.52
^{14}C × 10^4	1.05 ± 0.28	3.99 ± 0.59
Aorta, pooled (dpm)		
^{3}H	920	2160
^{14}C	88	198
Feces		
Grams/day	32.6 ± 6	7.5 ± 3
Neutral steroid		
^{3}H × 10^6	18.8 ± 10.4	3.8 ± 1.3
^{14}C × 10^3	10.8 ± 4.2	5.1 ± 1.8
Acidic steroid		
^{3}H × 10^5	1.6 ± 0.9	9.5 ± 2.2
^{14}C × 10^3	0.4 ± 0.1	3.8 ± 1.2

[a] After Kritchevsky et al., 1975a).

[b] Rabbits fed diets for 6 months. Three days before end of study each animal received 10 μ Ci of [1,2-^{3}H]cholesterol (exogenous cholesterol) and 0.5 μ Ci of [2-^{14}C]mevalonic acid (endogenous cholesterol). Semi-purified diet as described in Table 18.1. Fiber-cellulose.

[c] Numbers in parentheses indicate number of animals.

group was given the semi-purified diet plus alfalfa for 18 months. In this group the serum cholesterol levels had fallen to 163 mg/dl, the lipoprotein ratio had risen to 0.79 and the atherosclerosis regressed to a grade of 1.8.

E. Mechanism of action

Portman and Murphy (1958) were the first workers to examine the mechanism of the hypocholesterolaemic action of fibre. They found that rats fed a commercial ration excreted 37 mg of cholic acid/kg/day and 75.4 mg of digitonin-precipitable steroids. When the rats were placed on a semi-purified diet containing sucrose, excretion of acidic and neutral steroids fell to 8 and 44 mg/kg/day, respectively. Replacing one-third of the sucrose with cellulose resulted in increased bile acid excretion (23 mg/kg/day) but a further decrease in neutral steroid excretion to 30 mg. Portman (1960) studied bile acid turnover in rats fed commercial ration or the same ration after ethanol extraction. Bile acid half-life and excretion were the same on both diets. Rats fed a semi-purified diet exhibited a doubling of bile acid turnover time and 67% decrease in bile acid excretion compared to the controls. Addition of the extracted lipids to the semi-purified diet decreased bile acid turnover time but did not affect excretion.

Kritchevsky *et al.* (1975a) compared metabolism of endogenous and exogenous cholesterol in rabbits fed a commercial ration or a semi-purified diet containing 15% cellulose (Table 18.2). It is evident that less cholesterol (endogenous or exogenous) was absorbed and more was excreted by rabbits fed the commercial ration.

Leveille and Sauberlich (1966) found that rats fed pectin excreted more faecal bile acids than rats fed cellulose. Fisher *et al.* (1966) reported that chickens fed 0.6% cholesterol and pectin excreted 32% more lipid and 30% more cholesterol than chickens fed cellulose.

Barichello and Fedoroff (1971) speculated that alfalfa inhibited cholesterol absorption by forming unabsorbable complexes in the intestine. Alfalfa enchanced faecal excretion of neutral steroids but not of bile acids in cholesterol-fed rats (Kritchevsky *et al.*, 1974c). Malinow *et al.* (1979) reported that alfalfa decreased cholesterol absorption in rats by 38% but had no such effect when its saponins were extracted.

Dietary fibre may exert its hypolipidaemic and anti-atherogenic effect by decreasing absorption of cholesterol (Hyun *et al.*, 1963; Vahouny *et al.*, 1978) or by increased faecal excretion of bile acids (Kay and Truswell, 1980). Dietary fibre has been shown to bind bile acids (Eastwood and Hamilton, 1968; Story and Kritchevsky, 1976) as well as other lipids (Vahouny *et al.*, 1980) *in vitro*.

F. Man

There are no studies specifically relating fibre intake to atherosclerosis in man although Kromhout *et al.* (1982) observed a group of men for 10 years and found that those ingesting a high-fibre diet exhibited less atherosclerosis and other degenerative diseases. There are two types of human populations one can investigate—vegetarians, whose dietary lifestyle includes more fibre-rich foods or persons participating in experiments involving addition of fibre to the diet. Vegetarians habitually ingest a high-fibre diet (Hardinge *et al.* 1958). Sacks *et al.* (1975) determined plasma cholesterol, triglyceride and lipoprotein levels in 115 pairs of vegetarians and matched controls. Their data showed that the vegetarians had significantly lower levels of cholesterol and LDL. Burslem *et al.* (1978) also found vegetarians to have lower plasma total and LDL cholesterol levels than controls. They also found that vegetarians had significantly lower levels of apolipoproteins A1 and B. Knuiman and West (1982) determined serum cholesterol and lipoprotein levels in macrobiotic, vegetarian and non-vegetarian men. Lacto-ovo-vegetarians exhibited serum cholesterol levels that were 15% below non-vegetarian controls

(181 vs. 212 mg/dl) and higher HDL-cholesterol levels. Men on macrobiotic diets had even lower cholesterol levels (147 mg/dl) and their HDL-cholesterol/total cholesterol ratios were 40% above that of the non-vegetarians. Burr and Sweetnam (1982) conducted a study in which 10,943 subjects were questioned concerning their dietary habits and mortality was determined from National Health Service records. They found a significant negative association between vegetarianism and mortality from ischaemic heart disease. No significant associations were found with fibre. Kelsay (1978) reviewed effects of fibre on lipids in man and found pectin, rolled oats, guar gum and legumes to be hypocholesterolaemic, whereas wheat bran, bagasse and cellulose had no effect. Durrington *et al.* (1976) fed pectin (12 g/day) to 12 subjects and observed no significant changes in plasma lipoproteins. Jenkins *et al.* (1980) found that the feeding of guar crispbread (13 g/day for 2 to 8 weeks) caused reductions in total and LDL cholesterol levels. Oat bran (Kirby *et al.*, 1981) caused a 13% reduction in total cholesterol and a 13% fall in LDL cholesterol. There were no changes in HDL-cholesterol levels. Pectin (9 g/day) reduced total cholesterol by 8% and VLDL + LDL cholesterol by 11% (Nakamura *et al.*, 1982). This regimen led to greater increases in faecal excretion of neutral steroid than bile acid which is at variance with the findings of Kay and Truswell (1977) and Miettinen and Tarpila (1977).

Increases in faecal bulk are not correlated with hypocholesterolaemic effect. Jenkins *et al.* (1979) fed pectin, guar, bran, carrot, cabbage and apple. Only the first two of these exerted a hypocholesterolaemic effect but they caused the smallest increase in faecal weight (Table 18.3). Ullrich *et al.* (1981) studied faecal steroid excretion on diets low (21 g/day) or high (59 g/day) in fibre. There were no differences in total steroid excretion. The ratios of primary (cholic and chenodeoxycholic) to secondary (deoxycholic and lithocholic) acids were 0.025, 0.013 and 0.460 in subjects fed control,

TABLE 18.3. Comparison of hypocholesterolemic and faecal bulking effects of fibres[a]

Fibre	Grams added	Serum cholesterol/mg/dl		HDL cholesterol/ total cholesterol		Increase in faecal weight (g)
		Before	After	Before	After	
Pectin	30.8	175 ± 13	152 ± 13[b]	0.23	0.26	19
Guar	17.2	180 ± 13	157 ± 11[b]	0.28	0.30	20
Bran	18.0	186 ± 18	183 ± 17	0.23	0.21	127
Carrot	20.1	160 ± 8	158 ± 8	0.29	0.24	59
Cabbage	18.3	163 ± 14	167 ± 16	0.25	0.23	67
Apple	21.9	161 ± 12	160 ± 13	0.28	0.27	40

[a] After Jenkins *et al.*, 1979.
[b] Before vs. after $p < 0.01$.

low-fibre or high-fibre diets, respectively. The ratios of cholesterol to coprostanol in the faeces were 0.46, 0.52 and 1.24 in the three groups.

Stasse-Wolthius *et al.* (1979) found that the effects of dietary fibre on cholesterolaemia and HDL-cholesterol levels were dependent, in part, on the cholesterol content of the diet, with the most striking effects being observed in subjects fed a high-fibre, low-cholesterol diet. The same group (Stasse-Wolthius *et al.*, 1980) examined the effects of vegetables and legumes, pectin or bran on serum total and HDL-cholesterol levels, faecal weight, transit time and faecal steroid excretion. None of the substances had a significant effect on HDL-cholesterol levels and only pectin reduced serum cholesterol significantly. Vegetables and bran increased faecal weight and reduced transit time significantly. In males, pectin increased faecal total steroid excretion, vegetables increased neutral steroid excretion and bran decreased bile acid excretion.

Certain types of dietary fibre are hypolipidaemic and hypolipoproteinaemic in man. The latter effect is usually exerted on the VLDL and LDL fractions of plasma. A vegetarian or high-fibre dietary lifestyle has been associated with relative freedom from ischaemic heart disease. Pectin, wheat straw and alfalfa have all been found to inhibit experimental atherosclerosis. The precise mode by which dietary fibre acts is still unclear. It may be a reflection of the effects which certain fibres exert on bile acid metabolism; it does not appear to be related to faecal bulk. We have yet to elucidate the mechanism(s) by which fibre lowers lipid levels and the particular aspects of fibre structure responsible for the observed effects.

Acknowledgements

This research was supported, in part, by a grant (HL-03299) and a Research Career Award (HL-00734) from the National Institutes of Health and by the Commonwealth of Pennsylvania.

References

BARICHELLO, A. W. and FEDOROFF, S. (1971). *Br. J. Exp. Pathol.* **52**, 81–87.

BARR, D. P., RUSS, E. M. and EDER, H. A. (1951). *Am. J. Med.* **11**, 480–493.

BERENSON, L. M., BHANDARU, R. R., RADHAKRISHNAMURTHY, B., SRINIVASAN, S. R. and BERENSON, G. S. (1975). *Life Sci.* **16**, 1533–1544.

BURR, M. L. and SWEETNAM, P. M. (1982). *Am. J. Clin. Nutr.* **36**, 873–877.

BURSLEM, J., SCHONFELD, G., HOWARD, M. A., WERDMAN, S. W. and MILLER, J. P. (1978). *Metab., Clin. Exp.* **27**, 711–719.

CHEN, W. L. and ANDERSON, J. W. (1979a). *Proc. Soc. Exp. Biol. Med.* **162**, 310–313.

CHEN, W. L. and ANDERSON, J. W. (1979b). *J. Nutr.* **109**, 1028–1034.

COOKSON, F. B., ALTSCHUL, R. and FEDOROFF, S. (1967). *J. Atheroscler. Res.* **7**, 69–81.

COREY, J. E., HAYES, K. C., DORR, B. and HEGSTED, D. M. (1974). *Atherosclerosis* **19**, 119–134.

DURRINGTON, P. N., MANNING, A. P., BOLTON, C. H. and HARTOG, M. (1976). *Lancet* **2**, 394–396.

EASTWOOD, M. A. and HAMILTON, D. (1968). *Biochim. Biophys. Acta* **152**, 165–173.

ERSHOFF, B. H. and WELLS, A. F. (1962). *Proc. Soc. Exp. Biol. Med.* **110**, 580–582.

FISHER, H., SOLLER, W. G. and GRIMINGER, P. (1966). *J. Atheroscler. Res.* **6**, 292–298.

GOFMAN, J. W., LINDGREN, F., ELLIOTT, H., MANTZ, W., HEWITT, J., STRISOWER, B., HERRING, V. and LYON, T. P. (1950). *Science* **111**, 166–171.

HARDINGE, M. G., CHAMBERS, A. C., CROOKS, H. and STARE, F. J. (1958). *Am. J. Clin. Nutr.* **6**, 523–528.

HOPKINS, P. N. and WILLIAMS, R. R. (1981). *Atherosclerosis* **40**, 1–52.

HOWARD, A. N., GRESHAM, G. A., JENNINGS, I. W. and JONES, D. (1967). *Prog. Biochem. Pharmacol.* **2**, 117–127.

HYUN, S. A., VAHOUNY, G. V. and TREADWELL, C. R. (1963). *Proc Soc. Exp. Biol. Med.* **112**, 496–501.

JENKINS, D. J. A., REYNOLDS, D., LEEDS, A. R., WALLER, A. L. and CUMMINGS, J. H. (1979). *Am. J. Clin. Nutr.* **32**, 2430–2435.

JENKINS, D. J. A., REYNOLDS, D., SLAVIN, B., LEEDS, A. R., JENKINS, A. L. and JEPSOM, E. M. (1980). *Am. J. Clin. Nutr.* **33**, 575–581.

KANNEL, W. B., DAWBER, T. R., KAGAN, A., REVOTSKI, N. and STOKES, J., III (1961). *Ann. Intern. Med.* **55**, 33–50.

KAY, R. M. and TRUSWELL, A. S. (1977). *Am. J. Clin. Nutr.* **30**, 171–175.

KAY, R. M. and TRUSWELL, A. S. (1980). *In* "Medical Aspects of Dietary Fiber" (G. A. Spiller and R. M. Kay, eds), pp. 153–173. Plenum, New York.

KELSAY, J. L. (1978). *Am. J. Clin. Nutr.* **31**, 142–159.

KIRBY, R. W., ANDERSON, J. W., SIELING, B., REES, E. D., CHEN, W. L., MILLER, R. E. and KAY, R. M. (1981). *Am. J. Clin. Nutr.* **34**, 824–829.

KIRIYAMA, S., OKAZAKI, Y. and YOSHIDA, A. (1969). *J. Nutr.* **97**, 382–388.

KNUIMAN, J. T. and WEST, C. E. (1982). *Atherosclerosis* **43**, 71–82.

KRITCHEVSKY, D. (1964). *J. Atheroscler. Res.* **4**, 103–105.

KRITCHEVSKY, D. and TEPPER, S. A. (1965). *Life Sci.* **4**, 1468–1471.

KRITCHEVSKY, D. and TEPPER, S. A. (1968). *J. Atheroscler. Res.* **8**, 357–369.

KRITCHEVSKY, D., SALLATA, P. and TEPPER, S. A. (1968). *J. Atheroscler. Res.* **8**, 697–703.

KRITCHEVSKY, D., TEPPER, S. A. and KITAGAWA, M. (1973). *Nutr. Rep. Int.* **7**, 193–202.

KRITCHEVSKY, D., DAVIDSON, L. M., SHAPIRO, I. L., KIM, H. K., KITAGAWA, M., MALHOTRA, S., NAIR, P. P., CLARKSON, T. B., BERSOHN, I. and WINTER, P. A. D. (1974a). *Am. J. Clin. Nutr.* **27**, 29–50.

KRITCHEVSKY, D., DAVIDSON, L. M., VAN DER WATT, J. J., WINTER, P. A. D. and BERSOHN, I. (1974b). *S. Afr. Med. J.* **48**, 2413–2414.

KRITCHEVSKY, D., TEPPER, S. A. and STORY, J. A. (1974c). *Nutr. Rep. Int.* **9**, 301–308.

KRITCHEVSKY, D., TEPPER, S. A., KIM, H. K., MOSES, D. E. and STORY, J. A. (1975a). *Exp. Mol. Pathol.* **22**, 11–19.

KRITCHEVSKY, D., TEPPER, S. A. and STORY, J. A. (1975b). *J. Food Sci.* **40**, 8–11.

KRITCHEVSKY, D., TEPPER, S. A., WILLIAMS, D. E. and STORY, J. A. (1977). *Atherosclerosis* **26**, 397–403.

KRITCHEVSKY, D., DAVIDSON, L. M., KIM, H. K., KRENDEL, D. A., MALHOTRA, S., MENDELSOHN, D., VAN DER WATT, J. J., DU PLESSIS, J. P. and WINTER, P. A. D. (1980). *Am. J. Clin. Nutr.* **33**, 1869–1887.

KRITCHEVSKY, D., DAVIDSON, L. M., KRENDEL, D. A., VAN DER WATT, J. J., RUSSELL, D., FRIEDLAND, S. and MENDELSOHN, D. (1981). *Ann. Nutr. Metab.* **25**, 125–136.

KROMHOUT, D., BOSSCHIETER, E. B. and DE LEZENNE COULANDER, C. (1982). *Lancet* **2**, 518–522.

LAMBERT, G. F., MILLER, J. P., OLSEN, R. T. and FROST, D. V. (1958). *Proc. Soc. Exp. Biol. Med.* **97**, 544–549.

LANG, C. M. and BARTHEL, C. H. (1972). *Am. J. Clin. Nutr.* **25**, 470–475.

LEVEILLE, G. A. and SAUBERLICH, H. E. (1966). *J. Nutr.* **88**, 209–214.

LITTLE, J. A., McGUIRE, V. and DERKSEN, A. (1979). *In* "Nutrition, Lipids and Coronary Heart Disease" (R. I. Levy, B. Rifkind, B. H. Dennis and N. Ernst, eds), pp. 119–148. Raven Press, New York.

MALINOW, M. R., McLAUGHLIN, P., NAITO, H. K., LEWIS, L. A. and McNULTY, W. P. (1978). *Atherosclerosis* **30**, 27–43.

MALINOW, M. R., McLAUGHLIN, P., STAFFORD, C., LIVINGSTON, A. L., KOHLER, G. O. and CHEEKE, P. R. (1979). *Am. J. Clin. Nutr.* **32**, 1810–1812.

MALMROS, H. and WIGAND, G. (1959). *Lancet* **2**, 749–751.

MIETTINEN, T. A. and TARPILA, S. (1977). *Clin. Chim. Acta* **79**, 471–477.

MILLER, G. J. and MILLER, N. E. (1975). *Lancet* **1**, 16–19.

MOORE, J. H. (1967). *Br. J. Nutr.* **21**, 207–215.

NAKAMURA, H., ISHIKAWA, T., TADA, N., KAGAMI, A., KONDO, K., MYAZIMA, E. and TAKEYAMA, S. (1982). *Nutr. Rep. Int.* **26**, 215–222.

PORTMAN, O. W. (1960). *Am. J. Clin. Nutr.* **8**, 462–470.

PORTMAN, O. W. and MURPHY, P. (1958). *Arch. Biochem. Biophys.* **76**, 367–376.

SACKS, F. M., CASTELLI, W. P., DONNER, A. and KASS, E. H. (1975). *N. Engl. J. Med.* **292**, 1148–1151.

STASSE-WOLTHIUS, M., HAUTVAST, J. G. A. J., HERMUS, R. J. J., KATAN, M. B., BAUSCH, J. E., REITBERG-BRUSSNARD, J. H., VELMA, J. P., ZONDERVAN, J. E., EASTWOOD, M. A. and BRYDON, G. R. (1979). *Am. J. Clin. Nutr.* **32**, 1881–1888.

STASSE-WOLTHIUS, M., ALBERS, H. F. F., VAN JEVEREN, J. G. C., WIL DE JONG, J., HAUTVAST, J. G. A. J., HERMUS, R. J. J., KATAN, M. B., BRYDON, G. B. and EASTWOOD, M. A. (1980). *Am. J. Clin. Nutr.* **33**, 1745–1756.

STORY, J. A. and KELLEY, M. J. (1982). *In* "Dietary Fiber in Health and Disease" (G. V. Vahouny and D. Kritchevsky, eds). pp. 229–236. Plenum, New York.

STORY, J. A. and KRITCHEVSKY, D. (1976). *J. Nutr.* **106**, 1292–1294.

STORY, J. A., BALDINO, A., CZARNECKI, S. K. and KRITCHEVSKY, D. (1981). *Nutr. Rep. Int.* **24**, 1213–1219.

ULLRICH, I. H., LAI, H. Y., VONA, L., REID, R. L. and ALBRINK, M. J. (1981). *Am. J. Clin. Nutr.* **34**, 2054–2060.

VAHOUNY, G. V., ROY, T., GALLO, L. L., STORY, J. A., KRITCHEVSKY, D., CASSIDY, M., GRUND, B. M. and TREADWELL, C. R. (1978). *Am. J. Clin. Nutr.* **31**, S208–S212.

VAHOUNY, G. V., TOMBES, R., CASSIDY, M. M., KRITCHEVSKY, D. and GALLO, L. L. (1980). *Lipids* **15**, 1012–1018.

WELLS, A. F. and ERSHOFF, B. H. (1961). *J. Nutr.* **74**, 87–92.

WELLS, W. W. and ANDERSON, S. C. (1969). *J. Nutr.* **68**, 541–549.

Chapter 19

Varicose veins, haemorrhoids, deep-vein thrombosis and pelvic phleboliths

DENIS BURKITT

I.   Varicose veins

The literature on this very common disorder has been so dominated by procedures of treatment that questions of causation and potential prevention have received too little serious attention. Writers on the subject in surgical textbooks have usually started from the erroneous assumption that this is a disease equally common to all mankind throughout the world, and have failed to realise that this is an uncommon disorder in other than affluent Western communities (Burkitt, 1976). As a consequence, hypotheses of causation

317

Dietary Fibre, Fibre-Depleted Foods
and Disease

have been postulated and perpetuated that are totally at variance with the epidemiological features of the disease, as will be shown below. The most commonly cited causes of varicose veins are man's upright posture, prolonged standing, hereditary factors, pregnancy and female sex. These may be contributory, but not primary, causative factors. Until recently the constrictive clothing worn by women was blamed, but it would be ludicrous to incriminate such a factor today. The assumption that varicose veins are universally common, with the inevitable deduction that the possibility of prevention must be discounted, was illustrated by an editorial in the *Lancet* (Editorial, 1975) which emphasised that the high and rising prevalence of this disorder called for more intensive efforts to devise improved treatment. There was no suggestion that the disorder might be preventable or that causative factors should be identified and minimised.

Conventional hypotheses will be examined, and an alternative suggested, after reviewing the epidemiological features of this condition.

A. *Epidemiology*

1. *Western countries*

The *Lancet* editorial referred to above declared that "varicose veins are probably the commonest disorder presented to general surgeons. It may be found in as many as 50% of an adult European population and occupies a similar proportion of the average surgical waiting list."

A detailed survey of a total population was undertaken in the state of Michigan, U.S.A. This revealed prevalences of 19% in all men over the age of 30 years, and of 23.5% and 42% in those over the ages of 40 and 50 years, respectively. The comparable figures for women in these groups were 44%, 54% and 64% (Coon *et al.*, 1973). There can thus be no doubt that this is indeed a very common complaint in the Western world. Moreover, the prevalence of varicose veins appears to be comparable in both black and white Americans today (Cleave, 1974). This has been confirmed by numerous personal discussions with American surgeons.

2. *Developing countries*

Most available evidence is in the form of personal impressions, but when this evidence is abundant and consistent and reflects long experience of competent observers, it must carry considerable weight. Moreover, in areas where specific surveys have been undertaken, the results have not been very different from what had been expected from clinical impressions, though figures have been somewhat higher. Burkitt (1976) questioned doctors in over 200 hospitals in nearly 50 countries through postal questionnaires and personal visits. Reports from 142 mainly rural hospitals in 19 countries in Africa indicate that in the course of a year 13% saw no cases, 52% saw 1–5, 27% saw

TABLE 19.1. Surveys of varicose veins prevalence rates (%)[a]

Source	Reference	Examined		Prevalence	
		Men	Women	Men	Women
Africans					
Egypt factor, women	Mekky et al. (1969)		467		6.0
Kenyan women near term	Burkitt (1976)				
Arab			66		1.5
African			156		3.2
Indian			72		9.7
Mali, W. Africa	Rougemont (1974)		469		10.9
Transvaal, S. Africa	Daynes and Beighton (1973)		297		7.7
Tanzania	Burkitt et al. (1975)	179	163	1.1	1.8
Asians					
Hong Kong, young adults	Alexander (1972)	1138	1112	4.6	0.8
Indians	Burkitt et al. (1975)	274	255	0.4	0.4
	Burkitt et al. (1975)	237	263	1.7	1.1
	Burkitt et al. (1975)	250	250	0.4	0.0
Pregnant women	Burkitt et al. (1975)		300		0.3
Pregnant women	Phillips and Burkitt (1976)		1000		1.1
Sweepers	Malhotra (1972)	1000		25.0 (North Indian)	
				6.8 (South Indian)	
South American					
Peru (little westernised)	Dalrymple and Crofts (1975)	2084 men and women			0.5

[a] From Burkitt (1976). Copyright 1976, American Medical Association.

5–19, and only 7% saw more than 20 patients with varicose veins. Figures from 20 rural hospitals in South America were slightly higher, with 50% estimating over 20 cases a year. Of 63 hospitals in Asia, only 18% estimated over 20 cases and 50% under 5 a year. The Asian hospitals were contacted over a period of 2 years by asking doctors through monthly postal returns to give particulars of any patients seen with varicose veins. In both Africa and Asia only a little over two patients were reported per hospital per year. Females predominated, as they do in hospital figures generally.

Results of specific surveys of population groups for the prevalence of varicose veins undertaken in Africa, Asia and Peru are tabulated in Table 19.1. These figures indicate somewhat higher prevalences than those suggested from previous enquiries, but much lower than those in affluent communities. They suggest that among communities with minimal contact with Western civilization, the age-standaridised prevalence rates of varicose veins are usually under 5% of the adult community, and that in Third World countries in general they seldom exceed 10%. Even when age distribution is taken into account, these are much lower than Western figures, although almost as many people who reach adult life in Third World countries survive to old age as in the West. The short life expectancy at birth is accounted for by the heavy childhood mortality (Walker, 1974).

It is particularly noteworthy that the carefully conducted study in the South Pacific islands and New Zealand by Beaglehole et al. (1975) indicated clearly that the main factor that affected the prevalence of varicose veins in these communities was the degree of contact with Western civilisation (Table 19.2). Thus, traditionally living communities like Tokelau and Pukapuka islanders had very low prevalences, but New Zealand Maori women, who belong to the same Polynesian ethnic group, had an even higher prevalence than New Zealand white women. These surveys reported higher rates in women than in men. They also showed that age was a risk factor in all groups, but that female sex and parity were risk factors only in westernized New Zealand Europeans and Maoris, but not among Polynesian islanders.

TABLE 19.2. Age-standardised varicose veins prevalence rates (%) in South Pacific Island Polynesians and Maoris, also New Zealand Maoris and Europeans

	Island Polynesians[a]		New Zealand	
	Tokelau	Pukapuka	Maoris[b]	Europeans
Males	2.9	2.1	33.4	19.6
Females	0.8	4.0	43.6	37.8

[a] Little westernisation of diet and lifestyle.

[b] Much westernisation of diet and lifestyle; they have descended from Island Polynesians. Adapted from Beaglehole et al., 1975.

B. Relationships to other diseases characteristic of modern Western civilisation

Epidemiological prevalences of varicose veins are related to the prevalences of the other characteristically Western diseases discussed in this volume. A more specific and positive relationship has been demonstrated in the case of diverticular disease of the colon. Latto *et al.* (1973) observed that the prevalence of varicose veins in British patients with radiologically demonstrated diverticular disease was approximately double that observed in age- and sex-matched controls; this suggested that these two disparate conditions shared some causative factor common to each.

C. Postulated aetiology

The epidemiological data outlined above render most of the conventional concepts of causation of varicose veins no longer tenable. If man's erect posture were the prime factor, then *major* disparities in geographical distribution and prevalence rates should not be apparent. Were prolonged standing of major importance, the condition should be less common amongst sedentary Western communities. The comparable prevalence rates in black and white Americans today (Stamler, 1958; Cleave, 1974), and the relationships to Western civilisation demonstrated by prevalence rates from the South Pacific communities (Prior and Tasman-Jones, 1981), appear to refute the claim for an important hereditary factor. Moreover, no evidence has yet been presented to support the contention of a supposed genetically inherited weakness in the walls of the veins. Different individuals and ethnic groups are admittedly more or less susceptible, but this susceptibility is only expressed in a particular environment.

There is nothing to support the contention that pregnancy is a primary factor. Although varicose veins may appear or become more prominent during pregnancy, Phillips and Burkitt (1976) found a prevalence of only 1.1% in 1000 pregnant women in India (Table 19.1). On a worldwide geographical basis, there is usually an inverse ratio between the prevalence of varicose veins in a country and the average number of pregnancies.

Although female sex appears an important risk factor in Western countries, this is by no means universal in the third world. In three out of four surveys in India the disorder was more common in men (Burkitt *et al.*, 1975). As with cholesterol gallstones—another environmentally dependent disease which is more common in women in the West—there may well be hormonal or other factors that modify environmental influences.

D. Alternative hypothesis of causation

It is generally agreed that varicosities of the leg veins result from incompetence of the valves that, when intact, ensure a one-way flow of venous blood, and are indispensable for the efficient working of the muscular venous pump that makes possible the return of blood, against gravity, to the heart. There has been diversity of opinion as to the cause of this incompetence. Most varicose veins are "idiopathic", i.e. of unknown cause, and these alone are considered here. The small proportion which are secondary to venous thrombosis may be considered virtually non-existent in Third World communities amongst whom, as will be described below, venous thrombosis is rare.

Any adequate hypothesis attempting to explain the pathogenesis of varicose veins must take into consideration the following observed facts:

1. The geographical variations of the disease and its relationship to Western civilisation.

2. The epidemiological relationships between this and other diseases characteristic of modern Western civilisation and in particular with diverticular disease of the colon.

3. The comparable prevalences in black and white Americans today.

4. Their progressive increase in prevalence with advancing age.

5. Their rarity in all animals.

In the past it has often been suggested that raised intra-abdominal pressures due to supposed factors such as pregnancy or obesity might contribute to the cause of varicose veins, but a different cause of increased pressure will be argued hereafter. It is doubtful whether suggested causes such as obesity, abdominal tumours or pregnancy significantly raise intraabdominal pressures. The only one that might be related to the prevalence of varicose veins is obesity, which might share common causative factors rather than there being a direct cause and effect relationship between these two diseases.

The activity that raises intra-abdominal pressures more than anything else is muscular straining as in the Valsalva manoeuvre or straining at stool, and these pressures have been demonstrated to be readily transmitted down the large veins draining blood from the legs. Edwards and Edwards (1940) demonstrated that in varicose veins the valves showed no evidence of disease but the stretching of the walls of the veins prevented the cusps from meeting one another, thus rendering the valves incompetent.

The hypothesis that varicose veins are related to raised intra-abdominal pressures transmitted to the venous trunks draining the lower limb, and thence down the limb as the successive valves become incompetent, is consistent with the findings of Folse (1970) using a bi-directional ultrasonic flow detector. His findings may be summarised thus:

1. Both the iliofemoral and saphenous veins above varicosities are always incompetent, and reverse blood flow precedes the development of varicosities.

2. Valve incompetence always proceeds from above downwards.

3. Varicosities below the knee almost invariably precede those above the knee but they are accompanied by incompetent veins above.

4. There can be incompetence without varices but never varices without incompetence.

5. Some valves can remain competent while others, subject to the same intravenous pressure, become incompetent.

Although these workers recognised the importance of raised intra-abdominal pressures in the pathogenesis of varicose veins, they did not appreciate the importance of straining at stool and the relationship between the condition and the consistency of stool voided.

It is important to emphasise that although straining at stool is postulated to be much the most important cause of raised intra-abdominal pressures, other causes may include such activities as trishaw riding in Southeast Asia, where this occupation has been shown to be associated with a higher prevalence of varicose veins.

E.   Varicose veins and diet

Communities with low prevalence rates of varicose veins appear invariably to pass large-volume soft-consistency stools. All communities with small volume, firm-consistency stools appear to have high prevalence rates of varicose veins. These epidemiological observations are consistent with the experimental evidence that relates the prevalence rates of varicose veins to raised intra-abdominal pressures.

The most important cause of the constipation which is so prevalent in Western communities and which necessitates abdominal straining, is a deficiency of fibre, especially cereal fibre, in the diet. Postulating this as a cause of varicose veins could also explain the relationships between this disorder and some other diseases characteristic of modern Westen civilisation.

II.   Haemorrhoids

New light on the nature of haemorrhoids has not only profoundly altered the therapeutic approach to the problem, but has also improved understanding of the possible causes of this disorder. Until the concept was challenged by Thomson (1975) it had been generally assumed, but with occasional dissenting voices, that haemorrhoids were varicosities of the anal veins analogous to varicosities of the leg, and to those of the lower end of the oesophagus consequent on portal hypertension. Thomson (1975), however, demonstrated that these structures were present at birth and were perfectly normal, highly vascular sub-mucosal cushions surrounding the upper part of the anal canal with the specific purpose of maintaining continence of both liquid faeces and gas. They cause no trouble unless damaged, and the cause of this damage is discussed in Section II,B.

A.   Epidemiology

The reported geographical distribution of hemorrhoids is in fact the geography of their complications, which may be bleeding, prolapse or occasionally thrombosis. Since the definition of haemorrhoids has been so imprecise, statements concerning rarity or frequent occurrence have often had little meaning. Almost any disorder or discomfort in the region of the anus may be attributed to so-called haemorrhoids.

The complications of a disease such as haemorrhoids are usually more readily recognised than the disease itself, and where these are not encountered the disease may be presumed to be rare, and vice versa. On the basis of this assumption, I endeavoured to obtain information on the frequency of these complications in Third World hospitals. My own experience and discussions with doctors working in rural hospitals throughout much of Africa and elsewhere indicated that in these situations surgery for haemorrhoids was a rare procedure. In contrast it has been estimated that approximately one in two Americans over the age of 50 suffer at some time from this disorder, which is one of the most common illnesses in the community after dental caries.

In order to confirm my clinical impressions of the relative rarity of haemorrhoids in Third World communities, questionnaires were sent monthly to over 100 hospitals in Africa and Asia asking for reports on any patients who suffered from bleeding or prolapsed piles. These hospitals were almost all in rural areas of developing countries. Over a period of $2\frac{1}{2}$ years, regular replies received from 77 of these hospitals indicated that fewer than three patients suffering from these complications were seen per hospital, per year in sub-Saharan Africa (Burkitt, 1975). By any standards this must be considered extremely rare compared to Western experience. The many American surgeons questioned by me concerning the prevalence of this disease in blacks and whites all affirmed that there was no obvious disparity in the United States.

As with varicose veins, haemorrhoids are exclusively confined to the human race and are much more prevalent in economically developed than in developing communities. Also, the prevalence of this disease, like that of varicose veins, appears to be directly related to the firmness, and inversely related to the size, of the motions commonly voided. All these factors must be taken into account when discussing possible aetiological factors.

B.   Postulated aetiology

In view of the revised concept of the nature of haemorrhoids outlined above, the causation of the disease means also the causation of the complications.

The most plausible hypothesis, and that which is most consistent with the epidemiological evidence is as follows. Straining at stool forces blood retrogradely down the inferior mesenteric veins, thus causing venous engorgement of the three vascular anal cushions. This makes them more vulnerable to the shearing stress exerted by the passage of firm faecal masses through the anal canal. These two factors, acting in combination, can damage the mucosa overlying the cushions causing the bright red blood that is characteristic of bleeding piles. The blood is obviously not from the piles themselves, or else it would be dark. It is believed to come from abrasions of the mucosa covering the piles. The shearing stress can also lead to rupture of the attachments of the cushions to the surrounding sphincter muscle, and this can lead to prolapse and to thrombosis of portions of the prolapsed tissue. The major cause of the abdominal straining and of the increased hardness of the faecal content is a low intake of fibre, especially cereal fibre, in the diet.

As in the case of varicose veins, no other hypothesis has been postulated that is consistent with the epidemiological features of the disease.

III.   Deep vein thrombosis

A.   Epidemiology

1.   Western countries

Deep vein thrombosis (DVT) is a common occurrence in Western countries. Kakkar et al. (1970) estimated that it occurred in 20 to 30% of all surgical patients and in 40 to 45% of older patients undergoing major surgery. Lambie et al. (1970), using ^{125}I-labelled fibrinogen, were able to demonstrate that nearly half of all "high-risk" surgical patients developed some venous thrombosis. Nicolaides et al. (1971) showed that it can be almost as common in severely ill medical patients of comparable age.

A great deal of DVT is not detected clinically, but clinical manifestations are recognisable often enough to be considered not uncommon findings. The most important complication of DVT is pulmonary embolism, and at least in severe cases this cannot easily be overlooked. The Registrar General's report for 1969 indicated that it was responsible for 2500 deaths annually in Britain. Davis-Christopher (Sabiston, 1972) estimated pulmonary embolism to be responsible for 5 to 9% of all hospital deaths, and Coon and Coller (1959) found pulmonary embolism in 14% of autopsies.

2.   Developing countries

All available evidence indicates that DVT, progressing to clinical manifestation, is rare throughout most of the Third World. Staff at more than half the 114 mission hospitals in rural Africa who replied to my questionnaires did not diagnose even one case of DVT annually. Replies to my monthly questionnaires specifically requesting statistics on DVT came from 99 rural hospitals in 14 countries in Africa; these indicated that less than one patient with clinical evidence of DVT was seen per hospital per year. Monthly returns from 13 Indian rural hospitals reported similar findings. The results of a prospective study in which doctors at 47 rural hospitals in Africa, who replied monthly to questionnaires asking particulars of any patients seen with clinical evidence of thrombosis, indicated a frequency of less than one patient per hospital per year (Burkitt, 1975). Previously, Dodd (1964) had reported only three patients with femoral thrombosis in a South African hospital over a period in which 11,000 patients, including 3000 for confinement, had been admitted.

The prevalence of post-partum clinical DVT in Chulalongkom Hospital in Thailand was found to be 1.7 per 10,000 deliveries, whereas the figure in a similar study at the Mayo Clinic was 134.7 per 10,000 deliveries (Chumni-jarakij, 1974). Such findings have been endorsed by autopsy studies. Thomas et al. (1960) contrasted the 2% autopsy incidence rate of thrombo-embolic phenomena found in Uganda Africans with the 24% and 22% rates in American whites and blacks, respectively. There is evidence that the discrepancy between DVT detected with the use of radioisotopes between more-developed and less-developed countries is less than that suggested on clinical grounds (Kallichurum, 1969).

It may be that the increased fibrinolytic activity, repeatedly demonstrated in Third World communities (Shaper, 1970; Shaper et al., 1966; Chakrabarti et al., 1968), dissolves clots before they increase to a size sufficient to produce clinical manifestations. The great rarity of pulmonary embolism in developing countries is further evidence that DVT is uncommon. Davies (1948), when reviewing autopsy records of 150 cases of sudden death in Africans in Uganda, found only a single case of fatal pulmonary emoblism. I remember no case of pulmonary embolism in my wards during 18 years of surgical practice in Uganda (1946–1964), and colleagues of mine with even longer experience report the same. At a similar period of time in Johannesburg, only three cases were seen following over 10,000 operations on African blacks (Barlow et al., 1953).

B.   Postulated aetiology

As in the case of varicose veins and haemorrhoids, the hypotheses of causation must be consistent with the epidemiological evidence, and particularly the rarity of the condition in developing communities and its virtual absence in veterinary surgery.

The enormous efforts currently being made to devise and develop improved drugs to reduce the risk of thrombosis, new innovations in controlled movement and the application of intermittent pressures appear almost to ignore the epidemiological features of the disease. The observations that fibrinolytic activity is similar in black and white Americans and that they are at comparable risk of developing DVT suggest that the causative factors must be largely environmental. An indication of a direction of investigation that might be followed comes from the observations of Latto (1979). He introduced the administration of ordinary bran pre- and post-operatively in his surgical wards as a prophylactic measure against constipation and other post-operative bowel complications. Not only did this prove extremely successful to the extent of virtually dispensing with laxatives, but after some 7 years it became apparent that clinically detectable DVT had almost disappeared and that during this period pulmonary embolism had not been diagnosed in any patient.

These clinical observations were succeeded by a prospective study of 50 patients over the age of 50 years undergoing the type of surgery that carried a high risk of DVT, many of them being prostatectomies. Using ^{125}I-labelled fibrinogen, their legs were examined at many levels each day post-operatively. Although 22% developed evidence of thrombosis, the clots disappeared within 72 h and in no case did clinical evidence of DVT appear. This suggests that diet may play some role in the pathogenesis of DVT, and that its action may be related to an increase in fibrinolytic activity. Simpson and Mann (1982) observed a reduction in blood clotting factors in patients fed high-fibre diets. Further studies of this nature may help to elucidate the problem of why DVT is predominantly a disease of Western civilisation.

IV. Pelvic phleboliths

A. Epidemiology

Pelvic phleboliths are calcified blood clots in the pelvic veins. During my long surgical experience in Africa, I had failed to recognise their rarity in radiographs of the pelvis, and it was not until I returned to the United Kingdom that I was introduced to the paper of Scott–Brown (1943) which emphasised the rarity of pelvic phleboliths in Africa. This led to the initiation of a study of the phenomena on a geographical basis (Burkitt et al., 1977). Whereas phleboliths are usually apparent on pelvic X-ray film in 30 to 60% of adults in Western countries and in white South Africans, they were only seen in 10 to 20% of adults in developing countries. Moreover, they were observed to be only one-third as common in black as in white South Africans (Kloppers and Fehrsen, 1977), yet as common in black as in white Americans (W. B. Ward and J. E. Reinhardt, personal communication, 1979). As with varicose veins and DVT, their prevalence increases with age. They are not observed in veterinary radiology.

B. Postulated aetiology

Both their increased frequency in Western nations compared to developing countries, and their localisation in the pelvic veins demand explanation.

The increased risk of DVT in developing countries has been discussed. The reason for localisation in the pelvic veins might be explained by the observations of Shemilt (1972). He measured pressures within the bladder through an inserted catheter, and assumed that these would approxiamtely reflect intra-abdominal pressures. At the same time he measured the pressures in catheterised pelvic veins, and found that during a Valsalva manouevre the pressures within the veins rose more steeply than did those within the abdomen. From this he postulated that cracks in the endothelium resultant on over-stretching might initiate clots.

As argued in connection with varicose veins, a low-fibre diet is the most common cause of abdominal straining, which, as emphasised above, might contribute to the pathogenesis of phleboliths. Not only may the prevalence of pelvic phleboliths be an indication of the frequency of DVT in a community, but Janvrin *et al.* (1980 provided evidence suggesting that the absence of pelvic phleboliths in an individual indicates a lower risk of developing post-operative DVT.

References

ALEXANDER, C. J. (1972). *Med. J. Aust.* **1**, 215–218.

BARLOW, M. D., GINSBERG, H. and GOTTLICH, J. (1953). *S. Afr. Med. J.* **27**, 242–246.

BEAGLEHOLE, R., PRIOR, I. A. M., SALMOND, C. E. and DAVIDSON, F. (1975). *Int. J. Epidemiol.* **4**, 295–299.

BURKITT, D. P. (1975). *Can. J. Surg.* **18**, 483–488.

BURKITT, D. P. (1976). *Arch. Surg.* (*Chicago*) **111**, 1327–1332.

BURKITT, D. P., JANSEN, H. K., MATEGAONKER, D. W., PHILLIPS, C., PHUNTSOG, Y. C. and SUKHNANDAN, R. (1975). *Lancet* **2**, 765.

BURKITT, D. P., LATTO, C., JANVRIN, S. B. and MAYO, M. B. (1977). *N. Engl. J. Med.* **296**, 1387–1389.

CHAKRABARTI, R., HOCKING, E. D., FEARNLEY, G. R., MANN, R. D., ATTWELL, T. H. and JACKSON, D. (1968). *Lancet* **1**, 987.

CHUMNIJARAKIJ, T. (1974). *Br. Med. J.* **1**, 245–246.

CLEAVE, T. L. (1974). "The Saccharine Disease", p. 45. John Wright, Bristol.

COON, W. W. and COLLER, F. A. (1959). *Surg, Gynecol. Obstet.* **109**, 259–269.

COON, W. W., WILLIS, P. W. and KELLER, J. B. (1973). *Circulation* **48**, 839–846.

DALRYMPLE, J. and CROFTS, T. (1975). *Lancet* **1**, 808–809.

DAVIES, J. N. P. (1948). *East Afr. Med. J.* **25**, 322–326.

DAYNES, S. G. andBEIGHTON, P. (1973). *Br. Med. J.* **3**, 354.

DODD, H. (1964). *Lancet* **2**, 809.

Editorial (1975). *Lancet* **2**, 311.

EDWARDS, J. E. and EDWARDS, E. A. (1940). *Am. Heart J.* **19**, 338–351.

FOLSE, R. (1970). *Surgery* **68**, 974–979.

JANVRIN, S. B., DAVIES, G. and GREENHALGH, R. M. (1980). *Br. J. Surg.* **67**, 690–693.

KAKKAR, V. V., HOWE, C. T., NICOLAIDES, A. N., RENNY, J. T. G. and CLARKE, M. B. (1970). *Am. J. Surg.* **120**, 527–530.

KALLICHURUM, S. (1969). *S. Afr. Med. J.* **43**, 358–363.

KLOPPERS, P. J. and FEHRSEN, G. S. (1977). *S. Afr. Med. J.* **21**, 745–746.

LAMBIE, J. M., MAHAFFY, R. G., BARBER, D. C., KARMODY, A. M., SCOTT, M. M. and MATHESON, N. A. (1970). *Br. Med. J.* **2**, 142–143.

LATTO, C. (1979). *In* "Haemorrhoids: Current Concepts on Causation and Management" (C. Wood, ed.), pp. 31–34. Royal Society of Medicine, London.

LATTO, C., WILKINSON, R. W. and GILMORE, O. J. (1973). *Lancet* **1**, 1089–1090.

MALHOTRA, S. L. (1972). *Int. J. Epidemiol.* **1**, 177–183.

MEKKY, S., SCHILLING, R. S. and WALFORD, J. (1969). *Br. Med. J.* **2**, 591–595.

NICOLAIDES, A. N., KAKKAR, V. V., FIELD, E. S. and FISH, P. (1971). *Br. J. Surg.* **59**, 713–717.

PHILLIPS, C. and BURKITT, D. P. (1976). *Br. Med. J.* **1**, 1148.

PRIOR, I. and TASMAN-JONES, C. (1981). *In* "Western Diseases: Their Emergence and Prevention" (H. C. Trowell and D. P. Burkitt, eds), pp. 227–267. Edward Arnold, London.

Registrar General (1969). Her Majesty's Stationery Office, London.

ROUGEMONT, A. (1974). *Lancet* **1**, 870.

SABISTON, D. C. (ED.) (1972). "Davis-Christopher Textbook of Surgery", 10th edition, pp. 1600–1623. Saunders, Philadelphia.

SCOTT BROWN, J. (1943). *East Afr. Med. J.* **20**, 122–123.

SHAPER, A. G. (1970). *In* "Atherosclerosis. Proceedings of Second International Symposium" (R. J. Jones, ed.). pp. 314–320. Springer-Verlag, Berlin.

SHAPER, A. G., JONES, K. W., KYOBE, J. and JONES, M. (1966). *J. Atheroscler. Res.* **6**, 313–327.

SHEMILT, P. (1972). *Br. J. Surg.* **59**, 695–700.

SIMPSON, H. C. R. and MANN, J. I. (1982). *Br. Med. J.* **284**, 1608.

STAMLER, J. (1958). *J. Natl. Med. Assoc.* **50**, 161–200.

THOMAS, W. A., DAVIES, J. N. P., O'NEAL, R. M. and DIMAKULANGAN, A. A. (1960). *Am. J. Cardiol.* **5**, 41–47.

THOMSON, W. H. F. (1975). *Br. J. Surg.* **62**, 542–552.

WALKER, A. R. P. (1974). *Postgrad. Med. J.* **50**, 29–32.

Chapter 20

Growth of Third World children

ALEXANDER WALKER and HARRY STEIN

I. The problem

If one enquires into the effects of diet (whether that of western or Third World populations) on growth and associated health, account must be taken of the following.

1. In Western countries, children now grow far more rapidly than in former years (Eveleth and Tanner, 1976). Diets, which have changed enormously, now contribute more energy, fat and protein, but less of fibre-containing foodstuffs (Hollingsworth, 1974).

2. In Third World countries, growth is slower. From babyhood to early adolescence, large proportions (Richardson, 1978, 1979; Anderson, 1979; Kotze *et al.*, 1982) fall below the respective third percentiles (weight/age, height/age) of Western reference standards (Vickers and Stuart, 1943; Stuart and Meredith, 1946). Habitual diet is relatively low in energy, fat and protein, but high in fibre-containing foods (den Hartog, 1980).

Dietary Fibre, Fibre-Depleted Foods
and Disease

3. In Third World populations, with urbanization, rise in privilege, or with migration to more prosperous countries, rate of growth increases (Eveleth and Tanner, 1976; Walker and Walker, 1977a). It is associated with increased consumptions of fat and sugar, and also animal protein, but decreased consumption of fibre-containing complex carbohydrates (Manning *et al.*, 1974).

4. As to health status in Third World populations, high morbidity and mortality from infections are experienced, particularly among the very young. This is due both to overcrowding, which in many situations leads to increased exposure, and to reduced immunity to infections associated with malnutrition (Geefhuysen *et al.*, 1971). In some centres, situations are improving (Stein and Rosen, 1980). A very important aspect, however, is that slower growth and the associated variables are possibly related to relatively low mortalities from degenerative diseases in adulthood (Trowell and Burkitt, 1981). In Western populations the converse prevails, i.e. the context of more rapid growth includes low mortalities from infections, but higher mortalities from accidents and malignant disease, and subsequent very high mortalities from degenerative diseases.

Several questions arise:

1. To what extent is slower growth due to (a) genetic reasons: (b) insufficient food consumption: (c) pattern of diet consumed: and (d) environmental non-dietary reasons?

2. Slower growth is regarded by most as essentially undesirable, deleterious or even pathological. Many equate markedly slower growth with malnutrition. To what extent are such beliefs warranted? Are they valid at all stages of youth? Are deleterious effects, e.g. greater proneness to infection, linked with dietary or non-dietary factors, or both?

3. Is it possible that growth in developed Western communities is now faster than optimal, and, rather than being deleterious, slower growth conceivably could be even beneficial in terms of health experience? An example of a situation where this is thought to apply is in relation to the size of the foetuses of black women whose pelvises are smaller than those of white women, and the fact that black neonates on average are 250–500 g smaller than white neonates as a result of slower foetal growth, is advantageous in terms of deliveries of these babies.

4. The questions raised require answers for at least two reasons. First, because slower growth, characteristic of the huge bulk of the world's population, is likely to remain so. Accordingly, it should be known whether slower growth, now or in later years, is or is not of meaningful public health importance. Second, because of population increase and the need to make more economical use of land, there will soon perforce have to be greater reliance on plant foods (associated with slower growth), not only by Third World popu-

TABLE 20.1. Mean weights and heights of a series of children aged 13 years

Population[a]	Boys		Girls	
	Weight (kg)	Height (cm)	Weight (kg)	Height (cm)
Germany[1] (1911)				
Poor class	32.3	133.3		
Middle class	33.3	137.7		
Wealthy class	34.7	140.4		
Scotland[1] (1926)				
Glasgow	33.4	135.6	34.5	139.8
Ayr	39.8	135.6	39.5	147.3
Iowa[2] (1946)	42.2	155.0	44.9	157.1
London[3] (1966)	43.0	155.1	46.5	155.2
Oslo[4] (1975)	44.2	156.4	46.8	158.4
Third percentile (Iowa)[5]	32.7	142.2	32.8	143.7
South African Populations				
Rural blacks (1938)[6]	31.8	140.1	33.0	141.5
Rural blacks (1983)[7]	37.0	144.5	38.3	147.6
Urban blacks (1983)[7]	39.5	148.5	41.7	149.9
Indians (1983)[7]				
Poor	37.2	151.2	41.2	151.6
Better class	41.1	153.6	43.5	154.0
Coloureds (1983)[7]				
Poor	34.8	148.4	38.5	149.1
Better class	36.8	150.0	42.2	151.7
Whites (1981)[8]	44.1	156.3	46.8	157.1
Other African Populations				
Tanzania (1971)[9]	32.5	137.5	36.0	143.0
Lagos (1972)[9]	33.7	143.8	38.9	147.3
Ivory Coast (1980)[10]	34.5	144.3	41.1	147.3

[a] References: 1. Paton and Findlay (1926); 2. Stuart and Meredith (1946); 3. Tanner and Whitehouse (1976); 4. Brundtland et al. (1975); 5. Vaughan (1969); 6. Walker and Walker (1977a); 7. Walker et al. (unpublished); 8. Walker et al. (1978); 9. Eveleth and Tanner (1976); 10. Haller and Lauber (1980).

lations, but by increasing proportions of Western populations. Hence, we must know to what extent slower growth matters.

II. Anthropometry in schoolchildren

Past and present data on weights and heights of a series of schoolchildren aged 13 years are given in Table 20.1. Because of pupils' readier availability, data are limited to them.

Attention is drawn to (1) the tremendous rises in weight and height in Western schoolchildren; (2) the fact that current data on schoolchildren of the same age in Western populations are closely similar; and (3) the observation that in South African black children, and also in other similarly placed children, percentages below the respective third percentiles of reference standards are high.

Although not depicted, the percentage of those below the third percentile rises from infancy to puberty, and then falls sharply by mid-adolescence. The huge majority of school pupils have 90% or more of reference weight-for-height. Percentages who exhibit *wasting* (as opposed to *stunting*), i.e. below 80% of weight-for-height, are very small (Davies and Mbelwa, 1974: Stewart and Ellis, 1975; Walker and Walker, 1977a,b; Kotze *et al.*, 1982).

The data given are considered fairly representative of anthropometric situations in Western and Third World populations.

III.   What causes slower growth?

A.   Genetic propensity

Young children from elite segments of most ethnic groups grow at much the same velocity (Habicht *et al.*, 1974; Graitcer and Gentry, 1981), although there are exceptions. Asian children grow more slowly, even those from well-off families; moreover, children, especially girls, reach maximum height relatively early (Rao and Sastry, 1977; Ulijaszek *et al.*, 1979; Walker and Segal, 1981; Trowbridge, 1982). There are also genetic differences regarding ultimate height attained, e.g. Italians compared with Swedes, and, in Africa, Pygmies compared with Tutsi.

B.   Insufficiency of food intake

This certainly occurs, but is not solely responsible for slower growth. For example, in families of black teachers and others in regular employment in South African rural areas, children have been found to be only slightly heavier and taller (usually non-significantly) than the average. Furthermore, many pupils walk several miles to attend school; yet, they have the same mean anthropometric data as those who live nearby, i.e. the extra energy needed must be available from the family's meals (Walker *et al.*, 1978). As already indicated, the huge bulk of Third World children, 95% or more, have normal weight-for-height as stressed by others (Fagundez-Neto *et al.*, 1981). In urban centres, with a rise in socio-economic state and a measure of change in diet, children of parents in regular employment are significantly taller and heavier than the average (Kahn and Freedman, 1959).

C. Pattern of diet

The type of diet consumed, linked possibly with the high bulk associated with a near-vegetarian diet, is believed to be the factor primarily responsible for slower growth. In Western populations, strict vegetarian or vegan children, who subsist on high intakes of plant foods, are shorter and lighter than average. Moreover, frequencies of obesity in vegan babies, children and adults are lower than average (Purves and Sanders, 1980; Bergan and Brown, 1980). When consumers of traditional Third World diets are given supplementary food, the weight gain both in cases of children (Orr and Gilks, 1931) and adults (Prentice et al., 1980; Walker et al., 1981) is usually much less than would be expected should insufficiency of food be characteristic.

D. Non-dietary factors, maternal education

This component is now emerging as perhaps the single most significant determinant of child health and even of mortality (Caldwell, 1981). Cecily Williams (1954) maintained that there would be far less kwashiorkor had mothers a better understanding of how to make the best use of foods at hand.

1. Parasitic infections

In Kenya, removal of intestinal parasites enhanced the growth of previously infected children, i.e. non-nutritional interventions (improved sanitation and anti-helminthic campaigns) may significantly affect children's anthropometric status (Stephenson et al., 1980)

2. Size of family

Growth rate drops with increase in family size; this phenomenon, however, also prevails in Caucasian families.

Many factors therefore influence growth rate, and to attribute slower growth almost exclusively to poverty and insufficient food intake is simplistic and incorrect.

IV.   Growth standards: are they applicable universally?

The Iowa (Vickers and Stuart, 1943) and Boston (Stuart and Meredith, 1946) growth standards were based on weights and heights of a series of well-circumstanced Caucasian children. Their data differ little from those reported from London (Tanner and Whitehouse, 1976), Oslo (Brundtland et al., 1975), and Johannesburg (Walker and Walker, 1977b).

Recently, the U.S. National Center for Health Statistics (Hamill et al., 1979) compiled percentiles "which may be used to improve identification of potential health and nutritional problems and to facilitate the epidemiological comparison of one group of children with others". While the information presented is an advance compared with that given in the classical reference standards, the newer figures have little bearing on the issues under discussion.

In studies on pre-school children in different ethnic groups in the United States and Central America, Habicht *et al.* (1974) found that children in respective upper classes grew at much the same rate. This has already been noted with urban black children in Johannesburg (Kahn and Freedman, 1959). Similar findings were also presented in a more recent study (Graitcer and Gentry, 1981). Ethnicity was thus deemed of minor importance compared with the role of environmental factors, chiefly diet. Accordingly, growth standards were regarded as applicable to all, regardless of race. Evidence on the slower growth of children in some Asian populations [although not Japanese (Eveleth and Tanner, 1976)] was ignored (Rao and Sastry, 1977; Ulijaszek *et al.*, 1979; Walker and Walker, 1977b; Eusebio and Nube, 1981; Walker and Segal, 1981; Trowbridge, 1982). Trowbridge (1982) has pointed out that contrary to the conclusions of Habicht *et al.* (1974), "The weight-for-age growth of well-off Indian, Sri Lankan, and Philippine children in some studies falls below Western reference standards, the difference increasing with age . . .". He emphasized "For these reasons the alternative suggestion of using . . . appropriately adjusted cut-offs of an international standard to define levels of growth considered 'low' for a given population seems far preferable to the development of local standards". This approach would cause fewer complications than earlier FAO/WHO Recommendations (1975); "For target purposes weight-for-age of children should be derived preferably from suitable local anthropometric data, less acceptably from suitable data on comparable genetic groups and, possibly least acceptably, from the Harvard–Iowa standards. For assessment purposes, standard weights for actual heights should be derived".

There are, therefore, limitations to the universal application of reference standards.

V.   Does failure to comply with standards essentially denote inferiority in health?

What evidence is there that children with growth levels lower than those of Western standards, but short of being obviously malnourished, have inferior health? And do they need food supplements?

A.   Field studies

In Third World populations, among the very young, up to 2 years of age, those under the third percentile of weight-for-age have significantly increased morbidity and mortality. For such, dietary supplementation has been found to be rewarding (Kielmann and McCord, 1978; Martinez and Chavaz, 1979). Among children 3–5 years, information is less clear-cut. Hansen (1979) maintains that pre-school children under the third percentile "suffer more from severe forms of malnutrition and have a higher morbidity and mortality rate." However, the handicap is less well documented than that at up to 2 years. The greater proneness of very slow growers to infections is well known (Scrimshaw et al., 1968; Special Report, 1982) although there are limitations. In Nigeria, in a study on anthropometric assessment of energy protein malnutrition and subsequent risk of mortality among pre-school children, results indicated that it was only the *severely* malnourished who experienced substantially higher mortality risk. The normal and moderately malnourished children experienced the same reduced risk. Also in Nigeria, at Malumfashi, frequency of diarrhoea was not increased in underweight (75% weight/age) or stunted (90% height/age) children. But those who were wasted (80% weight/height), experienced 47% more episodes of diarrhoea than those not wasted (Tompkins, 1981). In Bangladesh, in a retrospective investigation on risk of diarrhoeal diseases according to nutritional status of children, results failed to demonstrate that nutritional status defined by anthropometry was associated with the subsequent risk of diarrhoeal diseases (Chen et al., 1980, 1981). Interestingly, in a study carried out in Tanzania, where very slow growth is usual, serum IgE levels were found to be extremely high, "suggesting that the immune mechanisms were not retarded by undernutrition" (Meakins et al., 1981). According to Reddy (1979), stunted children compared with controls do not have impaired immune responses. Clearly, there are insufficiencies of knowledge on the handicaps of slower growth in later pre-school years.

At school-going ages, disabilities linked with markedly slower growth are least well defined. In South Africa, one-third to one-half of rural black school pupils up to late puberty lie below the third percentile of reference weight-for-age. In comparison with moieties above and below this percentile, in different regions we have found either no differences or only very minor differences regarding school attendance (which is excellent), prowess in examinations, ability to traverse long distances to school, in serum albumin concentrations, and in several other variables, including death rate (Walker et al., 1978). This good health experience is not unexpected, for, as Jeanneret and Raymond (1976) averred, school pupils of all populations, developed and developing, have very low morbidity and mortality rates.

What of brain damage due to severe malnutrition and undernutrition? Only in the very young, up to 2 years of age, may damage occur (Stoch and Smythe, 1976; Evans et al., 1980; Richardson, 1980; Dobbing, 1981). Malnutrition, generally, is not regarded as a major cause of mental retardation. Toward the end of World War II, there was a period of 4.6 months of almost complete starvation in Holland. Yet there appears to have been no evidence that the cohort of very young children who were exposed evidenced brain damage in their later years (Brozek, 1979). Currently, according to Waterlow (1981b) "there is debate about the extent to which mental impairment is a direct result of an episode of malnutrition at a vulnerable time, or an indirect result of the social deprivation and poverty which are associated with malnutrition". The foregoing concerns an area (undernutrition, malnutrition, brain damage) where there is much speculation, but where definitive information is lacking.

What of dietary intervention? In very young slow growers, dietary supplementation decreases morbidity and mortality rates. In very slow growing preschoolchildren, some have reported beneficial results. Among schoolchildren, an increase in growth rate often occurs, especially where undernutrition and malnutrition have been common. Yet under less severe conditions, some trial results have proved disappointing (Baertl et al., 1970; Lieberman et al., 1976). Because of lack of response in the former study made in Peru, it was concluded that "this tends to cast doubt on the value of school lunch programs, the most common form of supplementation throughout the world."

In Western populations, the importance of school meals and breakfast, to health, have been questioned (Bender, 1981; Dickie and Bender, 1982). Aware of uncertainties, a joint FAO/WHO Expert Committee on Nutrition (1976) emphasized that "value systems need to be established to assess the comparative benefits by various intervention programmes". Another WHO report, entitled "Supplementary feeding programme: need for a fresh look" (World Health Organization, 1976), averred "there is a feeling that feeding programes have been unsuccessful or unrealistic, but sometimes the need for them is evident and urgent". None, of course, would dispute this.

There are numerous other growth–health–disease situations where knowledge is defective. For example, in a contribution on mortality of low birth weight infants in England and Wales from 1953 to 1979, it was concluded that "There is a serious lack of representative data on rates of handicap in the survivors" (Pharaoh and Alberman, 1981). A series of "healthy breast-fed Australian infants had weight increments in the second 3 months of infancy which were well below standard figures for normal weight reported from Britain, and more closely resembled data from developing countries" (Hitchcock et al., 1981). The authors thus doubted whether current U.K. figures "represent optimum, or even desirable goals. The present study highlights the need for more longitudinal studies of growth and feeding practices in healthy infants".

Clearly, much further investigation is required concerning the sequelae of growth that is much slower than that which prevails in privileged populations.

B.   Views of authorities on slower growth

Cathcart (1940) asked, "Should we aim, as some enthusiasts would have us do, at feeding children in such a way so as to produce that maximum growth and development of which each child is capable? If we succeed in this, are we sure that we have benefited the child? Does maximum growth make for health and longevity? There is certainly some evidence that it does not". More forcibly than Cathcart, Garrow (1967) questioned, "is the normal growth for a North American child necessarily optimal? Are children who are smaller necessarily malnourished? . . . we urgently need facts rather than opinions". Goldstein (1974) contended "there is no necessary reason why, say, a 7-year-old child from an impoverished (poor growth) environment should be assessed against standards for children living in an economically well-off environment on the grounds that the latter standards represent the actual growth potential of the former. The poorer child, whatever his genetic endowment, has a growth pattern related to his environment, which may in fact be optimal."

Waterlow and Rutishauser (1974) regard a child under height-for-age to the extent of 90% or less of Boston standards as *stunted* or retarded, and if under weight-for-height to the extent of 80% or less of expected weight-for-height, as *wasted*. They have questioned whether a stunted child, *ipso facto*, requires nutritional intervention. But if stunted *and* wasted, intervention is called for. They do not consider "children as malnourished just because their weight-for-age is low".

Goldstein and Tanner (1980a, b), in correspondence over their paper on ecological considerations in the creation and use of child growth standards, emphasized, "We were at pains to point out that the idea of 'equal genetic potential', even if it could be sustained in reality, could not be considered separately from the existing environment . . . and that a better definition of optimal (environment) would be the level of nutrition and medical care associated with . . . the lowest mortality and morbidity rates".

Many have emphasized that reference anthropometric standards must be used with caution. According to Keller *et al.* (1976), "Although cases of clinical malnutrition usually exhibit a very low weight-for-age index . . . this index would be expected also to classify as malnourished a considerable number of small but healthy children . . .". According to Waterlow (1981a) "If children who are stunted but not wasted are removed from the category of 'malnourished,' the prevalence of malnutrition in pre-school children in many countries would be reduced by a factor of 5 or more". Furthermore, in the United States where the National Center for Health Statistics pooled skinfold thickness measurements of some 20,000 children aged 1–17 years, it was emphasized "that the percentiles describe the skinfold thickness of

American children and adolescents and should *not* be considered 'norms' or 'standards'" (Owen, 1982).

Jelliffe and Jelliffe (1974) broadened the question at issue and underlined the dilemma over the fact that "growth standards from Western industrialized countries are themselves changing—often upwards. An unsolved question is—which to select? Which standard represents the optimum as regards present and future health and survival, and which the over-nourished with potential of actual risks of obesity"? Others have written similarly (Walker and Richardson, 1973).

Obviously, the use of reference growth standards, and the making of interpretations and drawing of conclusions, require enormous discretion.

VI. Could rapid growth be even detrimental?

A patent weakness of reference growth standards is that little if anything is known of the subsequent health of pupils in adulthood. Was the health status of the very small proportion of very slow growers actually prejudiced then or in the future? Which percentile had the best long distance track record in relation to proneness to degenerative diseases—the fiftieth or below?

Experimentally, early studies by McCay *et al.* (1939) indicated that slower growth in rats is associated with delayed senescence and greater longevity. Masoro *et al.* (1982) reported that severely restricted rats lived a median of 1047 days, compared with a median of 714 days when the same diet was fed to appetite. Ziegler (1966) maintained that "animal experiments have proved that *ad libitum* access to energy rich food leads to maximal, but not necessarily optimal, growth acceleration and weight gain, but is also associated with increased rates of diseases later on . . . such as neoplastic and cardiovascular degenerative diseases". Studies have shown that experimental animals fed high- compared with low-fibre diets are less responsive to chemical carcinogens in respect of bowel and breast tumours (Cummings, 1981).

In the human situation it is interesting that in Western populations, earlier menarche, associated with more rapid growth of girls, is one of the risk factors for breast cancer, which now affects 1 of 11 women in the United States (Miller, 1981). It is also of significance that earlier menarche—about 3 years earlier than a century ago—has made earlier childbearing in Western populations possible. In Third World populations the somewhat earlier menarche has permitted greater numbers of children to be born than in the past, with an increasing survival rate and attendant problems of overcrowding. This has promoted, *inter alia,* psychological problems arising from earlier sexual maturity but delayed emotional maturity associated with prolonged parental dependence, due to longer years of schooling and increased attendance at universities.

A further aspect has been stressed by Stini (1981). In studying the association of early growth patterns with the process of ageing, he concluded, *inter alia*, "Growth-maximizing diets have their greatest impact on male children. The connection between male responsiveness to environmental influences during early growth and vulnerability in the later years is significant to the understanding of the ageing process".

Hence, in terms of proneness to degenerative diseases in later life, it could be argued that rapid growth, usual to Western children and urged by some for Third World children, may not be altogether as meritorious as some insist. Indeed, it is contended that intervention in Third World contexts to promote more rapid growth could even be perilous (Goldstein and Tanner, 1980a; Suwanwela *et al.*, 1981). To advocate the attainment of maximum growth is out of harmony with current exhortations to the young to restrict intakes of fat and sugar (and hence their energy intake) with a view to combating future cardiovascular and other diseases (Walker, 1982).

All the foregoing concern a poorly researched area of biology, yet could be of tremendous importance to public health.

VII. Conclusions

1. Consumption of Western diets, with associated non-dietary contexts, conduces to: (a) more rapid growth in the young, increased height at maturity, but a high frequency of obesity; (b) low rates of infections in the young (and older populations); (c) high frequencies and mortalities from degenerative diseases—principally diabetes, coronary heart disease, stroke and certain types of cancer (colon and breast); and (d) low infant mortality rate, high expectation of life at birth, although indifferent expectation of life at middle-age.

2. Consumption of Third World diets, with associated non-dietary contexts, conduces to the converses of the characteristics enumerated in (a) to (d).

3. The situations described in 1 and 2 are regulated by numerous factors, dietary and non-dietary. This plurality of influencing factors clearly demands the exercising of caution both over criticisms of, as well as praises of, Western and Third World diets.

4. As to the disadvantages of slower growth in very young children (up to 2 years) in the Third World, very slow growth is linked unquestionably with highly increased morbidity and mortality rates. In such contexts dietary supplementation is mandatory. There is the possibility of brain damage in the very young when exposed to severe malnutrition and undernutrition. However, definitive knowledge in this field is lacking. In Third World preschool children, e.g. 3–5 years, low weight-for-age can be, yet is not essentially, associated with increased morbidity and mortality. Certainly, when

stunting *and* wasting are present, dietary intervention is required, although usually the proportion affected with this combination of features is very small. In Third World schoolchildren from 6 to about 15 years, very low weight-for-age prevails in very large proportions, i.e. up to 50% or more, although normal weight-for-height is almost characteristic. The proportion with wasting is extremely low. The disabilities linked with slower growth are not obvious; indeed, this period is the most healthful in the life span. By mid-adolescence, proportions under the third percentile have fallen tremendously, without intervention, especially in the case of girls.

5. The conclusion is reached that, apart from extreme deficits, slower growth associated with consumption of traditional high-fibre, low-fat intakes is not essentially deleterious. Indeed, in its contextual association with relatively low frequencies of degenerative diseases in later life, slower growth could well be optimal.

6. As numerous authorities have urged, the ramifications of differing rates of growth on subsequent as well as current health require extensive investigation through retrospective and longitudinal studies.

References

ANDERSON, M. A. *(1979)*. *Am. J. Clin. Nutr.* 32, 2339–2345.

BAERTL, J.M., MORALES, E., VERASTEGUI, G. and GRAHAM, G. G. (1970). *Am. J. Clin. Nutr.* 23, 707–715.

BENDER, A. E. (1981). *In* "Preventive Nutrition andSociety" (M. R. Turner, ed.), pp. 109–119. Academic Press, London.

BERGAN, J. G. and BROWN, P. T. (1980). *J. Am. Diet, Assoc.* 76, 151–155.

BROZEK, J. (1979). Discussion *In.* "Malnutrition in South Africa" (R. D. Griesel, ed.), p 147. University of South Africa, Pretoria.

BRUNDTLAND, G. H., LIESTOL, K. and WALLOE, L. (1975). *Acta Paediatr. Scand.* 64, 565–573.

CALDWELL, J. C. (1981). *World Health Forum* 2, 75–78.

CATHCART, E. P. (1940). *Lancet* 1, 533–537.

CHEN, L. C. CHOWDHURY, A. K. M. A. and HUFFMAN, S. L. (1980). *Am. J. Clin. Nutr.* 33, 1836–1845.

CHEN, L. C., HUG, E. and HUFFMAN, S. L. (1981). *Am. J. Epidemiol.* 114, 284–292.

CUMMINGS, J. H. (1981). *Proc. Nutr. Soc.* 40, 7–14.

DAVIES, C. T. M. and MBELWA, D. (1974). *East Afr. Med J.* 51, 382–387.

DEN HARTOG, A. P. (1980). *Voeding* 41, 292–302, 334–342, 348–357.

DICKIE, N. H. and BENDER, A. E. (1982). *Br. J. Nutr.* 48, 483–496.

DOBBING, J. (1981). *Lancet* 1, 836.

EUSEBIO, J. S. and NUBE, M. (1981). *Lancet* 2, 1223.

EVANS, D., BOWIE, M. D., HANSEN, J. D. L., MOODIE, A. D. and VAN DER SPUY, H. I. J. (1980). *J. Pediatr.* 97, 358–363.

EVELETH, P. B. and TANNER, J. M. (1976). "Worldwide Variation in Human Growth." Cambridge University Press, London.

FAGUNDES-NETO, U., BARUZZI, R. G., WEHBA, J., SILVESTRINI, W. S., MORAIS, M. B. and CAINELLI, M. (1981). *Am. J. Clin. Nutr.* 34, 2229–2235.

FAO/WHO Recommendations (1975). *Food Nutr.* **1**, 11.

FAO/WHO Expert Committee on Nutrition (1976). "Food and Nutrition Strategies in National Development", WHO Tech. Rep. Ser. No. 584, p. 58. World Health Organization, Geneva.

GARROW, J. S. (1967). *Lancet* **1**, 278–279.

GEEFHUYSEN, J., ROSEN, E. U., KATZ, J., IPP, T. and METZ, J. (1971). *Br. Med. J.* **4**, 527–529.

GOLDSTEIN, H. (1974). *Lancet* **1**, 1051–1052.

GOLDSTEIN, H. and TANNER, J. M. (1980a). *Lancet* **1**, 582–585.

GOLDSTEIN, H. and TANNER, J. M. (1980b). *Lancet,* **2**, 35.

GRAITCER, P. L. and GENTRY, E. M. (1981). *Lancet,* **2**, 297–299.

HABICHT, J.-P., YARBOROUGH, C., MARTORELL, R., MALINA, R. M. and KLEIN, R. E. (1974). *Lancet* **1**, 611–615.

HALLER, L. and LAUBER, E. (1980). *Acta Trop.* **37**, 63–73.

HAMILL, P. V. V., DRIZD, T. A., JOHNSON, C. L., REED, R. B., ROCHE, A. F. and MOORE, W. M. (1979). *Am. J. Clin. Nutr.* **32**, 607–629.

HANSEN, J. D. L. (1979). Discussion. *In* "Malnutrition in South Africa" (R. D. Griesel, ed.), pp. 29–30. University of South Africa, Pretoria.

HITCHCOCK, N. E., GRACIE, M. and OWLES, E. N. (1981). *Lancet* **1**, 64–65.

HOLLINGSWORTH, D. (1974). *Nutr. Rev.* **32**, 353–359.

JEANNERET, O. and RAYMOND, L. (1976). *WHO Chron.* **30**, 101–107.

JELLIFFE, D. B. and JELLIFFE, E. F. P. (1974). *Lancet* **2**, 47.

KAHN, E. and FREEDMAN, M. L. (1959). *S. Afr. Med. J.* **33**, 934–936.

KELLER, W., DONOSO, G. and DEMAEYER, E. M. (1976). *Nutr. Abstr. Rev.* **46**, 591–609.

KIELMANN, A. A. and McCORD, C. (1978). *Lancet* **1**, 1247–1250.

KOTZE, J. P., VAN DER MERWE, G. J., MOSTERT, W. P., REYNDERS, J. J., BARNARD, S. O. and SNYMAN, N. (1982). *J. Diet. Home Econ.* **10**, 77–81.

LIEBERMAN, H. M., HUNT, I. F., COULSON, A. H., CLARK, V. A., SWENDSEID, M. E. and HO L. (1976). *J. Am. Diet. Assoc.* **68**, 132–138.

McCAY, C. M., MAYNARD, L. A., SPERLING, G. and BARNES, L. L. (1939), *J. Nutr.* **18**, 1–13.

MANNING, E. B., MANN, J. I., SOPHANGISA, E. and TRUSWELL, A. S. (1974). *S. Afr. Med. J.* **48**, 485–497.

MARTINEZ, C. and CHAVAZ, A. (1979). *Nutr. Rep. Int.* **19**, 307–314.

MASORO, E. J., YU, B. P. and BERTRAND, H. A. (1982). *Proc. Natl. Acad. Sci. U.S.A.* **79**, 4239–4241.

MEAKINS, R. H., HARLAND, P. S. E. G. and CARSWELL, F. (1981). *Trans. R. Soc. Trop. Med. Hyg.* **75**, 731–735.

MILLER, A. B. (1981). *Cancer* **47**, 1109–1113.

ORR, J. B. and GILKS, J. L. (1931). "The Physique and Health of Two African Tribes", MRC Spec. Rep. Ser. No. 155. Her Majesty's Stationery Office, London.

OWEN, G. M. (1982). *Am. J. Clin. Nutr.* **35**, 629–638.

PATON, D. N. and FINDLAY, L. (1926). "Poverty, Nutrition and Growth" MRC Spec. Rep. Ser. No. 101. Her Majesty's Stationery Office, London.

PHARAOH, P. E. D. and ALBERMAN, E. D. (1981). *Arch Dis. Child.* **56**, 86–89.

PRENTICE, A. M., ROBERTS, S. B. WATKINSON, M., WHITEHEAD, R. G., PAUL, A. A., PRENTICE, A. and WATKINSON, A. A. (1980). *Lancet* **2**, 886–888.

PURVES, R. and SANDERS, T. A. B. (1980). *Proc. Nutr. Soc.* **39**, 79A.

RAO, D. H. and SASTRY, J. G. (1977). *Indian J. Med Res.* **66**, 950–956.

REDDY, V. (1979). *In* "Nutrition in Health or Disease and International Development" (A. H. Harper and G. K. Davis, eds), pp. 227–235. Alan R. Liss Inc., New York.

RICHARDSON, B. D. (1978), *S. Afr. J. Sci.* **74**, 246–249.

RICHARDSON, B. D. (1979). *Trans. R. Soc. Trop. Med. Hyg.* **71,** 210–216.

RICHARDSON, S. A. (1980). *In* "Nutrition in Childhood" (B. Wharton, ed.), pp. 163–176. Pitman, London.

SCRIMSHAW, N. S., TAYLOR, C. E. and GORDON, J. E. (1968). "Interaction of Nutrition and Infection." World Health Organization, Geneva.

Special Report (1982). *Nutr. Rev.* **33,** 119–128.

STEIN, H. and ROSEN, E. W. (1980). *S. Afr. Med J.* **58,** 1030–1032.

STEPHENSON, L. S., CROMPTON, D. W. T., LATHAM, M. C., SCHULPEN, T. W. J., NESHEIM, M. C. and JANSEN, A. A. J. (1980). *Am. J. Clin. Nutr.* **33,** 1165–1172.

STEWART, A. M. and ELLIS, B. P. B. (1975). *Cent. Afr. J. Med.* **21,** 45–49.

STINI, W. A. (1981). *Fed Proc. Fed. Am. Soc. Exp. Biol.* **40,** 2588–2594.

STOCH, M. B. and SMYTHE, P. M. (1976). *Arch. Dis. Child.* **51,** 327–336.

STUART, H. C. and MEREDITH, H. V. (1946). *Am. J. Public Health* **36,** 1365–1386.

SUWANWELA, C., POSHYACHINDA, V., THASANAPRADIT, P. and DHARMKRONG-AT, A. (1981). *World Health Forum* **2,** 222–224.

TANNER, J. M. and WHITEHOUSE, R. H. (1976). *Arch. Dis. Child.* **51,** 170–179.

TOMPKINS, A. (1981). *Lancet* **1,** 860–862.

TROWBRIDGE, F. L. (1982). *Lancet* **1,** 232.

TROWELL, H. C. and BURKITT, D. P. (1981). "Western Diseases: Their Emergence and Prevention." Edward Arnold, London.

ULIJASZEK, S., EVANS, E. and MUMFORD, P. (1979). *Lancet* **1,** 214.

VAUGHAN, V. C. (1969). *In* "Textbook of Pediatrics" (W. E. Nelson, V. C. Vaughan and R. J. McKay, eds), 9th edition, pp. 15–56. Saunders, Philadelphia.

VICKERS, V. S. and STUART, H. C. (1943). *J. Pediatr.* **22,** 155–170.

WALKER, A. R. P. (1982). *S. Afr. Med. J.* **61,** 126–129.

WALKER, A. R. P. and RICHARDSON, B. D. (1973). *Am. J. Clin. Nutr.* **26,** 897–900.

WALKER, A. R. P. and SEGAL, I. (1981). *Br. Med. J.* **2,** 63.

WALKER, A. R. P. and WALKER, B. F. (1977a). *S. Afr. Med. J.* **51,** 707–712.

WALKER, A. R. P. and WALKER, B. F. (1977b). *J. Trop. Med. Hyg.* **80,** 119–125.

WALKER, A. R. P., BHAMJEE, D., WALKER, B. F. and RICHARDSON, B. D. (1978). *J. Trop. Med. Hyg.* **81,** 2–8.

WALKER, A. R. P., METZ, J., LOWTHER, A. B. and LINNETT, P. J. (1981). *Lancet* **1,** 1054.

WATERLOW, J. C. (1981a). *Lancet* **1,** 100–101.

WATERLOW, J. C. (1981b). *Proc. Nutr. Soc.* **40,** 195–207.

WATERLOW, J. C. and RUTISHAUSER, I. H. E. (1974). *In* "Early Malnutrition and Mental Development" (J. Cravioto, L. Hambraeus and B. Valquist, eds), p. 5. Almqvist and Wiksell, Stockholm.

WILLIAMS, C. (1954). *Lancet* **1,** 323–325.

World Health Organization (1976). *PAG Bull.* **6,** 41.

ZIEGLER, E. (1966). "Die Ursache der Akzeleration." Schwabe, Basel.

Chapter 21

Renal stone

NORMAN BLACKLOCK

I.   Introduction

A. *Renal stone*

The dramatic rise in incidence of calcium stones of the kidney within the last 100 years resembles that of other conditions which are now recognised as the diseases of Western civilisation. More than 80% of those who have stones in the kidney may justifiably be regarded as having this additional disease which is characteristic of affluent modern societies. The idiopathic renal stone consists predominantly of calcium oxalate with or without calcium phosphate. This composition has been confirmed on a worldwide basis.

Every large series of kidney stone cases produces a small number in whom there is either a specific disorder of metabolism or an anatomical abnormality, or an infection. However, all of these conditions together constitute less than 20% of any group of kidney stone formers whether these are in Europe, North America, Australasia or Japan (Ljunghall and Hedstrand, 1975; Coe and Kavalach, 1974: Yoshida, 1979).

Within the technically advanced and affluent communities of the world, therefore, the predominant kidney stone—occurring in more than 80%— is a stone unaccompanied by detectable metabolic or other abnormality; hence the term *idiopathic stone*. Its cause is not yet clearly defined but is probably

345

Dietary Fibre, Fibre-Depleted Foods
and Disease

resultant on the coincidence of a number of contributory factors, intrinsic and environmental. The latter factors appear closely associated with the dietary lifestyle of affluence. Epidemiological studies within the past decade, coupled with experimental studies in man and in animals, have begun to define certain dietary associations which are probably causative. This has introduced a new concept concerning the cause of this idiopathic disease in susceptible phenotypes, it has begun to redirect research and it is altering the treatment of patients.

B.   Bladder stone

The urinary stone of history was the idiopathic bladder stone—a childhood problem predominantly afflicting the male. Whilst quite common in western Europe and England some hundreds of years ago, it is now a rarity in the Western world but still occurs commonly in the "endemic stone areas" of northeast Thailand, Indonesia, northwest India and some areas of the Middle East and Egypt. Field studies have implicated poor maternal nutrition as the main aetiological factor—the effects of poor or inadequate maternal milk taken by an already frail infant—and also the specific features of very early substitute feeds high in carbohydrate and low in protein. Interestingly, the evidence has been found for exactly similar circumstances in association with bladder stone in England some hundreds of years ago.

In mainland China at the turn of the century, there was the problem of bladder stone similar to that in the other endemic stone areas. Following the establishment of the Peoples Republic in 1949, malnutrition has progressively disappeared and with it the bladder stone problem. Nevertheless, as the incidence of bladder stone has diminished so has the incidence of idiopathic renal stone increased, although overall incidence rates of the latter are significantly lower than those in Japan, Europe and North America (Ku, 1978).

II.   Epidemiology of renal stone

When Grossman (1938) observed the great rise in hospital incidence of renal stone in Central Europe after World War I, he called the phenomenon "the stone wave". Whilst this rise might only have been apparent as the result of better diagnostic methods, the extent of the rise noted—100% in Finland between 1907 and 1954 (Sallinen, 1959) and 200% in Norway between 1920 and 1960 (Andersen, 1966)—indicates clearly that there has been a real increase. A similar course of events was observed in Japan from after the termination of the war in 1945 (Inada et al., 1958) (Fig. 21.1). Although graphs of incidence of renal stone have shown a progressive rise in Europe and Japan during the present century, this rise was interrupted during the war years when there was an actual diminution in the incidence of the condi-

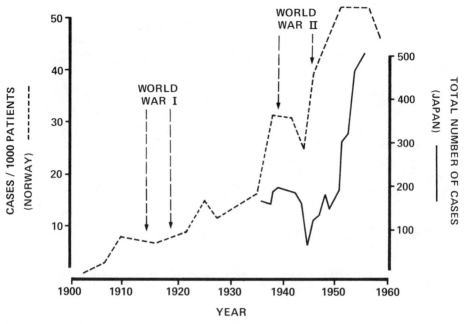

FIG. 21.1. Change in incidence of renal stone in patients of Oslo City Hospital, Norway, 1900–1960 (from Andersen, 1966) and in Japan 1935–1955 (from Inada *et al.,* 1958).

tion in Europe (Andersen, 1973). Necropsy statistics in Germany (Schumann, 1963) also provide further confirmation of a marked increase in renal urolithiasis (Fig. 21.2) and interestingly show, too, a diminished incidence during both World War I and World War II. Since both World Wars produced a major impact on food availability for the populace of both sides, it is likely that the diminished incidence of calcium stone of the kidney at those times was related to the changes in the diet.

The incidence rates of idiopathic stone per 100,000 people were 164 in the United States (Sierakowski *et al.,* 1978), 111 in Hungary (Rosdy, 1982), 82 in the United Kingdom (Currie and Turner, 1979) and 70 in Japan (Yoshida, 1979). Most of these figures have been obtained from hospital admission records and probably underestimate the true occurrence of the condition since Ljunghall and Hedstrand (1975) found that only 25% of stone patients were ever admitted to hospitals in Sweden. Prevalence rates from population studies give further perspectives concerning the extent of the problem. Ljunghall and Hedstrand (1975) found that the prevalence in a Swedish population was 13.7% and this compared with 12% in Denmark. Ljunghall and Hedstrand (1975) and Norlin *et al.* (1976) considered from their evidence that renal stone prevalence rates were still rising in Sweden at the time of their surveys. In the United States, Finlayson (1974) found a prevalence

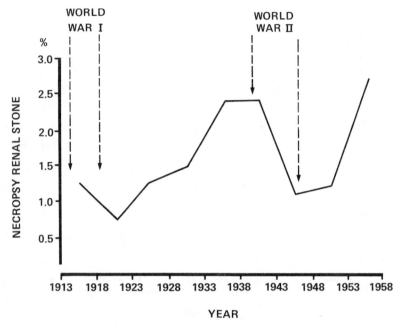

FIG. 21.2. Incidence of renal stone at necropsy in Leipzig, Germany between 1913 and 1958. From Schumann (1963).

rate around 12% and estimated that the direct medical cost of the disease was in excess of 47 million dollars per year.

In contrast to the figures of high and rising incidence rates in affluent communities, those in developing communities of the world remain low. Modlin (1969) noted that renal stones had not been reported in the South African Bantu living under tribal conditions. Reaser (1935) reported a relative immunity of the U.S. blacks at the time of his survey but this was less obvious some years later and after World War II (Quinland, 1945). By this time there was greater affluence of the U.S. blacks and the adoption by them of a lifestyle more like that of the whites.

In Nigeria, Esho (1979) reported very low rates of incidence from renal stone and only seven cases had been found in 100,000 hospital admissions in Lagos. There is a further example of how a previously low incidence rate in a specific community can be influenced by greater affluence. In West Germany, Boshamer (1961) observed that immigrant workers from southeast Europe—Turkey and the Balkans, where stone is uncommon—became kidney stone formers a year or two after their arrival to work in the more affluent conditions of industrial Germany. A further relationship with the affluent lifestyle is the very high incidence of this condition in the Arabian Peninsula, although other important factors, such as dehydration, are involved.

A familial predisposition to stone has been found, and this implicates genetic factors. This may be connected with familial idiopathic hyper-calciuria which has been described by Coe *et al.* (1979). However, White *et al.* (1969) found that the spouses of some hypercalciuric stone formers also had hypercalciuria, which suggested the influence of a domestic factor that is most likely a dietary one.

Apart from eating habits, other environmental conditions are known to influence the risk of stone formation, not least a hot climate. This has two effects. First, it produces a more concentrated urine if hydration is inade-quate and, second, there is a greater rate of sunshine-induced synthesis of vitamin D_3 precursor in the skin which increases intestinal calcium absorp-tion and hence calcium excretion in the urine (Parry and Lister, 1975). Whilst an indigenous population may be put at risk by excessive fluid loss in hot climatic conditions when hydration is insufficient, it is usually at least partially protected from the ill effects of excess vitamin D synthesis by the dark skin pigmentation and/or keratinisation; these modify the rate of syn-thesis (Macleod and Blacklock, 1979a).

In summary, from being virtually unknown in historic times, renal stone has become significant as a morbid condition in the affluent, westernised countries within the last 100 years whilst remaining rare in the Third World communities where the people live in poorer conditions. The association with affluence is further strengthened by the observations of Andersen (1973) and Robertson *et al.* (1979) who found the disease more prevalent in men in the higher socio-economic groups; their data also showed a strong correlation between the occurrence of stone and the level of affluence as defined by annual income and expenditure on food.

Idiopathic renal stone presents with the same characteristics in affected communities in all parts of the world. The peak age of occurrence in men is 35 years and in women there is a double peak—one at 30 and the second at 55 (Robertson *et al.*, 1979). This second peak may be associated with the hyper-calciuric bone loss observed to occur after the menopause (Nordin *et al.*, 1972). Idiopathic renal stone is increasingly common now in childhood (Ghazali *et al.*, 1973). The incidence in women is one-quarter of that in men during the reproductive years. Blacklock (1969) and Lavan *et al.* (1971) observed an association between idiopathic stone and overweight. Renal stone is a recurrent condition with recurrence rates as high as 75% (Williams, 1963; Blacklock, 1969).

III. Pathogenesis of renal stone

A. *Physico-chemical factors*

Calculi are predominantly crystalline substances and their formation in the urinary tract is attributable to precipitation from supersaturated solution

(Robertson and Nordin, 1976). Solutes in the urine are usually in a metastable zone of saturation between solubility and what is known as "formation limits". In metastable saturation, spontaneous formation of crystals is unlikely to occur, but if a nucleus of crystalline or organic material is present, then crystallization may take place on this to form an aggregate of crystals which may thereafter grow to form a small stone or microlith. If the urine exceeds the formation limit of saturation and becomes oversaturated, spontaneous crystallization may take place in the absence of any other factor. This may be modified, however, by inhibitors in the urine and it has been suggested that lack of these inhibitory factors may be a factor in calcium stone formation. Since the idiopathic renal stone is calcium oxalate, with or without calcium phosphate, the conditions that can lead to a state of oversaturation of the urine with these salts include (1) increase in urinary excretion rate of calcium; stone risk is increased six times with increase of urinary calcium excretion from 300 to 600 mg daily (Nordin *et al.*, 1976); (2) increase in urinary oxalate excretion; and (3) change of pH to alkalinity in the presence of hypercalciuria in the case of calcium phosphate crystallization.

Robertson and Peacock (1978) described six main urinary risk factors involved in the formation of calcium-containing stones which include urine volume, pH and the excretion rates of calcium, oxalate, uric acid and also glycosaminoglycans (GAGS), which are crystallization inhibitors in respect of calcium oxalate. These factors directly or indirectly affect the relative saturation of the urine with calcium salts. From these factors, the risk of calcium stone formation can be determined in each case (Robertson and Nordin, 1976). Risk factors are higher in stone formers than in normal subjects and are correlated with the severity of the disease and the rate of recurrence.

Hypercalciuria (a high rate of calcium excretion in the urine) increases the risk of stone formation and occurs in about 40% of stone formers compared with 10% of normal subjects (Robertson and Morgan, 1972). The excretion rate of calcium, however, is normal in most hypercalciuric subjects after overnight fasting.

In association with hypercalciuria there is increase in intestinal absorption of calcium. This was found in approximately 70% of solitary stone formers and 90 per cent with multiple, recurrent stones (Blacklock and Macleod, 1974). Nordin *et al.* (1976) found the stone risk to increase sixfold with a rise in the rate of radio-calcium absorption from 0.5 of the dose to 1.2 of the dose per hour. Increased absorption may be associated with increased ingestion of calcium, its greater availability in absorptive form, and the greater mucosal stimulus to absorption from increased formation of vitamin D.

Increase in the rate of urinary oxalate excretion has a greater risk effect per unit of increment in comparison with urinary calcium excretion. Calcium stone formers in general excrete more oxalate than non-stone formers; this is related to the greater rate of calcium absorption from the intestine. The probable mechanism is the relatively smaller residue of calcium left within the intestinal lumen as the result of the increased absorption rates; this leaves more dietary oxalate in a soluble form and therefore absorbable (Dobbins *et al.*, 1981).

The negative correlation between renal stone and water hardness—which is largely a manifestation of its calcium content—reported in the United Kingdom by Rose and Westbury (1975) and in the United States by Sierakowski *et al.* (1978)—may be due to this effect; dietary oxalate is precipitated as insoluble calcium oxalate during cooking, rendering it unavailable for absorption. Increase in urinary oxalate also occurs in association with a rise in uric acid excretion on a high-purine diet (Zarembski and Hodgkinson, 1969).

Uric acid is a risk factor in the urine for the reasons of its poor solubility which is further diminished in acid urine and its interference with natural crystallization inhibitors in the urine. Hyperuricosuria is found in calcium oxalate stone formers and in one series occured in 26% with or without hypercalciuria; it is more prevalent in those with recurrent calculi (Coe and Kavalach, 1974). These investigators also found that the purine consumption of calcium stone formers was significantly greater than those with no history of stone.

In summary, there are well recognised physico-chemical factors in respect of idiopathic stone formation associated with increased excretion rates of calcium, oxalate and uric acid. Whilst increased rates of excretion occur in approximately 60% of stone formers, the extent of this is only such that the abnormal values lie mainly at the upper levels of normal. Because of this, the disease has been described as "idiopathic". However, urinary electrolyte excretion is known to be influenced by food ingestion. Andersen (1973) was the first to suggest that dietary composition provided the baseline of stone incidence within a community by influencing urinary risk factors towards oversaturation with the salts of the commonly occurring stone, that is with calcium oxalate and calcium phosphate.

Whilst the urinary contents of the various risk factors involved in oversaturation are of major importance, the kinetics of crystal formation are such that this is unlikely to take place during the transit time of the glomerular filtrate through the nephron (Finlayson and Ried, 1978). However, if there is a fixed focus of calcification within the course of the nephron this will provoke crystallization on it from the tubular urine in transit. The predisposition to this will increase if the urine becomes more saturated with stoneforming salts. This is the basis of the fixed particle mechanism propounded by Finlayson and Reid (1978), a calcified deposit in the tubular cell being an essential pre-requisite for the development of nephrolithiasis. Anderson (1969) and others have noted the significantly greater incidence of nephrocalcinosis in a stone-forming population, which may be relevant in

this regard. Furthermore, Burry *et al.* (1976) found increasing incidence of
nephrocalcinosis with age in their necropsy series. The notable feature of
their findings was that calcification was already present in 60% of adolescents
under the age of 20 in Australasia. The cause of this focal calcification is of
major importance in the overall consideration of idiopathic stone. A possible
mechanism for it, and its relation to sucrose ingestion, is discussed later.
There may be further significance in such foci of renal tubular cell damage in
respect of their role in the local release of prostaglandin E_2, which has been
found significantly to increase the rate of calcium excretion in the urine (Buck
et al., 1981).

B.   Dietary factors

i.   Dietary change with affluence

Differences in the present Western world diet compared with that of 200
years ago, when renal stone was uncommon, are similar to the dietary differences which exist between the poor and affluent communities of today
(Périssé *et al.*, 1969) (Fig. 21.3). Affluent diets contain three to five times
more fat and animal protein and five times more sugar (Andersen, 1973).
Cleave (1974) drew attention to the progressive and considerable increase in
sugar consumption in the United Kingdom between 1850 and 1960, the
steady rise being interrupted by rationing in the two World Wars (Fig. 21.4).

Inada *et al.* (1958) noted the considerable increase of renal stone in the
Japanese since about 1945. When the war ended reconstruction and the post-
war boom commenced (Fig. 21.1). Kagawa (1978) reported a dramatic

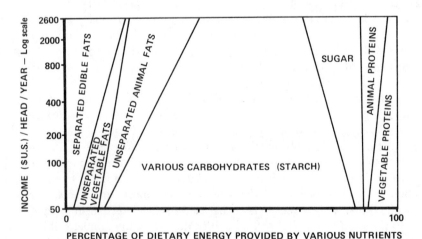

FIG. 21.3. Energy derived from fats, carbohydrates and proteins as percentages of the total
according to the income of 85 countries From Périssé *et al.* (1969). Copyright by the Food and
Agriculture Organization of the United Nations.

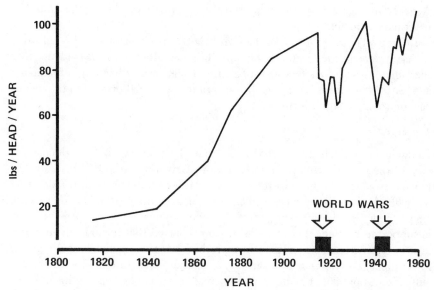

FIG. 21.4 Increased sugar consumption per head in Britain, 1815–1955 From Cleave (1974).

change in the Japanese dietary style that occurred during these years. Thus, sugar consumption increased twofold, meat, poultry and eggs increased sevenfold and dairy products by a factor of fifteen. At the same time there was a considerable reduction in the consumption of rice, wheat, barley, potatoes and vegetables.

2. *Animal protein*

Robertson *et al.* (1979) reported that additional animal protein increased significantly urinary excretion rates of calcium oxalate and uric acid so that there would be a greater likelihood of spontaneous calcium oxalate crystallization. Increased uric acid excretion also interferes with the inhibition of calcium oxalate crystallization by glycosaminoglycan. Coe and Kavalach (1974) found that the urate excretion rate was influenced by the consumption of purine-containing foods such as meat, fish and poultry, and also by the endogenous production of urate, itself increased by animal protein consumption. They observed that stone formers ate more meat, fish and poultry and less bread.

Animal protein, therefore, increases significantly three of the risk factors of calcium oxalate stone formation. It increases excretion of calcium (Anand and Linswiler, 1974), oxalate (Marshall *et al.*, 1972) and uric acid (Coe and Kavalach, 1974; Robertson *et al.*, 1976).

Meat eating can also adversely affect urine pH. Hadzija (1969) observed a significantly lower urine pH in animal protein supplemented diets in West

Africa. Any increase in acidity has the effect of further reducing the solubility of urinary uric acid.

Robertson *et al.* (1981) found a significantly lower incidence of renal stone in vegetarians in the United Kingdom. This, together with the evidence that meat increases the risk factors for calcium oxalate crystallization in the urine, suggests the need for reduction of the amount of animal protein in the diet of calcium oxalate stone formers.

3.   *Sugar*

Hodgkinson and Heaton (1965) and others have observed that glucose increases the rate of urine calcium excretion. Lemann *et al.* (1969) found that glucose exaggerates an existing hypercalciuria in known calcium stone formers besides provoking increased calciuria in a group of normal people. This suggested a disorder of carbohydrate metabolism in some stone formers. This is supported by Scholz *et al.* (1981), who reported that normo-calciuric and absorptive hypercalciuric stone formers had a higher gastrin, insulin and a lower glucagon response to a carbohydrate-rich meal compared with normal subjects and patients having renal hypercalciuria. Higher fasting insulin and glucagon, together with a greater and more prolonged insulin response after a glucose test meal, have also been noted by Rao *et al.* (1982) in 60% of recurrent calcium oxalate stone formers.

These findings suggest that a proportion of stone formers are maladapted to a high consumption of sucrose such as that found in a Western diet; they respond to this by significantly increased rates of calcium excretion. This effect is probably mediated by insulin which is calciuretic (De Fronzo *et al.*, 1975).

Even in a normal population, studies have also shown that sucrose or sucrose-containing products, when added as supplements to a standard diet, increase the frequency and magnitude of diurnal peaks of urinary calcium concentration in a majority of persons. Urinary oxalate excretion and concentration are increased concomitantly and the formation product of calcium oxalate is exceeded with the risk of spontaneous crystallization (Thom *et al.*, 1978, 1980).

Kang *et al.* (1977) observed that ingestion of sucrose by laboratory animals may result in a diffuse intercapillary glomerulosclerosis and that urinary excretion of N-acetyl-β-glucosaminadase, an indicator of renal tubular cell damage (Dance and Price, 1970), is significantly greater during and after sucrose feeding. Oxley *et al,* (1979) observed that rats which were fed sucrose developed nephrocalcinosis within a few weeks of commencement of sugar ingestion. The possibility that ingested sucrose produces damage in tubular cells is of great importance in view of the observations of Anderson (1969) and others of nephrocalcinosis and microcalculi in histological studies of human renal biopsies and resection specimens from calcium stone formers, as already noted. These are located both within the lumen of the tubule and in the tubular cells: they therefore could provide the calcified lesion, postulated by Finlayson and Reid (1978), as an essential prerequisite of a fixed particle mechanism for stone formation. These lesions have been produced in laboratory animals after sucrose feeding, and are associated with increased rates of urinary excretion of N-acetyl-β-glucosaminadase.

Yudkin et al. (1980) have also observed that a high sugar intake in 14 healthy male subjects significantly increased urinary excretion of N-acetyl-β-glucosaminadase and this persisted even after sugar ingestion ceased. The results of this study suggest that a high sugar intake can cause kidney damage in men and that it might, therefore, ultimately lead to the nephropathy and nephrocalcinosis comparable to that found in rats. The findings of Burry et al. (1976) to which reference has already been made, are more significant because of their observations in Australia of the presence of nephrocalcinosis in 10% of children under the age of 10 and 60% of adolescents under the age of 20. Serious consideration must now be given to the possible effects on the kidney in early life of the ingestion of excessive amounts of sugar as a factor in the production of a nephropathy, leaving the legacy of a predisposition to renal stone.

Sucrose also can induce a significant increase in the rate of calcium absorption from the intestine (Macleod and Blacklock, 1979a). Both normal subjects and idiopathic calcium stone formers showed increased calcium absorption following a sucrose meal; the increase, however, was proportionately less in stone formers in view of their spontaneously high basal rate of absorption. The greater induced calcium absorption from the upper intestine leaves a smaller calcium residue to combine with dietary oxalate in the lumen of the gut. More oxalate, therefore, remains soluble and absorbable and this may be the explanation of the increased urinary oxalate excretion found following sugar ingestion.

In summary, sucrose can influence adversely certain factors in the urine, i.e. calcium and oxalate content, to the extent of oversaturation and the possibility of spontaneous crystallization while at the same time increasing the uptake of calcium from the intestine. Furthermore, a proportion of renal stone formers have shown evidence of maladaptation to sucrose in having an exaggerated insulin response to glucose and resultant hypercalciuria. Finally, there is now evidence to suggest that sucrose can produce a nephropathy and therefore an initial renal lesion, or fixed focus, on which crystallization and crystal aggregation can subsequently take place.

4. *Dietary fibre*

African peasants eat a high-fibre, high-carbohydrate (starch) diet, often containing 80–120 g dietary fibre per day. Western adults eat a low-fibre, low-carbohydrate (starch) diet, often containing 15–25 g dietary fibre per day (p.

100). (Dietary fibre figures, some three to five times those for crude fibre, are replacing the latter data.) Dietary fibre exerts both a physical and physico-chemical effect in the alimentary tract. It absorbs water, increases stool bulk and in this way shortens intestinal transit time. This may influence oxalate absorption.

Haber, et al. (1977) showed that cereal fibre can trap and slow the absorption of nutrients, such as sugar. Wheat bran improves glucose tolerance and reduces plasma glucose in diabetics (Jeffreys, 1973). Kiehm et al. (1976) found that a high-fibre, high-carbohydrate diet diminished the requirement of sulphanylureas and insulin in diabetic patients. Miranda and Horwitz (1978) observed a lower mean serum glucagon with high-fibre diets. These effects of dietary fibre in diminishing the insulin and glucagon response to energy-dense nutrients are of considerable significance in calcium stone disease in view of the probable mediation of insulin and glucagon in renal function and urinary electrolyte excretion (De Fronzo et al., 1975). An abnormal insulin and gastrointestinal hormone response of some stone formers to a glucose meal has been reported by Scholz et al. (1981) and Rao et al. (1982).

Wheat bran has been observed to diminish calcium absorption from the intestine in a group of normal subjects by as much as 50%; this also negated the sucrose-induced increase in calcium absorption (Macleod and Blacklock, 1979b). This may have resulted either from the cereal fibre trapping the nutrient (sugar) *and slowing its absorption* or specifically absorbing the calcium, or a combination of both. Reduced plasma levels of gastrointestinal hormones observed by Miranda and Horwitz (1978), accompanying high-fibre diets, may also influence absorption rates. In practical application of these observations, Shah et al. (1981) reported that urinary calcium levels of hypercalciuric stone formers had been reduced merely by the addition of wheat bran to the diet.

IV.   Conclusions

The epidemiology of idiopathic kidney stone and the evidence from metabolic studies of idiopathic stone formers confirm the suspicion that diet plays a large part in the pathogenesis of this disease. The hypothesis of Andersen (1973) appears largely to have been substantiated by the research work herein described. It has been shown that the diet typical of the affluent westernised countries increases the likelihood of calcium oxalate crystallization in the urine and reduces the activity of acid mucopolysaccharide inhibitors (GAGS) of this crystallization. These diets provide a reason for the frequency of stone formers in westernised communities. Further, the finding of a subset of stone formers, whose minimal aberrations of metabolism are aggravated by sucrose, suggests there may be an unknown number of such individuals in a general population who are maladapted to a high-sucrose, low-fibre diet and are at increased risk of idiopathic renal stone and other diseases of civilization. There are, therefore, grounds for postulating that the dietary changes that have occurred in westernised countries during the past 100 years are responsible for the recent greatly increased incidence of renal stone—the "stone wave".

The implication of these observations is that idiopathic calcium urolithiasis, whatever the minor metabolic abnormalities which are present, should be diminished significantly in incidence by the appropriate change of diet. Rao *et al.* (1982), in a clinical application of the lessons of both the epidemiology and the recent research work, have now shown in a series of idiopathic stone formers that those who complied with dietary instructions—more than 60%—showed significant diminution in the urinary excretion rates of calcium, oxalate and uric acid, with resultant lowering of saturation indices for calcium oxalate. The prescribed diet contained less meat, fat and sugar, but more dietary fibre.

However, the long latent interval that often occurs between one stone incident and another means that a long time may pass before statistical proof can be obtained of the efficacy of this change of diet. Available epidemiological and experimental studies strongly suggest that a decreased recurrence of renal stone will occur. More research along these lines is anticipated.

References

ANAND, C. R. and LINSWILER, H. M. (1974). *J. Nutr.* **104**, 695–700.

ANDERSEN, D. A. (1966). *J. Oslo City Hosp.* **16**, 101–147.

ANDERSEN, D. A. (1973). *In* "Urinary Calculi" (D. L. Cifuentes, A. Rapado and A. Hodgkinson, eds), Proc. Int. Symp. Renal Stone Res., pp. 130–134. Karger, Basel.

ANDERSON, C. K. (1969). *In* "Renal Stone Research Symposium" (A. Hodgkinson and B. E. C. Nordin, eds), pp. 133–136. Churchill, London.

BLACKLOCK, N. J. (1969). *In* "Renal Stone Research Symposium" (A. Hodgkinson and B. E. C. Nordin, eds), pp. 33–48. Churchill, London.

BLACKLOCK, N. J. and MACLEOD, M. (1974). *Br. J. Urol.* **46**, 385–392.

BOSHAMER, K. (1961). *Handb. Urol.* **10**, 34–50.

BUCK, A. C., SAMPSON, W. F., LOTE, C. J. and BLACKLOCK, N. J. (1981). *Br. J. Urol.* **53**, 485–491.

BURRY, A. F., AXELSON, R. A., TRULOVE, P. and SALL, J. R. (1976). *Hum. Pathol.* **7**, 435–449.

CLEAVE, T. L. (1974). "The Saccharine Disease", p. 7. John Wright, Bristol.

COE, F. L. and KAVALACH, A. G. (1974). *N. Engl. J. Med.* **300**, 337–340.

COE, F. L., PARKES, J. H. and MOORE, E. S. (1979). *N. Engl. J. Med.* **300**, 337–340.

CURRIE, W. J. C. and TURNER, P. (1979). *Br. J. Urol.* **51**, 337–342.

DANCE, N. and PRICE, R. G. (1970). *Clin. Chim. Acta* **27**, 87–92.

DE FRONZO, R. A., COOKE, C. R., ANDRES, R., FALOONA, G. R. and DAVIS, P. J. (1975). *J. Clin. Invest.* **55**, 845–855.

DOBBINS, J., COOPER, K., LANG, R., SMITH, L. H., BINDER, H. J. and BROADUS, A. E. (1981). *In* "Urolithiasis" (L. H. Smith, W. G. Robertson and B. Finlayson, eds), Proc. Int. Symp. Urolithiasis Res., pp. 775–779. Plenum, New York.

Esho, J. O. (1979). *Trop. Geogr. M. ed.* **30,** 477–481.

Finlayson, B. (1974). *Urol. Clin. North Am.* **1,** 181–212.

Finlayson, B. and Reid, F. (1978). *Invest. Urol.* **15,** 442–448.

Ghazali, S., Barratt, T. M. and Williams, D. I. (1973). *Arch. Dis. Child.* **48,** 291–295.

Grossman, W. (1938). *Urology* **10,** 46–54.

Haber, G. B., Heaton, F. W., Murphy, D. and Burroughs, L. F. (1977). *Lancet* **2,** 679–682.

Hadzija, B. W. (1969). *Pharmacology* **21,** 196–197.

Hodgkinson, A. and Heaton, F. W. (1965). *Clin. Chim. Acta* **11,** 354–362.

Inada, T., Miyazaki, S., Omori, T., Nihira, H. and Hind, T. (1958). *Urol. Int.* **7,** 150–165.

Jeffreys, D. B. (1973). *Proc. Nutr. Soc.* **33,** 11–12.

Kagawa, Y. (1978). *Prev. Med.* **7,** 205–217.

Kang, S. S., Price, R. G., Bruckdorfer, K. R., Worcester, N. A. and Yudkin, J. (1977). *Biochem. Soc. Trans.* **5,** 235–236.

Kiehm, T. G., Anderson, J. W. and Ward, K. (1976). *Am. J. Clin. Nutr.* **29,** 895–899.

Ku, F. L. (1978). *Chin. J. Surg.* (in Chinese) **16,** 323–326.

Lavan, J. N., Neale, F. C. and Posen, S. (1971). *Med. J. Aust.* **2,** 1049–1061.

Lemann, J., Piering, W. F. and Lennon, E. J. (1969). *N. Engl. J. Med.* **280,** 232–237.

Ljunghall, S. and Hedstrand, H. (1975). *Acta Med. Scand.* **197,** 439–445.

Macleod, M. A. and Blacklock, N. J. (1979a). *J. R. Nav. Med. Serv.* **65,** 75–78.

Macleod, M. A. and Blacklock, N. J. (1979b). *J. R. Nav. Med. Serv.* **65,** 143–146.

Marshall, R. W., Cochran, M. and Hodgkinson, A. (1972). *Clin. Sci.* **43,** 91–99.

Miranda, P. M. and Horwitz, D. L. (1978). *Ann. Intern. Med.* **88,** 482–486.

Modlin, M. (1969). *In* "Renal Stone Research Symposium" (A. Hodgkinson and B. E. C. Nordin, eds), pp. 49–54. Churchill, London.

Nordin, B. E. C., Peacock, M. and Wilkinson, R. (1972). *Clin. Endocrinol. Metab.* **1,** 169–183.

Norlin, A., Lindell, B., Granberg, P. O. and Lindvall, N. (1976). *Scand. J. Urol. Nephrol.* **10,** 150–153.

Oxley, J. A., Bruckdorfer, K. R. and Yudkin, J. (1979). *Proc. Nutr. Soc.* **38,** 85A.

Parry, E. S. and Lister, I. S. (1975). *Lancet* **1,** 1063–1065.

Périssé, J., Sizaret, F. and Françoise, P. (1969). *FAO Nutr. Newsl.* **7,** 1–9.

Quinland, W. S. (1945). *J. Urol.* **53,** 791–804.

Rao, P. J., Gordon, C., Davies, D. and Blacklock, N. J. (1982). *Br. J. Urol.* **54,** 575–577.

Reaser, E. F. (1935). *J. Urol.* **34,** 148–155.

Robertson, W. G. and Morgan, D. B. (1972). *Clin. Chim. Acta* **37,** 503–508.

Robertson, W. G. and Nordin, B. E. C. (1976). *In* "Scientific Foundations of Urology" (D. I. Williams and G. D. Chisholm, eds), Vol. 1, pp. 254–267, Heinemann, London.

Robertson, W. G. and Peacock, M. (1978). *In* "Proceedings of the 7th International Congress of Urology" (R. Barcelo, ed.), p. 363. Karger, Basel.

Robertson, W. G., Knowles, C. F. and Peacock, M. (1976). *In* "Urolithiasis Research" (H. Fleisch, W. G. Robertson, L. H. Smith and W. Vahlensieck, eds), Proc. Int. Symp., pp. 331–334. Plenum, New York.

Robertson, W. G., Peacock, M., Heyburn, P. J., Speed, R. and Hanes, F. (1978). *In* "Pathogenese and Klinik der Harnsteine, Symposium, 6th" (W. Vahlensieck and G. Gasser, eds), Vol. 14, pp. 5–14. Dietrich Steinkopff Verlag, Darmstadt.

Robertson, W. G., Peacock, M., Hanes, F. A., Heyburn, P. J., Rutherford, A., Clementson, E., Swaminathan, R. and Clark, P. B. (1979). *Br. J. Urol.* **51,** 427–531.

Robertson, W. G., Peacock, M., Heyburn, P. J., Hanes, F. A., Ouimet, D., Rutherford, A. and Sergeant, V. J. (1981). *In* "Urolithiasis (L. H. Smith, W. G., Robertson and B. Finlayson, eds), Proc. 4th Int. Symp. Urolithiasis Res., pp. 359–362. Plenum, New York.

ROSDY, E. (1982). *In* "Proceedings of the 18th Congress of the International Society of Urology", pp. 345–356. Medicina, Budapest.

ROSE, G. A. and WESTBURY, E. J. (1975). *Urol. Res.* **3**, 61–66.

SALLINEN, J. (1959). *Acta Chir. Scand.* **118**, 479–487.

SCHOLZ, B., SCHWILLE, P. O. and SIGEL, A. (1981). *In* "Urolithiasis" (L. H. Smith, W. G. Robertson and B. Finlayson, eds), Proc. 4th Int. Symp. Urolithiasis Res., pp. 795–800. Plenum, New York.

SCHUMANN, H. J. (1963). *Zentralbl. Allg. Pathol. Anta.* **105**, 88–94.

SHAH, P. J. R., WILLIAMS, G. and GREEN, N. A. (1981). *Br. J. Urol.* **52**, 426–429.

SIERAKOWSKI, R., FINLAYSON, B., LANDES, R. R., FINLAYSON, C. E. and SIERAKOWSKI, N. (1978). *Invest. Urol.* **15**, 438–441.

THOM, J. A., MORRIS, J. E., BISHOP, A. and BLACKLOCK, N. J. (1978). *Br. J. Urol.* **50**, 459–464.

THOM, J. A., MORRIS, J. E., BISHOP, A. and BLACKLOCK, N. J. (1980). *In* "Proceedings of the International Urinary Stone Conference, Perth, 1979" (G. Brockis and B. Finlayson, eds), pp. 103–105. P. S. G. Publishing Co., USA.

WHITE, R. W., COHEN, R. D., VINCE, F. P. WILLIAMSON, G., BLANDY, J. and TRESSIDDER, G. C. (1969). *In* "Renal Stone Research Symposium" (A. Hodgkinson and B. E. C. Nordin, eds), pp. 289–296. Churchill, London.

WILLIAMS, R. E. (1963). *Br. J. Urol.* **35**, 416–437.

YOSHIDA, O. (1979). *In* "Epidemiology of Urolithiasis in Japan," Proc. 18th Congr. Int. Soc. Urol. (author's translation). *Nippon Hinyokika Gakkai Zasshi* **70**, 975–982.

YUDKIN, J., KANG, S. S. and BRUCKDORFER, K. R. (1980). *Br. Med. J.* **281**, 1396.

ZAREMBSKI, P. M. and HODGKINSON, A. (1969). *Clin. Chim. Acta* **25**, 1–10.

Chapter 22

Mineral metabolism

ALEXANDER WALKER

I.   The practical problems at issue

A. *Third World populations*

Third World populations, characteristically, are habituated to high intakes of fibre-containing foods (cereals, tubers, legumes, vegetables), and low intakes

Dietary Fibre, Fibre-Depleted Foods
and Disease

of calcium and certain other mineral salts. Is this age-old general nutritional context—still common to the huge bulk of the world's populations—consistent with satisfactory mineral status? If not, what ameliorative measures may be suggested which would not at the same time promote development of degenerative disorders and diseases?

B.   Western populations

Western populations used to consume diets similar to those of most present-day Third World populations. Since last century there have been increases in intakes, *inter alia,* of certain mineral salts, particularly calcium. Simultaneously, there have been decreases in intakes of fibre-containing foods, principally cereals (Hollingsworth, 1974). Currently, to combat degenerative disorders and diseases, recommendations are being made to revert in measure to the diet of our ancestors. Authorities (U.S. Senate Select Committee on Nutrition and Human Needs, 1977; Truswell, 1980) urge reduced intakes of total energy, of animal protein, of fat, and of other components (sugar, salt, cholesterol, alcohol), but press for increased intakes of dietary fibre-containing foods, which imply an increased intake of phytic acid. On these accounts reservations are being expressed because some experimental studies on animals and humans have indicated that high intakes of fibre and phytic acid can have binding or precipitating effects on mineral salts in the gastrointestinal tract, thereby reducing their absorptions and utilizations, with consequent prejudice to mineral status. Are these misgivings warranted?

II.   Dietary situations

A.   Third World populations

Third World, compared with Western populations, eat diets of lower energy value, have relatively low intakes of total protein, especially animal protein, and of fat, especially animal fat. However, such populations have high intakes of fibre-containing foods, of phosphorus and usually of magnesium, yet low intakes of calcium and occasionally of iron. Intakes of dietary fibre are high, 35–70 g or more (Bingham and Cummings, 1980; Walker, 1981).

B.   Western populations

In Western populations, present-day intakes of dietary fibre are about 15–25 g (Gear *et al.*, 1979). Among strict vegetarians or vegans, intakes are higher, about 30–40 g (McKenzie, 1971). Yet in the past, intakes of Western populations were much greater than this amount; as examples, rural Scots used to consume oatmeal porridge often thrice daily, with a thick vegetable soup in the evening (Kitchin and Passmore, 1949). In the United Kingdom in 1880, consumption of bread, mainly unrefined, was very high (Leading Article, 1937)—three times or more higher than at present (Buss, 1979). Hence, any rise in dietary fibre intake among Western populations is grossly unlikely to reach previous high levels of consumption, or the present high consumptions of Third World populations.

The question is—in Western populations, will eating brown bread rather than white, the ingestion of 2 or 3 tablespoonsful of bran daily, and higher consumptions of vegetables and fruit cause mineral metabolism situations to deteriorate significantly, trivially, or not at all? Respecting calcium metabolism, will frequencies of rickets and osteomalacia, or of osteoporosis, increase? Will frequency of iron deficiency anaemia rise? Concerning zinc, will frequency of retarded growth or of other sequelae increase? Not least of the enquiries raised, will the disadvantages, if any, to mineral status, outweigh the advantages subsequent to eating more fibre-containing foods, respecting lesser pronenesses to, say, bowel diseases, and possibly other degenerative disorders and diseases?

III.   Avenues of approach to enquiries

In seeking elucidation, evidence must be assessed regarding (1) experimental studies on animals; (2) experimental studies on man; and (3) epidemiological observations.

What criteria for the presence of disorders or diseases due to *deficiency* or to *excess* of nutrients may be used for guidance? For identification of a deficiency disease, according to Yudkin (1961) there should be evidence of: (1) a low intake of the particular nutrient; (2) proof of metabolic involvement of the particular nutrient; (3) proof of benefit from an increased intake of that nutrient. These criteria probably apply equally in converse to a disease of nutritional excess. This list could be extended: (4) there should be evidence that the change effected is not a *placebo* effect; and (5) in the long-term there should be evidence that the changes accomplished in nutritional status are clinically meaningful.

IV.   Experimental studies on animals

Numerous investigations on animals on the effect of fibre foods or fibre-components on mineral metabolism have revealed a tendency for reduced absorptions and retentions to occur of calcium, magnesium, iron and zinc (Mellanby, 1949; Partridge, 1978; Kriek *et al.*, 1982).

A drawback in such studies is the often relatively short periods of observations. A more important reservation concerns the often excessively high dosage of the particular experimental component. For example, House *et al.*

(1982), using rats, used a 2% concentration of phytic acid in the rations. In humans this amount would correspond to the ingestion of about 10 g phytic acid daily, i.e. the amount contained in about 280 g bran—10 times the amount conceivably present in a Western diet.

V.   Experimental studies on humans

The earliest best known studies on man are those made during World War II by McCance and Widdowson (1942) on the effects of high intakes (450 g *per diem*) of brown and white breads on the metabolism of calcium, magnesium and iron. Most studies were undertaken on 10 volunteers for periods of 2 to 3 weeks. On the brown bread compared with the white bread regimen, balances of these elements became negative. These results were attributed to the interfering effect of the increased intake of phytic acid, which was only partially broken down during baking. Investigations made by others on various breads, legumes, vegetables and fruit, and on particular fibre components (pectin, cellulose, etc.) have tended to confirm the conclusions reached (Reinhold *et al.*, 1973; Ismail-Beigi *et al.*, 1977; Cummings *et al.*, 1979; Davies, 1979; Kelsay *et al.*, 1979; van Dokkum *et al.*, 1982) The investigations undertaken have limitations.

1. The intakes of fibre foods often bear little relationship to human dietary situations. As Rattan *et al.* (1981) pointed out, whereas in their series of subjects, habitually consumed bran supplements amounted to about 10 g *per diem*, in many experimental studies 20–60 g bran supplements have been employed.

2. Patterns of results are inconsistent; some studies indicate more marked interfering effects than others.

3. Studies very largely have been of short-term duration. Long-term investigations, e.g. those of Walker *et al.* (1948), Hegsted *et al.* (1952) and Malm (1958) suggest that adaptation occurs to a varying degree. Even in some short-term studies a measure of adaptation was apparent (Reinhold *et al.*, 1973).

In Third World populations balance observations have been carried out on individuals accustomed to high dietary fibre and low calcium intakes. Results have indicated that such regimens in the main do not significantly prejudice mineral salt balances and status. The percentage of absorptions noted were often exceptionally high, and subjects appeared in balance. This behaviour, regarding calcium, was reported many years ago by Basu *et al.* (1939), Nicholls and Nimalasuriya (1939), and more recently by Bhaskaram and Reddy (1979). The latter authors concluded, *inter alia,* "that high levels of phytate or calcium deficiency *per se* may not play a significant role in the aetiology of rickets" as seen occasionally in rural dwellers in India. Adaptation was also noted by the present writer when carrying out balance observations (unpublished) some years ago on six South African black prisoners aged 20–25 years whose prison diet closely resembled that of rural dwellers. Mean daily crude fibre intake was about 18 g, which, on calculation, becomes 50–60 g dietary fibre. It was derived primarily from whole maize, partially refined maize meal, brown bread, and beans. Mean daily intake of calcium was 275 mg. Percentage absorptions of calcium varied from 61 to 83%, i.e. far higher than the usual 20–30% which prevail with Western subjects. Results showed that regarding calcium, magnesium and iron, subjects were in balance.

The experimental studies described suggest that the drawbacks of habitually high fibre intakes and of low calcium and other mineral salt intakes of Third World dwellers may be of less significance to health than might be expected.

VI. Epidemiological observations with special reference to calcium

Since common potentially deleterious causes must give rise to common disorders or diseases, it would be argued that if the precipitating and binding effects of phytic acid and of fibre are as marked as some experimental studies aver, then, epidemiologically, there should be ample evidence of adverse metabolic and clinical effects in a variety of populations including (1) ancestors of Western populations; (2) rural populations in certain European countries who still consume large amounts of cereals; (3) segments in Western communities used to very high, compared with very low, consumptions of fibre foods; (4) strict vegetarians (although not vegetarians who consume macrobiotic diets); (5) immigrant Asians in the United Kingdom; (6) Third World populations generally; and (7) certain wartime populations who, from involuntary dietary changes, consumed increased intakes of brown bread and vegetables.

The situation regarding fibre foods and calcium status will be considered first; magnesium, iron and zinc will be discussed later.

A. Ancestors of Western populations and present-day descendants

In the United States and United Kingdom a century or more ago, in children who lived in urban areas, rickets was common and responsible for as much as one-third of total infant deaths (Aitken, 1870; Cheadle, 1902; Hess, 1929). The disease occurred more frequently in infants in higher social classes. While little historical inquiry has been pursued on rural dwellers, there is evidence that rural Scottish people were "big-boned and well developed" (Watson, 1907), had good teeth (Haddon, 1903), and that rickets, at least in the Highland child, was uncommon (Edie and Simpson, 1911).

At the present time, rickets, formerly common, is very uncommon. In the United States, studies on several large hospital populations have indicated that at each hospital there is often only one case per year on average (Bach-rach *et al.*, 1979; Rudolf *et al.*, 1980). Low intakes of fibre-containing foods are usual. Among the very young, a daily calcium intake of less than 400 mg (i.e. that of most rural dwellers in Third World populations) is consumed by as much as 8 to 15% of the population (National Center of Statistics, 1979). Yet, rickets remains rare, thereby indicating that a low calcium intake *per se* is not associated with proneness to rickets.

In the middle-aged and elderly, especially among post-menopausal wom-en, osteoporosis sequelae (vertebral body lesions and femoral fractures) are common and increasing (Horsman *et al.*, 1977; Riggs *et al.*, 1982).

B. Rural populations in Eastern Europe

Consumption of traditional diets in measure continues. In consonance, coro-nary heart disease has only one-third to one-half of its frequency in U.S. populations (Pisa and Uemura, 1982), and cancers of the colon and breast are less than half as common as in affluent Western populations (Hansluwka, 1978). Among these less socio-economically advanced populations, rickets appears rare.

In the Middle East, a population that has attracted considerable attention is that in Iran, where, at least in rural areas, the traditional bread contributes to a very high intake of phytic acid. However, calcium intake is high, about 1 g. Balance studies have indicated that the status of mineral salts—calcium, iron, zinc—is prejudiced (Reinhold *et al.*, 1973; Campbell *et al.*, 1976; Is-mail-Beigi *et al.*, 1977). A "high prevalence of rickets" was claimed (Re-inhold, 1976), yet no detailed data have been published on the diagnostic criteria used (e.g. biochemical rickets can have 10 times the frequency of radiological rickets) or the frequencies of rickets in various regions and in different populations. Indeed, rickets is not common. For instance, at Shiraz (300,000 population), from 1958 to 1967 an annual average of only two affected children were admitted to the hospital (Amirhakimi, 1973); the rate appears slightly higher in Teheran (Salimpour, 1975). Inferior mineraliza-tion was claimed. However, as with rickets, no telling data have been pub-lished on populations in different areas respecting cortical indices of metacar-pal, humerus, or other bones. Nor have epidemiological data been published on frequencies of osteomalacia or of osteoporosis (e.g. frequency of femoral fractures in the elderly). It is remarkable that the situation in Iran regarding the interfering effect of dietary fibre and phytic acid on mineral metabolism has been accorded worldwide publicity, despite the paucity of clear-cut epi-demiological information on the implied widespread sequelae of inadequate mineralization.

C. Communities in Western populations

There are no reports that rickets, or osteoporosis, is more common in the people with high, compared with low, intake of fibre-containing foods.

D. Strict vegetarians

Among vegans there are no reports that rickets is more common than among omnivorous eaters. Yet among vegetarians who consume macrobiotic diets (not necessarily high in fibre foods, moreover, unbalanced in other respects), infantile rickets does occur. The few cases reported have evoked inordinate publicity (Dwyer et al., 1979). However, it has been pointed out that even among segments of these particular populations among whom dietary circumstances are adverse, rickets is very uncommon (Finberg, 1979). This suggests that consumers of macrobiotic diets as a whole are not unduly susceptible to rickets.

E. Immigrant populations in the United Kingdom

The increase and, latterly, the decrease in the incidence of rickets in Asians in the United Kingdom was reviewed in the Department of Health and Social Security (DHSS) report on "Rickets and Osteomalacia" (DHSS Report, 1980). Whereas in young children and scholars, evidence of biochemical rickets was common (in some series as much as 50%), radiological abnormalities had a far lower frequency (Leading Article, 1979). Almost invariably the disease was mild and in no case a threat to life, thereby standing in gross contrast to the situation in Western populations in the past. As to causative factors, many have been blamed. Currently, the primary influencing factor is thought to be inadequate vitamin D status, due much more to insufficient exposure to available radiation, than to a low intake of the vitamin (DHSS Report, 1980). Some have blamed the high fibre and phytic acid intakes derived from chapattis (Robertson et al., 1977), yet Davies (1979) considers that "the precise role if any of phytate in the aetiology of 'Asian' rickets has yet to be established". No blame has been attached to a low calcium intake, which usually is unexpectedly high (O'Hara-May and Widdowson, 1976).

As to osteomalacia in the United Kingdom, while the disease in Asian adults, especially women, is uncommon, the incidence is not decreasing. Its occurrence is judged to be due almost wholly to inadequate exposure to radiation (DHHS Report, 1980).

This occurrence of rickets in Asian immigrants to the United Kingdom cannot therefore be regarded as a serious argument against the currently urged desirability of increasing intake of fibre-containing foods.

F.   Third World populations

In the DHSS report it was stated that rickets and osteomalacia occur among some populations in India, Africa and the Middle East. Cases were associated with "female seclusion (purdah); poverty, over-crowding, bad sanitation, sunless dwellings; frequent pregnancies, prolonged lactation, infant seclusion, late weaning, predominantly vegetarian diets, especially those based on coarsely milled wheat and pulses; generalized malnutrition and associated gastro-intestinal and chest infections, and worm infestations". In Johannesburg, South Africa, rickets in very young black children is now far less common than in the past (Stein and Rosen, 1980). In rural areas, characteristically, admissions to hospitals for rickets are rare. The reason why, in certain circumscribed regions, rickets (Pettifor et al., 1980) and other bone diseases (Fincham et al., 1981) occur remain obscure. Frequencies of bow legs and knock knees in pre-puberty and adolescent children appear much the same in black, Indian, Eur-African-Malay and white populations (Richardson and Walker, 1975). Mean indices of mineralization of bone in metacarpals in children in the four ethnic groups are similar (Walker et al., 1973), as are those of black and white subjects from youth to old age (Solomon, 1979). Mean data on black and white mothers who have had few or very many babies, respecting cortical indices in metacarpals and humerus, are also closely similar (Walker et al., 1972). Rural blacks have excellent teeth (Walker et al., 1981). Frequencies of osteoporosis stigmata are far less frequent and severe in black than in white adults (Dent et al., 1968; Solomon, 1979). Biochemically, in black children, somewhat low values for serum calcium and phosphorus, and elevated levels of serum alkaline phosphatase, are common (Pettifor et al., 1981). Such characteristics have also been noted in vegetarian children. However, the significances of these features in relation to proneness to bone disease, or to inferiority of mineralization, are not clear (DHSS Report, 1980).

Broadly, in Third World populations, bearing in mind the ubiquitousness of high-fibre, high-phytic acid and low-calcium intakes, it would seem that stigmata meaningful to health are very uncommon.

G.   Experience of wartime populations

In many countries during World War II, there were decreases in energy intake and in consumptions of animal foods, but increases in intakes of less refined cereal products and in vegetables and fruit. There were no reports of increases in rickets attributable to rises in intake of fibre-containing foods, with one exception. An increase occurred in Eire in 1942 to 1944 when wholemeal bread became the national staple. The higher intake of phytic acid was, and still is, blamed as the chief responsible factor (Jessop, 1950; Robertson et al., 1981). Several aspects remain unexplained (Walker, 1951; Walker and Burkitt, 1982). (1) There was no control population (Davidson, 1946). (2) Among babies, affected little or not at all by changes in bread composition, annual incidence of rickets was subject to even greater fluctuations than were observed in older children. (3) There were discrepancies in time-lag. The $82\frac{1}{2}$% extraction bread, with its far lower content of phytic acid, was introduced late in 1943; yet both in Dublin and Cork incidences of rickets were higher in 1944 than in 1943. (4) From the final report of the Dublin doctors (Walsh *et al.*, 1946), few conclusions can be reached about the responsibilities of the extraction rate of the flour, the intake of milk, and the intake of vitamin D.

VII.   Other influencing factors in calcium metabolism

A.   *Influence of dietary changes other than those concerning fibre and calcium intakes*

Osteoporosis stigmata are far more common in Western populations, despite their much higher calcium intakes, than in Third World populations. To combat attrition of bone, Western populations are being urged, by middle-age if not at youth, to increase their daily intake of the element to 1000–1500 mg (Recker *et al.*, 1977; Marcus, 1982), i.e. three to five times greater than that consumed in Third World populations. The higher requirement of calcium by Western populations is believed to be due in part to a much higher intake of protein, almost double that of Third World populations. In Western populations, even assuming that a rise in intake of fibre foods might slightly affect calcium absorption, the amount of the element ingested and available for metabolism would still remain much higher than that in Third World populations.

B.   *Influence of physical activity*

The anti-attrition effect of habitual physical activity on bone mass is well known. In one investigation, a high level of activity in post-menopausal women *increased* bone mass by 2.6% in 1 year; in a like series of sedentary women, bone mass *decreased* by 2.4% (Aloia *et al.*, 1978). Obviously, habitual activity, in individuals or in contrasting segments of populations, has a powerful influence on calcium metabolism.

C.   *Influence of pregnancy and lactation*

A mother contributes about 30 g calcium to the foetus and about 50 g during 8 months of lactation, i.e. about 80 g per child, or 320 g for four children. This amount is more than one-third of her total store of calcium. However, during pregnancy and lactation, absorption of the element takes place at a high rate. A recent study has underlined the excellent capacity of the body to rapidly make good the losses sustained in these physiological processes (Lamke *et al.*, 1977). In one group it was found that when lactation was continued for 3 months, there was a net *loss* of about 4% of body calcium; in another group, when lactation proceeded for 6 months, there was no loss of calcium. In the first group, 3 months after weaning, not only was the loss sustained made good, but there was a new gain of 7%.

In the aspects already considered, the proportions and amounts of calcium involved far transcend amounts possibly rendered unavailable due to a high or a moderately increased intake of dietary fibre. The phenomena underline the resilience of calcium status.

VIII.   Fibre foods and magnesium

As mentioned, experimental studies on animals (Seelig, 1964; Kelsay *et al.*, 1979) and man (McCance and Widdowson, 1942) have indicated that high-fibre diets and fibre components tend to lessen absorption and retention of magnesium. In Third World populations, somewhat low intakes and low values for serum magnesium are not uncommon. However, in our un-published studies on rural black adolescents, mean daily magnesium intake was 320 mg. Mean serum magnesium level was lower, but not significantly to that of a series of white adolescents. In the black subjects, moieties that had contrasting frequencies of defaecation and amounts of faeces voided daily, had the same mean levels for serum magnesium. In particular contexts in which maize is the staple, low serum magnesium levels have been considered to be involved in the aetiology of oesophageal cancer (van Rensburg, 1981). Obviously, further research is required. With regard to present-day en-treaties to Western populations to increase intake of dietary fibre, no reserva-tions appear to have been made over possible prejudicial effects on magne-sium metabolism.

IX.   Fibre foods and iron

In experimental studies on animals, a high-fibre diet tends to lessen absorp-tion and retention of iron (Morris and Ellis, 1976). In man, the pioneer studies of McCance *et al.* (1943) showed that brown compared with white bread decreased the absorption and retention of iron. Similar observations were reported by Dobbs and McLean Baird (1977). However, Sandstead *et al.* (1978) found an addition of 26 g bran (containing an extra 11–12 g dietary fibre) to be without appreciable effect on iron absorption. Third World populations, despite high intakes of dietary fibre, apart from the adverse effect of certain parasitic infections (malaria, schistosomiasis, ancylostomiasis), do not characteristically suffer from iron deficiency anaemia (Walker and Walker, 1977). Certainly some Indian populations, especially females, suffer more from this type of anaemia than most other populations; however, the extent of the responsibility borne by dietary fibre or phytic acid has not yet been elucidated (Bothwell *et al.*, 1979). In wartime Eire, a greater frequency of anaemia did not ensue when wholemeal bread became the staple (Saunders, 1944).

Possible prejudice to iron status due to a high intake of dietary fibre, as is usual with Third World populations, or to an increased intake as currently urged for Western populations, would seem of little moment to health.

X.   Fibre foods and zinc

Experimental studies carried out on animals on the effect of dietary fibre or phytic acid on zinc status, have demonstrated that in certain contexts zinc status is prejudiced (Davies, 1979). Long-term observations on the effect of simulated human diets high and low in fibre foods on zinc metabolism do not appear to have been undertaken. Experimental studies on man have shown that high-fibre diets tend to diminish absorption and retention of zinc (Reinhold *et al.*, 1973; Campbell *et al.*, 1976). According to Prasad (1978), chief stigmata of zinc deficiency are retarded growth and, acutely, testicular atrophy, hyperkeratosis, geophagia and iron deficiency anaemia. A primary or secondary deficiency of zinc has also been linked with adverse effects on wound healing, immune competence and sexual function (Tasman-Jones, 1980), retardation of foetal growth (Meadows *et al.*, 1981), and certain behavioural disorders (Gordon *et al.*, 1981).

In Third World populations, the extent to which a deficiency of zinc, primary or secondary, is a hazard to health obviously requires intensive study before recommendations of zinc fortification of staple foods be considered. In Western populations, an increase in dietary fibre intake would seem unlikely to prejudice zinc status and cause deficiency sequelae. In his review, James (1980) concluded that ". . . increasing the intake of fibre by 15-25 g is unlikely to affect zinc balance appreciably. Zinc balance seems less susceptible to interference by phytate and fibre than calcium balance".

XI.   Discussion and conclusions

Current interest on the influence of dietary fibre on mineral metabolism is due largely to the fact that present dietary recommendations to Western populations include increased consumptions of less refined cereal products, and legumes and vegetables. These changes imply increased consumptions of dietary fibre, and usually of phytic acid.

Some experimental studies on animals, although not all, and some short-term studies on humans, although not all, have demonstrated reductions in absorptions and retentions of calcium, magnesium, iron and zinc. Unfortunately, in such studies, many have used unphysiologically high dosages of fibre and phytic acid, thereby rendering interpretations of results more difficult.

Epidemiologically, as to calcium, convincing evidence on inferior mineralization of bone is lacking. Neither ancestors of Western populations, nor present-day European rural dwellers, nor strict vegetarians, nor Third World populations, all of whom were or are accustomed to high fibre intakes and low intakes of calcium and other mineral salts, were or are characterized by clinically meaningfully inferior mineral status. Moreover, within given communities, neither in Western nor in Third World contexts, is there satisfactory evidence that very high- compared with low-fibre consuming segments, are at a detectable inferior mineralization or clinical disadvantage.

Studies on Third World populations show that in the presence of a high fibre intake, utilization of their almost invariably low calcium intake is far better than would be expected. Cases of rickets do occur, but, characteristically, where there is exposure to available radiation, the disease is very uncommon. Among the low-calcium-eating moiety in Western populations, rickets is very rare. Of studies cited in favour of the reduced availability hypotheses—in Eire, during World War II when high extraction brown bread was introduced as the staple, and frequency of rickets increased—the specific culpability of brown bread was not proved. In Iran, high dietary fibre and phytic acid intakes, and high calcium intakes, are usual in some segments of the population. Yet, claims of a high frequency of rickets and of inferior mineralization of bone have not been supported by appropriate epidemiological evidence. In the United Kingdom, the increase, and latterly the decrease, in occurrence of rickets among Asian children has been attributed to many causes including inadequate vitamin D status and excessive dietary fibre and phytic acid intakes. The precise responsibility has not been resolved. But there appears to be no evidence that the children affected (with evidence of biochemical or clinical rickets) were accustomed to consuming more fibre or phytic acid, or had lower calcium intakes, than those not affected.

There appears to be no general evidence of *long-term* prejudicial clinical or other effects of habitually high dietary fibre intakes on the utilization of iron.

The situation regarding extent of interference of high fibre intake on magnesium status requires further study.

As to zinc, experimental studies on animals and man have demonstrated that high-fibre foods reduce absorption and retention of the element. Low zinc status has been associated with a great variety of stigmata. Whether, in a Third World community, those with evidence of zinc deficiency stigmata were accustomed to eating higher than average dietary fibre intakes, is not known. In Western populations, an increase in fibre intake would seem un- likely to prejudice zinc status.

As in all issues which concern important aspects of the everyday nutrition of the masses, research on the bearing of dietary fibre and phytic acid on mineral metabolism must continue. This is mandatory, if only for the added reason that world population is increasing at a rate faster than world food production, so that there will *have* to be progressively greater reliance on plant foods, due to the far more economical use of land in their production. It is therefore imperative that definitive information be obtained on the advan- tages, and on the possible disadvantages, of high fibre intakes on mineral metabolism in communities both in developed and developing populations.

In the meantime, the view is held that in Western populations, as a na- tional policy, available evidence does not warrant restriction in the intake of fibre-containing foods. Moreover, in Third World populations, while there is judged to be no call for a decrease in the intake of dietary fibre, certainly every effort should be made to encourage an increase in the variety of foods consumed. Finally, the potentially nutritionally negative characteristics of dietary fibre regarding mineral metabolism must not be regarded in isolation. The latter, in this writer's view, is far transcended by dietary fibre's potential benefits in relation to lesser proneness to bowel diseases (McLennan, 1977), diabetes (Anderson, 1980), coronary heart disease (Morris *et al.*, 1977) and possibly survival (Kromhout *et al.*, 1982).

References

AITKEN, W. (1870). *In* "A System of Medicine" (J. R. Reynold, ed.), Vol. I, p. 805. Mac- millan, London.

ALOIA, J. F., COHN, S. H., OSTUNI, J. A., CANE, R. and ELLIS, K. (1978). *Ann. Intern. Med.* **89**, 356–358.

AMIRHAKIMI, G. H. (1973). *Clin. Pediatr.* **12**, 88–92.

ANDERSON, J. W. (1980). *In* "Medical Aspects of Dietary Fiber" (G. A. Spiller and R. M. Kay, eds), pp. 193–222. Plenum, New York.

BACHRACH, S., FISHER, J. and PARKS, J. S. (1979). *Pediatrics* **64**, 871–877.

BASU, K. P., BASAK, M. N. and SIRCAR, B. C. R. (1939). *Indian J. Med. Res.* **27**, 471–499.

BHASKARAM, C. and REDDY, V. (1979). *Indian J. Med. Res.* **69**, 265–270.

BINGHAM, S. and CUMMINGS, J. H. (1980). *In* "Medical Aspects of Dietary Fiber" (G. A. Spiller and R. McPherson Kay, eds), pp. 261–293. Plenum, New York.

BOTHWELL, T. H., CHARLTON, R. W., COOK, J. D. and FINCH, C. A. (1979). "Iron Metabolism in Man." Blackwell, Oxford.

BUSS, D. H. (1979). *J. Hum. Nutr.* **33**, 47–55.

CAMPBELL, B. J., REINHOLD, J. G., CANNELL, J. J. and NOURMAND, I. (1976). *Pahlavi Med. J.* **7**, 1.

CHEADLE, W. B. (1902). *In* "A System of Medicine" (T. C. Allbutt, ed.), Vol. III, p. 108. Macmillan, London.

CUMMINGS, J. H., SOUTHGATE, D. A. T., BRANCH, W. J., WIGGINS, H. S., HOUSTON, H., JENKINS, D. J. A., JIVRAY, T. and HILL, M. J. (1979). *Br. J. Nutr.* **41**, 477–485.

DAVIDSON, L. S. P. (1946). *Proc. Nutr. Soc.* **4**, 47–48.

DAVIES, N. T. (1979). *Proc. Nutr. Soc.* **38**, 121–128.

DENT, C. E., ENGELBRECHT, H. E. and GODFREY, R. C. (1968). *Br. Med. J.* **4**, 76–79.

Department of Health and Social Security (DHHS) Report. (1980). "Rickets and Osteomalacia." Her Majesty's Stationery Office, LONDON.

DOBBS, R. J. and McLEAN BAIRD, I. (1977). *Br. Med. J.* **1**, 1641–1642.

DWYER, J. T., DIETZ, W. H., HASS, G. and SUSKIND, R. (1979). *Am. J. Dis. Child.* **133**, 134–140.

EDIE, E. S. and SIMPSON, G. C. E. (1911). *Br. Med. J.* **1**, 1421–1422.

FINBERG, L. (1979). *Am. J. Dis. Child.* **133**, 129.

FINCHAM, J. E., VAN RENSBURG, S. J. and MARASUS, W. F. O. (1981). *S. Afr. Med. J.* **60**, 445–447.

GEAR, J. S. S., WARE, A., FURSDON, P., MANN, J. I., NOLAN, D. J., BRODRIBB, A. J. M. and VESSEY, M. P. (1979). *Lancet* **1**, 511–514.

GORDON, E. F., GORDON, R. C. and PASSAL, D. B. (1981). *J. Pediatr.* **99**, 341–349.

HADDON, J. (1903). *Br. Med. J.* **1**, 1182.

HANSLUWKA, H. (1978). *World Health Stat. Rep.* **31**, 158–194.

HEGSTED, D. M., MOSCOSO, I. and COLLAZOS, C. (1952). *J. Nutr.* **46**, 181–201.

HESS, A. F. (1929). "Rickets, Including Osteomalacia and Tetany." Henry Kimpton, London.

HOLLINGSWORTH, D. (1974). *Nutr. Rev.* **32**, 353–359.

HORSMAN, A., GALLAGHER, J. C., SIMPSON, M. and NORDIN, B. E. C. (1977). *Br. Med. J.* **2**, 789–792.

HOUSE, W. A., WELSH, R. M. and VAN CAMPEN, D. R. (1982). *J. Nutr.* **112**, 941–953.

ISMAIL-BEIGI, F., REINHOLD, J. G., FARAJI, B. and ABADI, P. (1977). *J. Nutr.* **107**, 510–518.

JAMES, W. P. T. (1980). *In* "Medical Aspects of Dietary Fiber" (G. A. Spiller and R. McPherson Kay, eds), pp. 239–259. Plenum, New York.

JESSOP, W. J. E. (1950). *Br. J. Nutr.* **4**, 289–295.

KELSAY, J. L., BEHALL, K. M. and PRATHER, E. S. (1979). *Am. J. Clin. Nutr.* **32**, 1876–1880.

KITCHIN, A. H. and PASSMORE, R. (1949). "The Scotsman's Food." Livingstone, Edinburgh.

KRIEK, N. P. J., SLY, M. R., DU BRUYN, D. B., DE KLERK, W. A., RENAN, M. J., VAN SCHALKWYK, D. J. and VAN RENSBURG, S. J. (1982). *Br. J. Exp. Pathol.* **63**, 246–260.

KROMHOUT, D., BOSSCHIETER, E. B. and COULANDER, C. L. (1982). *Lancet* **2**, 518–522.

LAMKE, B., BRUNDIN, J. and MOBERG, P. (1977). *Acta Obstet. Gynecol. Scand.* **56**, 217–219.

Leading Article (1937). *Br. Med. J.* **2**, 752–753.

Leading Article (1979). *Br. Med. J.* **1**, 1744.

McCANCE, R. A. and WIDDOWSON, E. M. (1942). *J. Physiol. (London)* **101**, 44–85.

McCANCE, R. A., EDGECOMBE, C. N. and WIDDOWSON, E. M. (1943). *Lancet* **1**, 588–592.

McKENZIE, J. (1971). *Plant Foods Hum. Nutr.* **2**, 79–88.

McLENNAN, R. and JENSEN, O. M. (1977). *Lancet* **2**, 207–211.

MALM, O. J. (1958). "Calcium Requirement and Adaptation in Adult Man." Halden Press, Oslo University.

MARCUS, R. (1982). *Metab. Clin. Exp.* **31**, 93–102.

MEADOWS, N. J. RUSE, W., SMITH, M. F., DAY, J., KEELING, P. W. N., SCOPES, J. W., THOMPSON, R. P. H. and BLOXAM, D. L. (1981). *Lancet* **2**, 1135–1137.

MELLANBY, E. (1949). *J. Physiol. (London)* **109**, 488.

MORRIS, E. R. and ELLIS, R. (1976). *J. Nutr.* **106**, 753–760.

MORRIS, J. N., MARR, J. W. and CLAYTON, D. G. (1977). *Br. Med J.* **2**, 1307–1314.

National Center of Statistics (1979). "Dietary Intake Service Data. United States, 1971–1974," DHEW Publ. No. (PHS) 79-1221. 2,123-151 NCS, Bethesda, Maryland.

NICHOLLS, L. and NIMALASURIYA, A. (1939). *J. Nutr.* **18**, 563–577.

O'HARA-MAY, J. and WIDDOWSON, E. M. (1976). *Br. J. Nutr.* **36**, 23–36.

PARTRIDGE, I. G. (1978). *Br. J. Nutr.* **39**, 538–545.

PETTIFOR, J. M., ISDALE, J. M., SAHAKIAN, J. and HANSEN, J. D. L. (1980). *Arch. Dis. Child.* **55**, 155–157.

PETTIFOR, J. M., ROSS, P., MOODLEY, G. and SHUENYANE, E. (1981). *Am. J. Clin. Nutr.* **34**, 2187–2191.

PISA, Z. and UEMURA, K. (1982). *World Health Stat. Q.* **35**, 11–47.

PRASAD, A. S. (1978). "Trace Elements and Iron in Human Metabolism." Plenum, New York.

RATTAN, J., LEVIN, N., GRAFF, E., WEISER, N. and GILAT, T. (1981). *J. Clin. Gastroenterol.* **3**, 389–393.

RECKER, R. R., SAVILLE, P. D. and HEANEY, R. P. (1977). *Ann. Intern. Med.* **87**, 649–655.

REINHOLD, J. G. (1976). *Lancet* **2**, 1132–1133.

REINHOLD, J. G., LAHIMGARZADEH, A., NASR, K. and HEDAYATI, H. (1973). *Lancet* **1**, 283–288.

RICHARDSON, B. D. and WALKER, A. R. P. (1975). *Postgrad. Med. J.* **51**, 22–29.

RIGGS, B. L., SEEMAN, E., HODGSON, S. F., TAVES, D. R. and O'FALLON, W. M. (1982). *N. Engl. J. Med.* **306**, 446–450.

ROBERTSON, I., KELMAN, A. and DUNNIGAN, M. G. (1977). *Br. Med. J.* **1**, 229–230.

ROBERTSON, I., FORD, J. A., MCINTOSH, W. B. and DUNNIGAN, M. G. (1981). *Br. J. Nutr.* **45**, 17–22.

RUDOLF, M., ARULANANTHAM, K. and GREENSTEIN, R. M. (1980). *Pediatrics* **66**, 72–76.

SALIMPOUR, R. (1975). *Arch. Dis. Child.* **50**, 63–66.

SANDSTEAD, H., KLEVAY, L., MUNOZ, J., JACOB, R., LOGAN, G., DINTZIS, F., INGLETT, G. and SHUEY, W. (1978). *Fed. Proc. Fed. Am. Soc. Exp. Biol.* **37**, 254.

SAUNDERS, J. C. (1944). *Lancet* **1**, 516.

SEELIG, M. G. (1964). *Am. J. Clin. Nutr.* **14**, 342–390.

SOLOMON, L. (1979). *Lancet* **2**, 1326–1330.

STEIN, H. and ROSEN, E. U. (1980). *S. Afr. Med. J.* **58**, 1030–1032.

TASMAN-JONES, C. (1980). *Adv. Intern. Med.* **26**, 97–114.

TRUSWELL, A. S. (1980). *Food Tech. Aust.* **32**, 295–298.

U.S. SENATE SELECT COMMITTEE ON NUTRITION and Human Needs (1977). "Dietary Goals for the United States", 1st edition, Stock No. 052-070-03913-2. U.S. Government Printing Office, Washington, D.C.

VAN DOKKUM, W., WESSTRA, A. and SCHIPPERS, F. A. (1982). *Br. J. Nutr.* **47**, 451–460.

VAN RENSBURG, S. J. (1981). *JNCI, J. Natl. Cancer Inst.* **67**, 243–252.

WALKER, A. R. P. (1951). *Lancet* **2**, 244–248,

WALKER, A. R. P. (1981). *In* "Western Diseases: Their Emergence and Prevention" (H. C. Trowell and D. P. Burkitt, eds), pp. 285–318. Edward Arnold, London.

WALKER, A. R. P. and BURKITT, D. P. (1982). *Pediatrics* **69**, 130–131.

WALKER, A. R. P. and WALKER, B. F. (1977). *Lancet* **2**, 771–772.

WALKER, A. R. P., FOX, F. W. and IRVING, J. T. (1948). *Biochem. J.* **42**, 452–462.

WALKER, A. R. P., RICHARDSON, B. D. and WALKER, B. F. (1972). *Clin. Sci.* **42**, 189–196.

WALKER, A. R. P., DISON, E., DUVENHAGE, A., WALKER, B. F. FRIEDLANDER, I. and AUCAMP, V. (1981). *Commun. Dent. Oral Epidemiol.* **9**, 37–43.

WALKER, B. F. WALKER, A. R. P. and WADVALLA, M. (1973). *Trop. Geogr. Med.* **25**, 65–70.

WALSH, J. P., KIDNEY, W., COLLIS, W. R. F., PRINGLE, H., REYNOLDS, R. A., DOUGLAS, S. and JESSOP, W. J. E. (1946). *J. Med. Assoc. Eire* **19**, 156.

WATSON, C. (1907). *Br. Med. J.* **1**, 985–986.

YUDKIN, J. (1961). *Practitioner* **187**, 150–158.

Chapter 23

Cereals, milling and fibre

NATHAN FISHER

Cereals are valuable sources of dietary fibre (DF) as well as of other important nutrients in the diet. In this brief account of the structure, composition and properties of the main cereals and cereal foods available in the United Kingdom, much of the data used is summarized from work (to be published separately) carried out in the author's Research Group [by Dr. D. G. H. Daniels, Miss B. M. Bell, Miss A. Y. Harland and Mr. G. Gudmunsen (Chemistry) Dr. C. S. Berry and Mr. J. A. Gregory (Biology) at the Flour Milling and Baking Research Association (FMBRA) (1982a)].

I. Cereal crops

Cereals are the fruits of cultivated grasses belonging to the genus Gramineae. The main species grown for human food are wheat, maize, rice, barley, oats, rye, sorghum and millet (Kent, 1975). Grains of wheat, rye, maize and sorghum are naked caryopses, whereas those of oats, barley and rice are covered caryopses. Since the hull or husk of the latter grains is high in DF, the total DF content of any cereal product containing these grains will depend on the extent of incorporation of husk material. Oat husk is extremely abrasive and has been used for polishing metal castings! All the cereal grains

Dietary Fibre, Fibre-Depleted Foods
and Disease

ISBN 0-12-701160-9

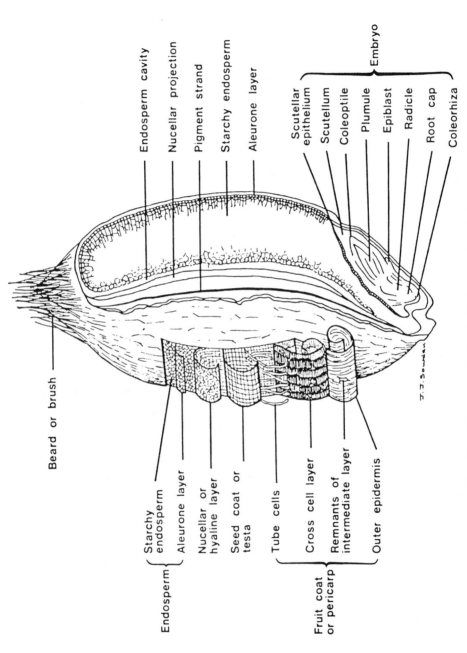

Endosperm cavity

Nucellar projection

Pigment strand

Starchy endosperm

Aleurone layer

Scutellar epithelium

Scutellum

Coleoptile

Plumule

Epiblast

Radicle

Root cap

Coleorhiza

Embryo

Beard or brush

Endosperm {
Starchy endosperm
Aleurone layer

Nucellar or hyaline layer

Seed coat or testa

Tube cells

Fruit coat or pericarp {
Cross cell layer
Remnants of intermediate layer
Outer epidermis

FIG. 23.1. The wheat grain, longitudinal section through the crease.

TABLE 23.1. Bran, germ and endosperm in different whole cereal grains (% w/w grain, 14% moisture basis)

	English wheat	CWRS[a] wheat	Rye	Maize	Sorghum
Bran	16.2	14.6	10.7	6.1	7.5
Germ	1.7[b]	2.3[b]	3.1[c]	10.5[c]	7.0[c]
Endosperm	68.0	69.1	72.2	69.5	71.6

[a] Canadian Western Red Spring.
[b] Embryo.
[c] Embryo + scutellum, as analysed in Table 23.3.

are basically similar in structure (Kent, 1975): Fig. 23.1 shows the structure of the wheat grain in longitudinal section taken through the crease.

It is important to realise that while the aleurone layer, a single layer of thick-walled cells, is botanically part of the endosperm, in milling practice it is included in the bran, of which it forms about half by weight. Commercial bran includes all layers from the aleurone layer to the outer epidermis. The embryo is usually called the germ.

II.   Fractionation of grain

Separation of grain into bran, germ and endosperm may be accomplished by hand dissection or various forms of milling. Yields of these fractions from various cereal grains are given in Table 23.1 (FMBRA, 1982a).

The relative weights of the fractions within any one cereal grain, and the differences in these proportions between grains, must be taken into account when considering the data for the *concentrations* of constituents such as DF within any one fraction.

III.   The milling of grain

In view of the importance of wheat to the national diet in the United Kingdom, most of the following discussion will concern wheat and wheat products, mainly flour and bread.

Wheat may be converted to wholemeal flour by simple impact methods (quern, mortar and pestle, ball mill, hammer mill), each of which produces some white (endosperm) flour that could readily be separated off if desired. However, because of the longitudinal crease, production of high yields of white flour demands more sophisticated methods. In these the moisture-conditioned grain is first sheared open and the endosperm scraped from the outer seed coats. These shearing and scraping processes are repeated and followed by the reduction of the larger particles to the consistency of flour, each fraction being separated into fine and coarse sub-fractions by the use of sieves. In the stone mill the grains are ground between stones constructed with complex systems of grooves, while in the roller mill the stones are replaced by two types of steel roller. Fluted steel "break rolls" open the grains, while smooth steel "reduction rolls" reduce the size of the particles thus produced. It is the differential in speed of rotation of stones or rollers which shears open the grain, and the main difference in the products of the different methods of milling is in the yields of white flours obtained. The roller mill is the more efficient in this regard, allowing more endosperm to be scraped off from the flattened bran without causing the colour of the flour to be significantly darkened. Roller milling does no more damage (indeed probably does less damage) to plant cell walls than stone milling. Neither the author nor those of his colleagues expert in milling and in the structure and composition of starch grains (D. J. Stevens, N. L. Kent, A. D. Evers, personal communications) know of any convincing evidence that distinguishes between the state or availability of starch in wholemeal flour and that in white flour.

Sifting of flour into whiter and darker fractions has been practised since ancient times (see pictures of sifting 2600 B.C., Stork and Teague, 1952; McCance and Widdowson, 1956; Anonymous, 1982). Later, before the Norman Conquest, flour was being sieved into "very fine flour" called "smedma" and "good flour" termed "grytt" (Stork and Teague, 1952). A fine hair sieve ("temes" or "temse") was in use at the time of the Conquest. Subsequently, large rotating cylindrical sieves of linen or cotton, later silk, were used. There is evidence (Pownall, 1795; Bennett and Elton, 1900; cited in Eastwood *et al.,* 1974) that in 1795, the main flour used for bread production in London was white with an extraction rate (yield from cleaned wheat) little different from that of present-day white flours.

IV.   Polysaccharides in ground whole grains

Recent comparative data (FMBRA, 1982a) for the starch and DF constituents of an English and a Canadian wheat, and for samples of rye, maize, sorghum and millet are given in Table 23.2 The wheat DF values are higher than those we have found in other studies in which the range was 9–12% at 14% moisture content.

V.   Polysaccharides in bran and germ

Corresponding values to those of Table 23.2 for bran and germ obtained from the same samples (excluding millet for which the separation was unsatisfactory) are given in Table 23.3.

TABLE 23.2. Polysaccharide contents of whole cereal grains[a]

	Wheat		Rye	Maize	Sorghum	Millet
	English	Canadian				
Starch	59.4	60.0	59.7	61.1	58.0	51.3
Non-cellulosic polysaccharides[b]	10.3	9.5	10.7	10.1	8.2	8.8
Cellulose	2.9	2.7	2.3	2.3	2.3	1.7
Lignin	1.8	1.5	1.7	0.1	0.4	1.0
Total DF	15.0	13.7	14.7	12.5	10.9	11.5

[a] Method of Southgate, 1976; % w/w ground grain, 14% moisture basis; duplicate determinations of single samples.

[b] Formerly called hemicelluloses.

Considerable variation between cereal species in DF composition is shown in Tables 23.2 and 23.3, but the values should be considered only in conjunction with those of Table 23.1 giving the contribution of each fraction to the total weight of the grain if a misleading impression of their potential as sources of dietary fibre is to be avoided. Certainly no suggestion is given that from the quantitative point of view, the *type* of cereal consumed in African countries, in addition to the *amounts* consumed, is implicated in the relative freedom of Africans from the diseases of Western civilisation, if this is indeed attributable to their DF intakes (Burkitt and Trowell, 1975).

The non-cellulosic polysaccharides of wheat consist mainly of arabino-xylans (Adams, 1955; MacArthur and D'Appolonia, 1980), i.e. polymers

TABLE 23.3. Polysaccharides of bran and germ fractions of various cereal grains[a]
(% w/w bran or germ, 14% moisture content)

	English wheat	CWRS wheat	Rye	Maize	Sorghum
Bran					
Starch	16.4	9.3	25.3	0.4	13.2
Non-cellulosic polysaccharides[b]	26.1	28.5	24.1	52.1	32.5
Cellulose	7.9	11.2	3.8	18.7	13.9
Lignin	4.8	4.5	3.6	1.1	5.6
Total DF[a]	38.8	44.2	31.5	71.9	52.0
Germ					
Starch	5.3	1.8	1.7	8.0	8.3
Non-cellulosic polysaccharides[b]	7.6	5.4	7.3	9.3	10.2
Cellulose	2.4	1.8	2.5	2.6	2.4
Lignin	0.6	0.6	0.5	1.2	0.6
Total DF	10.6	7.8	10.3	13.1	13.2

[a] The present state of dietary fibre determination is such that small differences should be regarded as unproven and ignored.

[b] Formerly termed hemicelluloses.

composed of the pentose sugars arabinose and xylose, the latter forming the backbones of the polymer molecules and arabinose forming the side chains. Some glucans are also present (Fincher, 1975), and smaller proportions of galactose, galacturonic acid and mannose are also found as constituents of the polymers. The different modes of action of bran and cabbage in the gut are attributed (Stephen and Cummings, 1980) to their different polysaccharide structures, the former being resistant to degradation by colonic bacteria, possibly owing to ester linkage with lignins (Ring and Selvendran, 1980), while the latter, containing a much higher level of uronic acid, is degraded and utilised for growth by gut bacteria. It is the resultant bacterial proliferation that causes the increased faecal output resulting from consumption of cabbage, while the same effect is produced by bran by virtue of the survival of the gross structure of the bran flakes during their passage through the gut. On reaching the colon, their structure and water-binding and retention capacities give the desired bulking effect (Stephen and Cummings, 1980).

It would be wrong to regard bran or any other food product derived from wheat simply as a source of DF, in view of the many other important ingredients that they contain. An overview (FMBRA, 1982a) of the composition of two wheat brans is given in Table 23.4.

Those prescribing bran should note particularly the variation in starch content between these samples, which is not atypical. These differences are not mainly due to the country of origin of the wheats but to their nature and the degree of separation used in preparing the bran. It is not possible to

TABLE 23.4. Composition of an English and a Canadian bran (% by weight dry matter)

	Bran	
Component	English	Canadian
Starch	22.0	12.4
NCP[a]	24.5	26.2
Cellulose	10.2	12.0
Lignin	4.3	4.4
Free sugars[b]	7.6	7.6
Protein	12.4	13.2
Non-protein, non-nucleic nitrogen-containing compounds	3.6	3.9
Nucleotides	0.2	0.4
Lipids	4.4	7.6
Ash	6.1	5.9
Phytate	4.0	3.7
Total recovered	99.3	97.3

[a] Non-cellulosic polysaccharides (hemicelluloses).

[b] These values from other brans.

TABLE 23.5. Particle size distributions of mill bran fractions and the coarsest fraction
of wholemeal wheat flour (percentage yield of bran)[a]

Component[b]	Sieve aperture (mm)								
	1.35	1.05	0.85	0.61	0.52	0.47	0.35	0.14	<0.14
Coarse bran[1]	54	14	14	12	3	1	2	0	0
Medium bran[2]	8	15	26	29	9	3	6	1	3
Fine bran[3]	0	0	0	10	17	11	40	6	15
Coarse fraction of wholemeal flour[4]	1	2	12	27	10	17	22	0	8

[a] Rounded to the nearest integer; values represent the percentage of the initial sample weight failing to
pass a sieve of the stated size.

[b] 1, "1st tails"; 2, "2nd tails"; 3, "3rd tails"; 4, pre-sieved wholemeal wheat flour, 92% of the finest
material having been removed.

prepare bran commercially with an endosperm content lower than about 10%
by weight, and some commercial products have far higher levels. The energy
value of bran varies with its available carbohydrate content and is given as
206 kcal/100g (Paul and Southgate, 1978). Different streams from the mill
give brans of varying particle sizes, as shown in Table 23.5.

Since the particle size of bran may influence its laxative action, the coarser
material being more effective (van Dokkum, 1978), the patient will need to
adjust the dosage to achieve the desired effect (cf. Painter, 1972). Fine
grinding of bran fed to rats caused a 30% reduction in faecal output (FMBRA,
1979). Cooking has also been reported to reduce the faecal bulking effect of
bran preparations (Wyman et al., 1976). No such effect was noted using rats
when bran was autoclaved at 15 psi for 60 min (FMBRA, 1979).

The mineral content of bran is given in Table 23.6; the data are drawn
from various literature sources. The wide ranges of values shown in this table

TABLE 23.6. Mineral composition of wheat bran
(% w/w bran with 14% moisture)

Element	Mean	Range
Potassium	0.98	0.61–1.32
Sodium	0.015	0.0043–0.026
Magnesium	0.32	0.035–0.622
Calcium	0.09	0.041–0.12
Manganese	0.017	0.009–0.043
Zinc	0.017	0.0064–0.048
Iron	0.012	0.0047–0.018
Copper	—	0.00134
Phosphorus	1.17	0.98–1.55
Sulphur	0.185	0.106–0.232
Chlorine	—	0.0332

again emphasise the variability of bran, the natural variability of which as a biological material is increased by the variability introduced by the different forms of grinding or milling by which it is prepared.

VI.   Bread as a source of dietary fibre and nutrients

The main cereal product consumed in the United Kingdom is bread, which is the major source of cereal dietary fibre in the national diet.

The earlier widespread belief that the bread consumed prior to the introduction of roller milling was wholemeal (Painter et al., 1972) has been shown to be erroneous (Eastwood et al., 1974). Nineteenth century flours were white and were estimated to have crude fibre (CF) (see Fisher and Hutchinson, 1973) contents of 0.2 to 0.5%, similar to present-day white flours (CF 0.1 to 0.2%). Reports of consumption published between 1841 and 1880 (Eastwood et al., 1974) gave values of 270–578 g flour/person/day, considerably in excess of the domestic consumption of 112 g/person/day in 1980 [National Food Survey (NFS) Committee, 1982].

The NFS monitors household consumption of foods, and the values for bread consumption in 1957 to 1981 are shown graphically in Figs. 23.2 and 23.3.

Non-domestic bread consumption in recent years has reached 20% of total bread production (N. Chamberlain, personal communication, 1982) and the graphs therefore seriously underestimate *total* bread consumption since about 1968. They do, however, illustrate the magnitude of the task of reversing the trend to lower bread consumption and of increasing the consumption of wholemeal and brown breads, as recommended by the recent report of the Panel on Bread, Flour and Other Cereal Products of the Committee on Medical Aspects of Food Policy (COMA, 1981). If the recommendation of the Panel on legalising the use of improvers in the commercial manufacture of wholemeal bread is adopted, wholemeal loaves with properties acceptable to a much wider section of the population will become available. In the meantime a profusion of breads and baked products with enhanced fibre contents is being marketed.

The nutrient concentrations in white, brown, germ and wholemeal breads as bought (*not* from identical grists) are summarised in Table 23.7 (Paul and Southgate, 1978; Panel on Bread, Flour and other Cereal Products, 1981).

From the general nutritional point of view, i.e. in the context of the average mixed diet consumed in the United Kingdom, there is little to choose between the different forms of bread. Indeed the report of the COMA Panel (Panel on Bread, Flour and other Cereal Products, 1981) indicated that supplementation of white flour with specified nutrients need no longer be legally mandatory. As regards their DF contents, recent evidence (FMBRA,

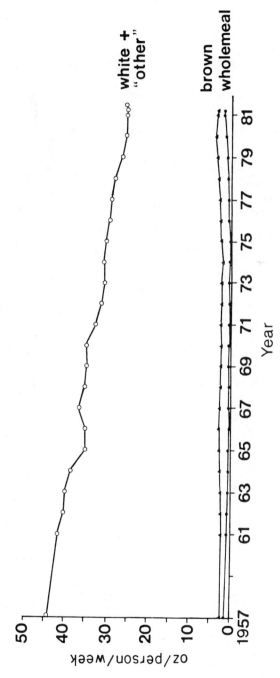

FIG. 23.2. Household bread consumption, 1957–1981 (NFS data).

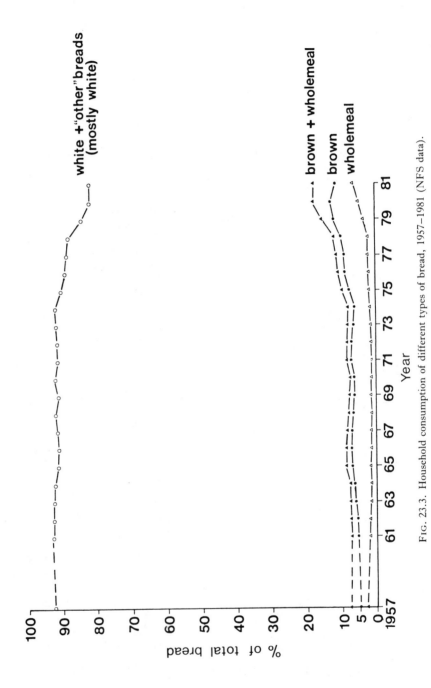

FIG. 23.3. Household consumption of different types of bread, 1957–1981 (NFS data).

TABLE 23.7. The nutrient composition of white, brown, germ and wholemeal breads (g/100 g as bought)

Nutrient	White	Brown	Germ[a]	Wholemeal
Water	39.0	39.0	40.0	40.0
Sugars	1.8	1.8	2.4	2.1
Starch and dextrins	47.9	42.9	42.7	39.7
Dietary fibre[b]	2.7 (4.3)	5.1 (6.4)	4.6 (5.8)	8.5 (8.5)
Energy (kcal)	233	223	228	216
Protein	7.8	8.9	9.7	8.8
Fat	1.7	2.2	2.2	2.7
Carbohydrate	49.7	44.7	45.1	41.8
Minerals (mg/100 g)				
Iron	1.7 (1.2)[c]	2.5 (1.7)[c]	4.5	2.5
Sodium	540	550	580	540
Potassium	100	210	210	220
Calcium	100	100	150	23
Magnesium	26	75	60	93
Phosphorus	97	190	190	230
(Phytic acid[d] as % of total P)[e]	1.2	55 (30)	38	43
Copper	0.15	0.23	0.18	0.27
Zinc	0.8	1.6	NA[g]	2.0
Chromium	0.026	NA	NA	0.06
Manganese	0.42	1.71	NA	4.0
Molybdenum	0.028	NA	NA	0.05
Selenium	0.04	0.067	NA	0.067
Vitamins/100 g				
Thiamin (mg)	0.18 (0.06)[c]	0.24 (0.17)[c]	0.52	0.26
Riboflavin (mg)	0.03	0.06	0.10	0.06
Nicotinic acid (mg)	1.4	2.9	3.9	3.9
Potential N. a. (mg)	1.6	1.8	2.0	1.7
Vitamin E (mg)	Trace	Trace	—	(0.2)[f]
Pyridoxin (mg)	0.04	0.08	0.09	0.14
Folic acid (μg)	27	36	20	39
Pantothenic acid (mg)	0.3	0.3	0.3	0.6
Biotin (μg)	1	3	2	6

[a] Proprietary brand.

[b] Parenthetical value calculated from Wenlock *et al.* (1983).

[c] Calculated for bread made from unfortified flour.

[d] Anti-nutrient.

[e] Daniels and Fisher (1981).

[f] Tentative value.

[g] Not available.

TABLE 23.8. Intakes of dietary fibre from bread,
1980 (g/person/day)

Bread	Intake	DF intake
White	103.5	2.8
Brown	16.2	0.8
Wholemeal	6.3	0.5

1982a; Wenlock, et al., 1983) indicates that the published value (Paul and Southgate, 1981) for white bread may be somewhat underestimated (see parenthetical values in Table 23.7), and in particular its pentose content, actually 2–3% by weight (dry matter basis), (Pomeranz, 1971; Neukom, 1976; Englyst et al., 1982; FMBRA, 1982a) has sometimes been considerably underestimated. Readers should also beware the "percentage trap"—a food containing a higher percentage of a nutrient may in practice be a less useful source of that nutrient than one with a lower percentage, if the latter is regarded as more palatable or more convenient by the public and is thus consumed in much greater quantities. This is illustrated in Table 23.8 for the DF supplied by the different forms of bread in 1980, using the published percentages of DF and the consumption data of the NFS.

VII.   Anti-nutrients in cereal products

As well as nutrients, bran and other cereal products also contain antinutrients, including phytate, oxalate and growth-inhibitory alkylresorcinols. Indeed, DF may also behave as an anti-nutrient in respect of the binding of essential minerals such as zinc, calcium, iron and magnesium. However, given commonsense moderation these properties of cereals should not prove a serious problem although those caring for potentially vulnerable individuals, such as the very young and the elderly, and any individuals consuming extreme diets, should be made aware of the possible hazards of *excessive* fibre intake, including obstruction of the small intestine (Allen-Mersh and de Jode, 1982) or of the large intestine (Kang and Doe, 1979; Guller and Reber, 1980).

The beneficial effects of cereal dietary fibre in the treatment of various diseases are covered in other chapters. A lifespan study of the effects of cereal DF on the development of diverticular disorders in rats has recently been successfully concluded at FMBRA, and preliminary results have been reported (FMBRA, 1982b). Based on post-mortem findings (subject to possible modification after completion of histopathological studies), a linear inverse relationship has been demonstrated between the incidence of diverticular and the percentage of DF in the diet consumed. However, the slope is such that a very large increase in DF would be required to produce a worthwhile reduction in incidence of diverticula. Notwithstanding this, beneficial effects of DF on the time of development of diverticula and on their size were observed and are to be studied in future work.

VIII. Coda

One need not, in the pursuit of increased fibre intake, insist on the elimination of refined foods in general, and white bread in particular, as was once demanded in the heat of controversy. The unique, mouthwatering aroma and taste of freshly baked crusty white bread will surely continue to delight the senses of the fortunate. In sensible diets, this experience will be supplemented and varied by the pleasures of brown, germ and wholemeal breads now available in many diverse forms, as well as other enjoyable foods containing forms of fibre with different desirable physiological effects.

Acknowledgements

The FMBRA work described formed part of research projects sponsored by the U.K. Ministry of Agriculture, Fisheries and Food to whom our thanks are due. The results of the research are the property of the Ministry of Agriculture, Fisheries and Food and are Crown Copyright.

References

ADAMS, G. A. (1955). *Can. J. Chem.* **33**, 56–67.

ALLEN-MERSH, T. and DE JODE, L. R. (1982). *Br. Med. J.* **284**, 740.

ANONYMOUS (1982). *Bakers' Millers' J.* April, p. 22.

BENNETT, R. and ELTON, J. (1900). "History of Corn Milling", Vol. III, p. 290. Simpkin Marshall, London.

BURKITT, D. P. and TROWELL, H. C. (1975). "Refined Carbohydrate Foods and Disease: Some Implications of Dietary Fibre." Academic Press, London.

DANIELS, D. G. H. and FISHER, N. (1981). *Br. J. Nutr.* **46**, 1–6.

EASTWOOD, M. A., FISHER, N., GREENWOOD, C. T. and HUTCHINSON, J. B. (1974). *Lancet* **1**, 1029–1033.

ENGLYST, H., WIGGINS, H. S. and CUMMINGS, J. H. (1982). *Analyst* **107**, 307–318.

FINCHER, G. B. (1975). *J. Inst. Brew.* **81**, 116–122.

FISHER, N. and HUTCHINSON, J. B. (1973). *In* "Molecular Structure and Function of Food Carbohydrate" (G. G. Birch and L. F. Green, eds), pp. 275–291. Applied Science Publishers, London.

Flour Milling and Baking Research Association (FMBRA) (1979). *Annu. Rep. Acc.,* p. 18.

Flour Milling and Baking Research Association (FMBRA) (1982a). To be published on completion. See also FMBRA (1982b).

FLOUR MILLING and BAKING RESEARCH ASSOCIATION (FMBRA) (1982b). *Annu. Rep. Acc.,* p. 13.

GULLER, R. and REBER, M. (1980). *Schweiz Med. Wochenschr.* **111**, 89–91.

KANG, J. Y. and DOE, W. F. (1979). *Br. Med. J.* **1**, 1249–1250.

KENT, N. L. (1975). "Technology of Cereals", 2nd edition. Pergamon, Oxford.

MACARTHUR, L. A. and D'APPOLONIA, B. L. (1980). *Cereal Chem.* **57**, 39–45.

McCANCE, R. A. and WIDDOWSON, E. M. (1956). "Breads White and Brown, Their Place in Thought and Social History." Pitman, London.

National Food Survey Committee (1982). "Household Food Consumption and Expenditure, 1980", Annu. Rep. Her Majesty's Stationery Office, London.

NEUKOM, H. (1976). *Lebensm.-Wiss. Technol.* **9**, 143–148.

PAINTER, N. S. (1972). *Practitioner* **208**, 669–670.

PAINTER, N. S., ALMEIDA, A. Z. and COLEBOURNE, K. W. (1972). *Br. Med. J.* **2**, 137–140.

Panel on Bread, Flour and other Cereal Products (1981). "Nutritional Aspects of Bread and Flour." Her Majesty's Stationery Office, London.

PAUL, A. A. and SOUTHGATE, D. A. T. (1978). "McCance and Widdowson's The Composition of Foods," pp. 43–45. Her Majesty's Stationery Office, London.

POMERANZ, Y. (1971). "Wheat Chemistry and Technology", 2nd edition, p. 359. American Association of Cereal Chemists, St. Paul, Minnesota.

POWNALL, T. (1795). "Three Tracts on the Corn Trade and Corn Laws." Court of Aldermen, London.

RING, S. G. and SELVENDRAN, R. R. (1980). *Phytochemistry* **19**, 1723–1730.

SOUTHGATE, D. A. T. (1976). "Determination of Food Carbohydrates", pp. 137–142. Applied Science Publishers, London.

STEPHEN, A. M. and CUMMINGS, J. H. (1980). *Nature (London)* **284**, 283–284.

STORK, J. and TEAGUE, W. D. (1952). "A History of Milling, Flour for Man's Bread." University of Minnesota Press, Minneapolis.

VAN DOKKUM, W. (1978). *Voedingsmiddelentechnologie* **11**, 18–21.

WENLOCK, R. W., SIVELL, L. M., KING, R. T. SCUFFAM, D. and WIGGINS, R. A. (1983). *J. Sci. Food Agric.* **34**, 1302–1318.

WYMAN, J. B., HEATON, K. W., MANNINGS, A. P. and WICKS, A.C.B. (1976). *Am. J. Clin. Nutr.* **29**, 1474–1479.

Chapter 24

Other nutritional implications: energy and micronutrients*

KENNETH HEATON

I. General considerations

Fibre-depleted plant foods differ in many important ways from their full-fibre counterparts quite apart from their lack of fibre. They look different, they feel different in the mouth and they taste different; they have different keeping qualities, different cooking qualities and different possibilities for skillful combination with other ingredients to make new foods. In consequence, they have revolutionised man's eating habits. Individually, each difference makes food easier to obtain or to eat. The combination of differences creates irresistible pressure to consume more food and to consume it more quickly.

Cleave was a visionary, and his unique vision was the awesome potential inherent in fibre-depleted foods (or, as he called them, refined carbohydrates) for causing overnutrition and for disrupting health. He particularly blamed sugar and sugar products because he saw that they were far more changed from sugar's parent materials (sugar beet, sugar cane) and from their sweet-tasting counterparts in a natural, lightly processed diet (fruits and vegetables) than is white flour in comparison with wholemeal.

* This chapter is dedicated to T. L. Cleave, who died while it was being written and who inspired many of its ideas.

391

Dietary Fibre, Fibre-Depleted Foods
and Disease

Some of the above statements about sugar (i.e. the fibre-depleted products of the cane and beet, which include brown sugars, syrup and molasses) are obvious and incontestable. Others require scientific verification. This chapter reports the results of several studies that verify these statements. But first, let some self-evident facts be stated:

1. The desire for sweetness is universal in mankind; breast milk is sweet.

2. Before man invented the mass production of sugar, this desire could be satisfied only with fruit (and occasionally honey), hence only in times and places where fruit was available. For long periods of the year, sweetness would be unobtainable.

3. Fruit is bulky and satisfying. Since it requires chewing, it cannot be consumed fast. Manufactured sugar-containing products require little or no chewing and sugar itself can be drunk.

4. In eating fruit one obtains a range of vitamins and minerals as well as energy.

5. White sugar provides no vitamins or minerals and brown sugar provides only trace amounts.

6. Artificially sweetened foods and drinks are very widely consumed and provide a substantial part of most people's energy intake in Western populations.

From these simple observations it could be predicted that, with *ad libitum* intake, a diet rich in fibre-depleted sugars would inflate energy intake above that obtained from a diet containing only full-fibre sugars (largely present in fruit). It could also be predicted that a fibre-depleted diet would provide less minerals and vitamins. Are these predictions borne out by the results of appropriately designed experiments?

II.   Energy intake and weight change

Mann *et al.* (1970) reported a study in which 17 middle-aged men, employees of a Cape Town insurance company, were instructed to cut out foods containing sucrose for 22 weeks. According to diet records they reduced their mean sucrose intake from 85 to 12 g/day. They were told to keep up their weight by eating more of other foods but failed to do so, their weight falling by an average of 2.8 lb. Two control groups, one asked to limit starch and the other to eat normally, both *gained* about 2 lb weight, so in effect the involuntary weight loss attributable to sucrose restriction was 4.8 lb. Rifkind *et al.* (1966) reported a similar unintentional weight loss in 11 post-myocardial infarction patients who were asked to follow a low-sucrose diet for 10 weeks. The weight loss was described as moderate but no figures were given. Energy intakes were not reported in either of these studies which were primarily concerned with blood lipid levels.

In Bristol, we have carried out three studies of *ad libitum* energy intake in which volunteers have excluded from their diet in one case all fibre-depleted carbohydrate foods, in another case mainly fibre-depleted starch, and in a third case only fibre-free sugars. The results enable a distinction to be made between the effects of fibre-free sugars and of partially depleted starch (white flour). (See Chapter 2, p. 27.)

The first experiment involved 13 subjects with asymptomatic gallstones (10 being women) who had volunteered for a study of the effects of refined and unrefined carbohydrate diets upon bile composition and bile acid metabolism (Thornton et al., 1983). Most of these subjects were overweight (mean relative weight 120% of ideal, range 86–149). No restriction was placed on the total amount of food eaten, nor on the amount or type of animal products. However, at the beginning of one 6-week period the subjects were instructed in the replacement of all fibre-depleted carbohydrate foods and drinks with unrefined or full-fibre foods. In the other 6-week period, they were told not to eat whole grain products, were limited in their intake of fruit and vegetables and were asked to take sugar in drinks and on breakfast cereals and to eat confectionery and other sweetened foods. Every sixth day in this and the subsequent two studies the subjects recorded on a specially designed form everything they ate or drank so that records were obtained of dietary intake on all 7 days of the week. An experienced dietitian interviewed each subject with her forms and estimated the amounts recorded in grams. Each day's intake was then analysed by computer using a specially prepared programme for energy and for the nutrients listed in McCance and Widdowson's standard food tables (Paul and Southgate, 1978). The results for energy, refined sugar, carbohydrate, protein, fat and dietary fibre are shown in Table 24.1. Mean energy intake was higher by 2.01 MJ, i.e. by 23% on the fibre-depleted diet. Mean body weight rose 1.6 kg on the fibre-depleted diet and fell 1.6 kg on the full-fibre diet.

The second experiment involved 15 diabetics (4 of whom were women) who were taking a traditional low-carbohydrate diabetic diet and who volunteered for a study of the effects of an *ad libitum* unrefined carbohydrate diet on the control of diabetes mellitus (Manhire et al., 1981). Seven men and 3 women were on insulin and the others were taking oral hypoglycaemic drugs. Most were not obese (mean relative weight 109%, range 92–148). In one 6-week period, they were simply reinstructed in their prescribed diet. This diet was, of course, already low in sucrose but it was still fibre-depleted since in all patients white bread was the main bread eaten. In the other 6-week period, the subjects were given the same instructions as those in the first experiment, i.e. to replace all fibre-depleted carbohydrate foods and drinks with unrefined or full-fibre foods. This involved mainly a change to wholemeal bread and the consumption of more vegetables and fruit. Sucrose intake fell further but by a biologically insignificant amount (13 g/day). As Table 24.1 shows in the two middle columns, there was *no* change in energy intake despite a substantial rise in dietary fibre. Weight was unchanged on both diets.

TABLE 24.1. Mean daily intake of energy, macronutrients and dietary fibre in three groups of subjects on *ad libitum* diets restricted or not restricted in fibre-depleted carbohydrate foods[a,b]

	All fibre-depleted foods (asymptomatic gallstones)		Fibre-depleted starches (diabetics)		Fibre-depleted sugars (asymptomatic gallstones)	
	Restricted	Unrestricted	Restricted	Unrestricted	Restricted	Unrestricted
Energy (MJ)	7.16	9.17**	9.35	9.42	6.33	7.88**
Refined sugar (g)	6	106**	8	21*	16	112**
Other carbohydrate (g)	152	160	193	180	139	137
Protein (g)	74	75	98	97	62	62
Fat (g)	86	93	118	118	72	75
Dietary fibre (g)	27	13**	34	19**	19	16*

[a] Heaton *et al.*, 1983; Werner *et al.*, 1984.
[b] Versus restricted *p < 0.01, ** p < 0.001.

Thus, replacing fibre-depleted with full-fibre starch made no difference to energy intake whereas replacing all fibre-depleted carbohydrate foods with their full-fibre equivalents significantly reduced energy intake and body weight. This suggests that the latter result was due to the differences in sugar content between the two diets. In fact, in that experiment there was a strong correlation between the weight lost on the unrefined, full-fibre diet and the reduction in the intake of refined sugar ($r = 0.88$, $p < 0.01$; Heaton, 1980).

This inference is supported by the results of the third experiment (Werner et al., 1984). This involved 12 subjects with asymptomatic gallstones (8 of whom were women) who volunteered for a study of the effects of sucrose upon bile composition and secretion. In one 6-week period they were asked to add sugar to drinks and to eat sweets, cakes, biscuits and other prepared foods sweetened with sucrose. To ensure that their daily sucrose intake exceeded 100 g, they were asked to drink one or two cans of proprietary soft drink every day, each containing 29–39 g sucrose. In the other 6 weeks the subjects were asked to use only saccharine as a sweetener, to avoid sugar-containing prepared foods and to drink one or two cans per day of soft drink of the same flavour as the sugar-containing one but sweetened with saccharine. Cans of soft drink were supplied free of charge. Other dietary changes were discouraged but subjects were told not to go hungry and were allowed to eat *ad libitum* of foods devoid of added sucrose, including fresh and dried fruit.

Energy intake was higher by 1.55 MJ/day or 24.5% on the sugar-rich diet and this was entirely accounted for by the higher intake of fibre-free sucrose (112 vs. 16 g/day) (Table 24.1, right-hand two columns). Body weight was 1.4 kg higher at the end of this diet than at the end of the low-sugar diet. All other dietary differences were minor and, in particular, there was no difference in starch or fat. There was a slight difference (3 g/day) in dietary fibre intake, attributable to the consumption of more fruit on the low-sugar diet, but this is not biologically significant.

It might be argued that the energy-inflating effect of sucrose is due simply to the greater palatability of sucrose-sweetened foods and drinks or, alternatively, that people used to a sugary diet will find a low-sugar diet unpalatable and so eat less. The last study does not support these suggestions since no subject complained of being unsatisfied on the low-sugar diet, saccharine was freely allowed and, in most subjects, their usual diet was not particularly rich in sucrose. However, the best evidence against these suggestions comes from a further study in which sucrose was replaced covertly by a highly palatable sweetener, aspartame.

III. Covert removal of sucrose from the diet

In this ingenious study (Porikos et al., 1982), the spontaneous food intake of six men was measured for 24 days while they lived in a metabolic unit. They

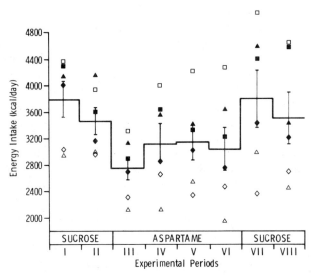

Fig. 24.1. Mean daily energy intake during eight 3-day experimental periods. During the middle four periods sucrose in the diet was covertly replaced with aspartame. The symbols show the data for each of the six volunteers. From Porikos *et al.* (1982).

were fed an attractive diet including two soft drinks per day and plenty of sweet foods such as cheesecakes and tarts, all foods being weighed surreptitiously before and after meals. Considerable effort was made to ensure that the subjects did not know that their food intake was being monitored or that their diet changed during the experiment. On days 7 to 18 sucrose was covertly replaced with aspartame, which reduced the energy density of the diet by 25%. The question was: Would the volunteers compensate, that is, increase their energy intake by eating more food? They did not, or, rather, they did so only partially (Fig. 24.1). During the 12 days when they ate sucrose *ad libitum,* their energy intake averaged 15.30 MJ/day (which the investigators considered excessive). With aspartame substitution, intake dropped immediately to 11.49 MJ/day. After 3 days it recovered to 13.00 MJ/day because the subjects ate more but it then remained stable at this reduced level during the remaining 9 days. Thus, replacing sucrose with a non-energy-supplying sweetener resulted in a 15% drop in energy intake, of which the subjects were quite unaware. Weight tended to rise with sucrose and fall with aspartame.

IV.   Mechanisms whereby fibre-free sugar inflates energy intake

Test meal experiments have revealed at least three mechanisms by which fibre-free sugar could inflate energy intake: (1) artificial ease and speed of ingestion; (2) reduced satiety compared with full-fibre equivalents; (3) rebound hypoglycaemia with earlier return of hunger.

Comparison of fibre-free with full-fibre sugar cannot be done meaningfully using cane-sugar or beet-sugar since nobody eats whole sugar cane or sugar beet. However, the comparison is accurately mimicked by using whole fruits and their fibre-free juices. Fruits and their juices contain other sugars besides sucrose but this does not make them less valid as a model.

Haber et al. (1977) asked 10 healthy volunteers to consume a standard meal of apples and the equivalent amount of apple juice as quickly as they comfortably could. The average time to finish the meals was 17.2 min for apples and 1.5 min for apple juice. Similarly, fibre-free sucrose added to beverages or incorporated in manufactured drinks slips in "abnormally" fast. This is simply because the solidity and chewiness associated with dietary fibre is absent. When the solidity of apples was removed partially by homogenising them into a puree, the average consumption time for the test meal was 5.9 min.

Satiety and hunger are subjective sensations and can be measured only by using a linear rating scale, for example a scale of 20 cm running from minus 10 for extreme hunger to plus 10 for extreme satiety. Such a scale was used by Haber et al. (1977) and by Bolton et al. (1981) to compare the satiety conferred by energy-equivalent meals of apples and apple juice, oranges and orange juice, and grapes and grape juice. In each case, the juice evoked considerably less satiety than the whole fruit (Table 24.2).

It is reasonable to assume that, if people eat to normal fullness and if their diet is changed to include foods with a lower satiating effect, then their energy intake will rise unconsciously. This being so, there is a need for more data on the energy/satiety ratio of different foods and, especially, on the effects of food processing upon this ratio. Meanwhile, the idea that a diet which requires less chewing will provide more energy is supported by a study in which 20 volunteers spent 5 days eating a high-fibre, low-sugar, low-fat diet requiring 17 min chewing time per day and 5 days eating a low-fibre, high-sugar, high-fat diet requiring only 12 min chewing per day (Duncan et

TABLE 24.2. Maximum level of satiety
on a 0–10 scale in 10 healthy, non-obese volunteers
after energy-equivalent meals of fruit
and fruit juices[a]

	Apples	Oranges	Grapes
Fruit	6.9 ± 0.3	6.4 ± 0.7	4.2 ± 1.1
Juice	1.4 ± 1.4	1.5 ± 1.3	0.8 ± 1.1
p	<0.01	<0.01	<0.01

[a] Haber et al., 1977; Bolton et al., 1981.

al., 1983). Energy intake averaged 1570 kcal/day on the chewy diet and 3000 kcal on the less chewy diet. The investigators noted that on the cake-and-Coke type of diet people tended to overeat, i.e. eat past the point of comfortable satiety.

Rebound hypoglycaemia with early return of appetite has been noted after test meals of apple juice and orange juice but not after whole apples and oranges (Haber *et al.*, 1977; Bolton *et al.*, 1981). With grapes and grape juice this difference was not observed, possibly because the grapes were extremely rich in sugars and low in fibre (Bolton *et al.*, 1981). The extent to which rebound hypoglycaemia occurs in a mixed diet containing sucrose in normally consumed amounts is uncertain, though it is widely accepted as occurring, at least in the United States (Schauss, 1980). There are certainly carbohydrate-sensitive people whose fasting serum insulin levels rise to abnormal levels on a sucrose-rich diet (Szanto and Yudkin, 1969; Reiser *et al.*, 1979, 1981).

V.   Micronutrient intake with full-fibre and fibre-depleted diets

It is well known that the refined or fibre-depleted foods are also depleted of vitamins and minerals. White sugar is 99.9% sucrose and contains no micronutrient whatever. Brown sugars, especially dark brown ones, contain appreciable amounts of minerals in the thin film of molasses which coats the sugar crystals and when large quantities are eaten the mineral intake may have nutritional significance (Brekhman and Nesterenko, 1983). However, brown sugars are consumed in small amounts. Vitamins and trace minerals are scanty or absent in confectionery, ice-cream, jellies, cakes, biscuits, pastries, etc.

The manufacture of white flour entails marked reductions in the content of all vitamins and minerals since these are concentrated in the germ and the bran. For example, in the milling of 70% extraction flour, 84% of the pyridoxine present in the wheat grain is lost. The figures for other vitamins are thiamine, 80%; nicotinic acid, 77%; riboflavine, 67%; pantothenic acid, 50%; biotin, 77%; folic acid, 68%; and vitamin E, 100% (Moran, 1959). Since World War II, British millers have been compelled by legislation to add thiamine and nicotinic acid (also iron and calcium) to white flour but at the time of writing, new legislation is in preparation to allow this to cease. In the meantime, Table 24.3 shows the micronutrient composition of wholemeal and white bread. Similar losses occur in the milling of white rice and, indeed, in the production of all fibre-depleted foods.

In poor populations which rely heavily on a single staple food, these losses of micronutrients can be disastrous. The classic example is beri-beri, caused

TABLE 24.3. Vitamin and mineral concentrations
in wholemeal flour and enriched 70% extraction white flour
(mg/100 g)

	Wholemeal	White
Vitamins		
Thiamine	0.46	[a]0.31 (0.10)
Riboflavin	0.08	0.03
Nicotinic acid	5.6	[a]2.0 (0.7)
Pyridoxine	0.50	0.15
Pantothenic acid	0.80	0.30
Biotin	0.007	0.001
Folic acid	0.025	0.014
Tocopherols	2.1	0.85
Minerals		
Sodium	3	3
Potassium	360	130
Calcium	35	[a]140 (15)
Magnesium	140	36
Iron	4.0	[a]2.2 (1.5)
Copper	0.40	0.22
Zinc	3.0	0.9
Phosphorus	340	130

[a] Raised by enrichment; figures in parentheses for un-
enriched flour. Data from Paul and Southgate, 1978.

by thiamine deficiency, which became endemic in the rice-eating areas of the world after the introduction of factory-milled white rice in the late nineteenth century. This problem has largely been solved by parboiling and enrichment (and by higher living standards and so a more varied diet) but it illustrates the potential dangers of large-scale food processing.

Three questions remain: (1) In the context of a mixed Western diet, what are the effects on vitamin and mineral intake of including refined, fibre-depleted foods in the diet? (2) Do reduced intakes result in sub-clinical deficiencies? (3) Do sub-clinical deficiencies reduce vitality or resistance to disease, whether infectious or degenerative? The last two questions are highly controversial and beyond the scope of this volume. Suffice it to say that there are data which purport to link magnesium and selenium deficiency with coronary heart disease, chromium deficiency with diabetes, deficiencies of zinc, pyridoxine and ascorbic acid with diseases of T lymphocyte dysfunction and trace element deficiencies with crime and delinquency. There is also considerable evidence linking a high Na/K ratio with essential hypertension.

On the first question, of the effects of refined, fibre-depleted foods on vitamin and mineral intake in a Western population, remarkably little work has been done. However, a recent study in Bristol (Heaton *et al.*, 1983) has

TABLE 24.4. Mean daily intake of 12 vitamins and 7 minerals in two groups of subjects on *ad libitum* diets restricted or not restricted in fibre-depleted foods[a,b]

	All fibre-depleted foods		Fibre-depleted starches	
	Restricted	Unrestricted	Restricted	Unrestricted
Thiamine (mg)	1.30 ± 0.12	1.27 ± 0.10	1.67 ± 0.12	*1.47 ± 0.15
Riboflavin (mg)	1.82 ± 0.14	1.78 ± 0.13	2.86 ± 0.27	*2.41 ± 0.24
Nicotinic acid equivalents (mg)	27.5 ± 2.5	28.3 ± 1.9	35.6 ± 2.5	38.9 ± 3.3
Vitamin B_6 (mg)	1.40 ± 0.10	***1.03 ± 0.07	1.80 ± 0.12	**1.50 ± 0.11
Pantothenic acid (mg)	4.73 ± 0.36	**3.97 ± 0.35	6.70 ± 0.49	**5.40 ± 0.38
Total folic acid (mg)	204 ± 14	***147 ± 11	275 ± 18	***213 ± 15
Vitamin B_{12} (μg)	10 ± 3.1	8.0 ± 2.6	13.8 ± 3.1	*6.9 ± 0.9
Biotin (μg)	30.4 ± 3.1	*24.1 ± 2.8	42.0 ± 4.1	***30.2 ± 2.7
Vitamin C (mg)	57.1 ± 4.8	**43.5 ± 3.2	81.7 ± 5.6	77.0 ± 7.6
Retinol equivalents (mg)	1981 ± 498	1488 ± 357	3476 ± 760	*1607 ± 268
Vitamin D (μg)	3.55 ± 0.84	2.51 ± 0.44	3.21 ± 0.57	3.32 ± 0.46
Vitamin E (mg)	5.01 ± 0.53	*3.93 ± 0.31	6.7 ± 0.6	**5.6 ± 0.5
Potassium (mg)	2739 ± 298	*2319 ± 181	3722 ± 228	***3047 ± 213
Calcium (mg)	702 ± 46	***897 ± 55	1155 ± 92	*1295 ± 130
Magnesium (mg)	328 ± 30	***206 ± 15	425 ± 28	***263 ± 18
Phosphorus (mg)	1351 ± 94	***1165 ± 71	1888 ± 126	***1591 ± 127
Copper (mg)	1.57 ± 0.15	**1.38 ± 0.16	2.84 ± 0.04	**1.55 ± 0.11
Iron (mg)	11.4 ± 1.1	10.9 ± 0.8	15.4 ± 1.0	***12.4 ± 1.0
Zinc (mg)	11.8 ± 1.0	***9.1 ± 0.6	15.8 ± 1.0	*14.0 ± 1.3

[a] Adapted from Heaton *et al.,* 1983.

[b] Versus restricted *$p < 0.05$, **$p < 0.01$, ***$p < 0.001$.

provided data on the micronutrient intake of 28 volunteers over two 6-week periods while they ate, alternately, a diet containing fibre-depleted carbohydrate foods in commonly consumed amounts and a diet virtually devoid of such foods. Further details of the subjects and the experimental design are given in Section II.

Table 24.4 shows that with refined foods in the diet there was, in one or both groups, a lower intake of 10 vitamins, that is, of all vitamins except nicotinic acid and vitamin D. There was also a lower intake of 6 out of 7 minerals, that is, of potassium, magnesium, phosphorus, copper, iron and zinc. It is possible that some of these minerals might be absorbed less efficiently from full-fibre foods, but this is only likely with cereal foods containing intact phytic acid, such as unleavened flour.

Temple (1983) has calculated the likely intake of certain vitamins and minerals on two diets—a typical British diet containing white bread, cornflakes and white sugar and an equicaloric one containing in their place whole wheat bread, a whole grain breakfast cereal and more vegetables including pulses. He found the following reductions on the fibre-depleted diet—selenium, 61%; folic acid, 54%; vitamin E, 45%; vitamin B6, 37%; choline,

29%; chromium, 15%; magnesium, 64%; zinc, 31%; manganese, 72%; copper, 48%; and potassium, 31%. He calculated that the Na/K ratio would be 1.73 on the fibre-depleted diet and 1.06 on the full-fibre diet. These theoretical figures are in reasonable agreement with the actual data obtained in the Bristol study.

If the intake of micronutrients obtained from a full-fibre diet is the physiological or optimum intake, then the intake derived from a diet rich in fibre-depleted foods is likely to be sub-optimal. It is unlikely that, in sensible educated people eating a mixed diet, the inclusion of fibre-depleted foods will lead to overt deficiencies. However, there are vulnerable groups such as the old, the depressed, alcoholics, and adolescents living away from home for the first time, in whom deficiencies could arise due to a higher than average intake of refined foods.

VI.   Summary

Fibre-depleted foods are changed physically and in other respects which would be expected to favour increased intake of energy. Studies of volunteers eating *ad libitum* diets rich and poor in fibre-depleted carbohydrate foods indicate that the consumption of fibre-free sucrose does considerably inflate energy intake and promotes weight gain. Fibre-depleted starch seems to have little or no effect on energy intake. Studies with model meals of fruit and fruit juice emphasise the lack of satiety produced by fibre-free sugars and their excessive ease and speed of ingestion.

Diets rich in fibre-depleted carbohydrate foods are not only deficient in fibre but also reduced in their contents of most vitamins and minerals. Micronutrient intake may well be sub-optimal in some people who eat much fibre-depleted food.

References

BOLTON, R. P., HEATON, K. W. and BURROUGHS, L. F. (1981). *Am. J. Clin. Nutr.* **34,** 211–217.

BREKHMAN, I. I. and NESTERENKO, I. F. (1983). "Brown Sugar and Health". Pergamon, Oxford.

DUNCAN, K. H., BACON, J. A. and WEINSIER, R. L. (1983). *Am. J. Clin. Nutr.* **37,** 763–767.

HABER, G. B., HEATON, K. W., MURPHY, D. and BURROUGHS, L. (1977). *Lancet* **2,** 679–682.

HEATON, K. W. (1980). *In* "Medical Aspects of Dietary Fiber" (G. A. Spiller and R. M. Kay, eds), pp. 223–238. Plenum, New York.

HEATON, K. W., EMMETT, P. M., HENRY, C. L., THORNTON, J. R., MANHIRE, A. and HARTOG, M. (1983). *Hum. Nutr.: Clin. Nutr.* **37C,** 31–35.

MANHIRE, A., HENRY, C. L., HARTOG, M. and HEATON, K. W. (1981). *J. Hum. Nutr.* **35,** 99–101.

MANN, J. I., TRUSWELL, A. S., HENDRICKS, D. A. and MANNING, E. (1970). *Lancet* **1,** 870–872.

MORAN, T. (1959). *Nutr. Abstr. Rev.* **29**, 1–16.

PAUL, A. A. and SOUTHGATE, D. A. T. (1978). "McCance and Widdowson's The Composition of Foods", 4th revised and extended edition of M.R.C. Spec. Rep. No. 297. Her Majesty's Stationery Office, London.

PORIKOS, K. P., HESSER, M. F. and VAN ITALLIE, T. B. (1982). *Physiol. Behav.* **29**, 293–300.

REISER, S., HANDLER, H. B., GARDNER, L. B., HALLFRISCH, J. G., MICHAELIS, O. E. and PRATHER, E. S. (1979). *Am. J. Clin. Nutr.* **32**, 2206–2216.

REISER, S., BOHN, E., HALLFRISCH, J., MICHAELIS, O. E., KEENEY, M. and PRATHER, E. S. (1981). *Am. J. Clin. Nutr.* **34**, 2348–2358.

RIFKIND, B. M., LAWSON, D. H. and GALE, M. (1966). *Lancet* **2**, 1379–1381.

SCHAUSS, A. (1980). "Diet, Crime and Delinquency." Parker House, Berkeley.

SZANTO, S. and YUDKIN, J. (1969). *Postgrad. Med. J.* **45**, 602–607.

TEMPLE, N. J. (1983). *Med. Hypotheses* **10**, 411–424.

THORNTON, J. R., EMMETT, P. M. and HEATON, K. W. (1983). *Gut* **24**, 2–6.

WERNER, D., EMMETT, P. M. and HEATON, K. W. (1984). *Gut* **25**, 269–274.

Chapter 25

A better Western diet: what can be achieved?

ALAN SILMAN and JEAN MARR

I. Introduction

A. Diet and disease: is prevention possible?

Epidemiological observations, laboratory experiments and analytical and intervention studies on human subjects in the area of nutrition and disease have as their ultimate goal, via the alteration of current nutritional habits, the achievement of either a reduction in disease incidence or its severity. The demonstration that, even in diseases with a multifactorial aetiology, diet plays a major causative role is of great potential significance to the community's health. Diet, in theory, should be amenable to whatever change is desirable, a situation not always possible in other environmental hazards not under con-

403

trol of the individual. A recurrent question posed by the previous chapters is that of whether the current Western diet is a major contributory factory in the pattern of disease seen in developed countries. Further, and more important, is the question whether alteration in diet would lead to a reduction in the incidence of the "diseases of modern civilisation". In the multifactorial model of disease aetiology, diet is but one factor of importance. From the demonstration that a particular component of the diet is associated with an increased risk for a particular disease, it does not follow that either: (1) All those with that pattern of diet will acquire this disease—the absolute risk even for those at the extremes of the distribution for the chosen dietary constituent are, for all the major diseases, low; or (2) those without the suspected dietary factor are likely to remain free of this disease.

It is perhaps more useful to consider dietary *attributable risk,* which can be defined as the increase in risk over and above the "background" risk and represents the increase in risk posed by possession of the dietary factor. The use of this measure in determining the implications of epidemiological studies is shown by considering the following example based on data of dietary fibre from cereals and coronary heart disease in men initially aged 30–67 by Morris *et al.* (1977).

1. Incidence of coronary heart disease per 1000 man-years in a prospective study was = 9.8 (i.e. total risk).

2. Incidence of coronary heart disease in men in the bottom third of the distribution for cereal fibre consumption per 1000 man-years = 17.1 (i.e. absolute risk in this group).

3. Excess of incidence of coronary heart disease for men in the bottom third of the distribution for cereal fibre consumption per 1000 man-years = 7.3 (i.e. attributable risk).

Thus, the attributable risk in this example is less than the baseline total population risk, i.e. the maximum community health benefit achievable by increasing the intake in this group would be to reduce their incidence by 43%.

Another widespread misconception is that following a demonstration of a potentially causative association, an alteration in diet would achieve the expected reduction in disease incidence; this may not be so for various reasons.

Intervention programmes often fail to produce the desired effect and the possible explanations for this are:

1. The dietary variable is in part confounding the effect of another more potent variable in disease terms, for example, genetic influences on both disease and nutrition.

2. For diseases with a long natural history, dietary alteration may have little effect if carried out at too advanced, or even at a sub-clinical stage. Primary prevention by dietary means of the chronic diseases of late adult life may need to commence in infancy or childhood.

3. A change in a single component of diet has effects on diet beyond that of the component. For example, a reduction in total fat intake results either in a reduction of total energy intake or an increase in energy intake from other sources (or a combination of both the above). These changes in themselves may mitigate or enhance the result of fat reduction.

4. If the effect of intervention is measured against a control group, then changes in the control group leading to a reduction in disease incidence may mask the success of the intervention strategy, a situation observed in the MRFIT study (1982).

It is therefore important to be cautious before advocating dietary changes as a mechanism for improving health.

B. Determinants of dietary behaviour

It has to be recognised that knowledge about food and health and the factors influencing dietary behaviour is minimal (Turner and Gray, 1982). This includes social custom (Turner, 1980), which is perhaps the most potent determinant of eating behaviour. A recent series of television commercials (sponsored by the Health Education Council of England and Wales) highlighted the social pressure to each, while the provision and acceptance of large quantities of food are socially desirable forms of behaviour. Body image is probably a more potent factor in limiting obesity than anxieties about health. The increasing availability and the use of convenience foods, take away ("fast") foods and eating out generally remove from the individual control over specific nutrient intake. In the United Kingdom such sources accounted for one-sixth of all expenditure on food (King, 1981), a proportion likely to be exceeded in the United States. The relationship between price, availability and commercial advertising to food consumption is strong but is beyond the scope of this chapter. Finally most of the population live in multi-person households where all members are influenced by the family diet. A dietary change advocated for a single individual, even though acceptable to him, may not be complied with if not acceptable to the other household members. A potent example of this is the advice to avoid the addition of salt in cooking as a measure in hypertension control.

II. Selecting the better diet

There is considerable controversy surrounding virtually all aspects of diet and disease and, perhaps with the exception of vitamin deficiency disorders, there is no unanimity on what might be achieved. There are many who argue that before dietary changes are advocated rigorous proof must be available that such changes would be effective (Ahrens, 1979). It has been pointed out, though, that the technical difficulties of mounting primary intervention trials of dietary change are such that evidence of benefit is unlikely to be obtained (Lewis, 1980) and that the balance of probabilities should dictate advice. There is, as Lewis argues, no rigorous proof that even stopping smoking is beneficial to health: attempted trials in this area have arrived at surprising results (Rose *et al.*, 1982). Isaksson (1978) showed too that many of the recommendations made were not followed by sections of the population. Too draconian alterations, such as those suggested by the McGovern Committee (U.S. Senate Select Committee, on Nutrition and Human Needs, 1977), have little chance of being adhered to. It is the basis of this book that there is a need to rectify the balance between refined and unrefined carbohydrate foods. It has already been mentioned that dietary change has to be considered as a totality and this fact underlies the remainder of this chapter. It is therefore our intention to consider several aspects of diet and assess what is desirable whilst remaining acceptable.

III.　Total energy intake

As a first stage in developing the ideal diet, an estimate of desirable total energy intake must be made. Previous dietary guidelines [U.S. Department of Agriculture, 1980; Department of Health and Social Security (DHSS), 1979] have concentrated on the relative contribution of the different nutrients in providing total energy intake but have given little consideration to absolute levels. A consequence of such an approach is that the recommended intakes of individual dietary components are determined in part by total energy requirements; this is an unsatisfactory situation.

In theory, it should be simple to calculate the appropriate energy intake for an individual on the basis of intake equals output: an excess of the former leading to an increase in body weight. There are two caveats, however. First, in cross-sectional studies the association is inconsistent: Keen *et al.* (1979) found a small negative association between energy intake and body mass index, whereas Morris *et al.* (1977) found a small positive association between energy intake, body weight and body mass index. It is possible, as the former group suggested, that in the static phase of obesity individuals will reduce their energy intake with the aim of achieving a reduction in body weight. Second, there has been a reduction in energy requirements over the past quarter century as witnessed by changes in the nature of occupations (Ministry of Agriculture, Fisheries and Food, unpublished data) (Fig. 25.1). The changes have been dramatic and as shown coincide with a decrease in total energy intake. This latter decrease, which amounts to a fall of some 14%, may have occurred either because of, or in spite of, changing requirements. This in its turn has had two consequences.

1. A reduction in total energy intake has been accompanied by a possible deleterious redistribution of sources of energy towards an increase in fat and a

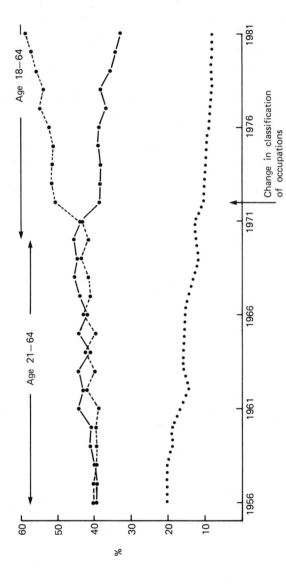

FIG. 25.1. Trends in activity of occupations for men in full time work (Ministry of Agriculture, Fisheries and Food, unpublished data). . . . , Much activity; ·······, little activity; —·—·, moderate activity.

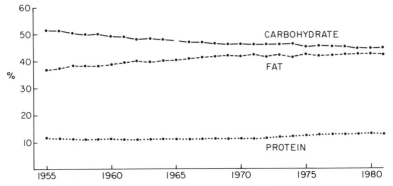

FIG. 25.2. Trends in percentage frequency distribution of nutrients to total energy intake
(Data from Ministry of Agriculture, Fisheries and Food, 1957–1982).

decrease in carbohydrates (Fig. 25.2). Such changes may indeed be consequent upon Western man's cultural drive for a reduction in energy intake.

2. There has been a reduction in total energy turnover. The physiological
significance of this is unknown but it has been suggested that such a change is
not beneficial to health and may even lead to an increase in coronary heart
disease (Morris et al., 1980). This is of potential considerable importance.

Energy intake and coronary heart disease

The role of diet in the aetiology of coronary heart disease has been studied
extensively. Many national dietary guidelines explicitly or implicitly are
guidelines primarily for the prevention of this condition. Though a direct
relationship between increasing body weight and risk of coronary disease has
been suggested (Hubert et al., 1982), it is not a simple one and Jarrett et al.
(1982) showed a J-shaped relationship with those in the lowest quarter of
body weight distribution are also at increased risk. One explanation for this
phenomenon is the possible inverse relationship between energy intake and
the risk of coronary heart disease. The Boston and Irish Brothers study
(Trulson et al., 1964) showed that the Irish siblings had a mean calorie intake
of some 500 cal greater than their Bostonian counterparts with two-thirds the
risk of coronary disease. Den Hartog and his colleagues (1965) showed an
inverse relationship between energy intake and serum cholesterol; a finding
also seen in the Framingham study (Kannel and Gordon, 1970). It was
suggested from the latter study that this may relate to a reduction in physical
activity. In a longitudinal study of men divided into thirds by energy intake,
there was an inverse relationship between energy intake and risk of developing coronary heart disease (Morris et al., 1977). Indeed Gordon et al. (1981),
reviewing three studies from the United States, showed similar results.

We conclude, therefore, by advising that total energy intake should match output provided that output is sufficient to maintain an adequate energy turnover for the average Western adult. In the British National Food Survey, the calculated energy intake from the foods purchased for home consumption averaged 9.4 MJ (2250 kcal) for the years 1978–1980, whereas in 1967–1969 the calculated consumption was around 10.4 MJ (2600 kcal) excluding any contribution from alcohol. The population should aim at returning to this higher level. Any excess in relation to output should be compensated by increased physical activity.

IV. Carbohydrates

Recommendations about carbohydrate content both quantitatively and qualitatively are considered by examining the three main dietary components of carbohydrate intake, i.e. sugar, starch and dietary fibre.

A. Sugar

All national dietary guidelines have called for a reduction in sugar (sucrose) intake (Canadian Committee on Diet and Cardiovascular Disease, 1977; Irish Agricultural Institute, 1977; U.S. Senate Select Committee on Nutrition and Human Needs, 1977; Comité Français d'Education, 1978; Isaksson, 1978; DHSS, 1979) though the amount of reduction varies. Sugar is the main dietary cause of dental caries (Newbrun, 1982) but is of little importance in the aetiology of diabetes (Kahn et al., 1977; Baird, 1972). Though a role in the aetiology of ischaemic heart disease was suggested (Yudkin and Roddy, 1964), longitudinal studies have not confirmed this association (Gordon et al., 1981). However, sugar contains no nutritional benefit, and though it is, for many, a cheap and convenient source of calories, its role in nutrition can be replaced by the inclusion of other foodstuffs. Sugar has thus been described as "empty calories" (Passmore et al., 1979) emphasising its lack of a unique physiological role. Sugar consumption has, in fact, decreased from high levels in the early 1960s, showing a gradual reduction over the following 20 years. A further reduction in intake may be difficult to achieve as many sugar-containing foods are considered as "luxury" or "reward" items and thus are not easily substituted by other foodstuffs. It is interesting to note (Périssé et al., 1969) that between countries there is an inverse relationship between sugar and starch consumption, the former increasing with increasing affluence. Thus, a pragmatic dietary policy, while accepting that sugar produces caries as well as being unnecessary for nutrition, would be unlikely to be successful if it attempted to limit all sugar. A more useful approach would be to combine the further development of safe and acceptable sugar supplements with attempts to change the status of sweet foods.

TABLE 25.1. Carbohydrate intake—changes in intake[a]

	1955–1957	1966–1968	1978–1980
Carbohydrate intake (g/person/day)	335	321	268
Change since 1955–1957 (%)	—	−4	−20
Contribution to total energy intake (%)		47	45

[a] Data from Ministry of Agriculture, Fisheries and Food Reports, 1957–1982.

B. Complex carbohydrate starches

In the United Kingdom there has been a dramatic and sustained fall in the relative contribution of carbohydrates to the national diet (Table 25.1). In the past quarter century their contribution to the national diet in the United Kingdom has fallen from 51% to 45%, representing a decrease from a mean daily consumption of 335 g to 268 g. The major reasons for the decrease have been a decline in bread consumption by 38% and potatoes by 24%. Such changes, quantitatively, are the most important in recent years in the Western diet.

The potential advantages of increasing the relative and absolute intake of these foods are: (1) They are replacement energy sources for more "harmful" sources such as fats and sugars; (2) foods high in starch carry other nutrients of value for example protein in bread and vitamin C in potatoes; and (3) they are major sources of dietary fibre. The recognition of these facts have led various policy-making bodies to suggest an unqualified increase in the consumption of these foods by up to 100% (U.S. Senate Select Committee on Nutrition and Human Needs, 1977). However, it is important to remember that no foods are consumed in isolation from other foodstuffs and starchy foods (particularly those high in dietary fibre) are probably unpalatable on their own (Silman, 1979) and their palatability is normally enhanced by the addition of either fat or sugar. However, the idea of bread as a healthy food is now being promoted (DHSS, 1981).

The Boston Brothers study (Trulson et al., 1964) highlighted the association that was observed in the Irish siblings, of a low risk of disease with a high intake of both bread and potatoes. It would be prudent therefore to recommend an increase in bread intake by 500 g/person/week to reach the 1500 g taken 25 years ago, a total intake equivalent to about five large slices of bread per day. Similarly potatoes could be increased by 400 g/person/week to reach the 1600 g 25 years ago. This is a total intake equivalent to about one large potato per day. Though it has been suggested that pulses are not of relevance to the Western diet (Passmore et al., 1979), this has been disputed (Grimble et al., 1979) and some substitution for the other starchy foods is taking place.

C.   Dietary fibre

The role of dietary fibre in disease aetiology and prevention has been considered in detail in previous chapters. There has been a substantial decline in consumption of dietary fibre over the past century both in the United Kingdom (Robertson, 1972; Southgate et al., 1978) and in the United States (Heller and Hackler, 1978). The decline has been due to a reduction in intake of dietary fibre from cereal sources as opposed to that from fruit and vegetables, the latter, with the exception of potatoes, having increased. Higher intakes of cereal fibre started during the Second World War in the United Kingdom with the introduction of the high-extraction, high-fibre National Flour Mandatory from 1942 to 1953, then low-fibre, low-extraction white flour replaced the wartime flour and thus cereal fibre consumption dropped. Although among many populations of the world there is evidence of an inverse relationship between wealth and unrefined carbohydrate consumption (Périssé et al., 1969), within Western countries the picture is more complex. In the United Kingdom the consumption of dietary fibre in the highest income group is between 21 and 28 g/day compared with a range of 27 to 31 g in the lowest income group. This tendency for increasing fibre intake with decreasing income is perhaps explained by the increased contribution of bread in the diet. The Department of Health and Social Security report on Nutritional Aspects of Bread and Flour (DHSS, 1981) suggested that the reluctance to change from white to wholemeal bread is due to the Bread and Flour Regulations of 1963 which did not allow the addition of ingredients that would improve texture and palatability to wholemeal bread but were added to white bread. Grimes and Gordon (1978) suggested that it is likely that, especially as wholemeal bread increased satiety, more white bread would be consumed by a given individual. A consequence of this might be that diets high in fibre might reduce total energy intake (Heaton, 1973). This, however, was not reported by Morris et al. (1977) who observed a positive relationship between total energy and cereal fibre intakes. There also does not appear to be any relationship between body weight and cereal fibre intake (Silman, 1979).

There are large differences in individual dietary fibre intake, there being a 10-fold difference between the highest and the lowest consumers. This is evidence that volunteers can be encouraged to increase their consumption of dietary fibre, for example, Wright et al. (1979), but no evidence of what may happen when unselected individuals are similarly encouraged. The range of dietary fibre consumption in a population in a village in Cambridge was found to vary from 8 to 32 g/day with a mean of 20 g (Bingham et al., 1979); dietary fibre from cereal sources provided only 30% of this total, i.e. about 6 g/day. An average intake of 9 g/day has been shown in other studies (Sil-

TABLE 25.2. Proposed changes in dietary fibre content of Western diet

Source of fibre	Current diet, dietary fibre (g/day)[a]	Approximate increase (%)	Proposed diet, dietary fibre (g/day)
Cereals			
Bread			
White	2.4	40	3.4
Brown	0.8	100	1.6
Wholemeal	0.5	100	1.0
Other breads	0.4	Nil	0.4
Breakfast cereals	1.5	50	2.3
Biscuits, cakes, crispbreads, etc.	4.4	Nil	4.4
Total from cereals	10.0	31	13.1
Fruit and vegetables			
Potatoes	3.6	50	5.4
Vegetables	4.8	50	7.2
Fruit	2.8	25	3.5
Total from fruit and vegetables	11.2	40	16.1
Total dietary fibre	21.2	38	29.2

[a] Data from Ministry of Agriculture, Fisheries and Food Reports, 1957–1982; data 1980.

man, 1980). These figures are very low compared with the total dietary fibre of 55 to 150 g/day estimated to be eaten by African blacks (see Chapter 5). However, with a return to higher levels of bread consumption, which would be a realistic and acceptable modification to the Western diet, it should be possible to increase total dietary fibre from 20 to 30 g/day, of which half would come from cereals (Table 25.2).

That many epidemiological studies have failed to show an association within a Western population between dietary fibre and disease may be explained by the fact that the overwhelming majority of the Western population is in the high-risk (low-intake) area. Perhaps the changes we propose may be too modest to achieve an effect though it is unlikely that an increase in excess of what we propose would be acceptable. However, Walker and his colleagues (1982) commented that the wartime improvement in health in Switzerland resulted from a daily fibre intake only slightly more than that outlined above.

V.   Other nutrients

A.   Fats

More has been written on the relationship of dietary fats and ischaemic heart disease than all other aspects of diet and disease. There is still lack of agreement on what is the exact relationship between dietary fats, serum cholesterol

TABLE 25.3. Percentage contribution of different foods
to fat intake[a]

Food	All fats	SFA	PUFA
Milk and cream	14.0	19.0	3.6
Cheese	4.8	6.4	1.2
Meat	27.4	25.4	17.4
Eggs	2.7	1.9	2.8
Fish	1.1	0.4	3.3
Margarine	11.9	9.3	20.3
Butter	12.8	17.1	3.3
Other fats and oils	11.9	9.2	22.6
Fruit, vegetables	2.6	1.8	6.0
Bread and flour	2.6	1.1	7.9
Cakes, pastry, biscuits	5.8	6.4	6.2
Other foods	2.4	2.0	5.4
	100	100	100
Total consumption (g/day)	105.6	46.8	11.3

[a] Data from Ministry of Agriculture, Fisheries and Food,
1957–1982; data 1980.

and the incidence of ischaemic heart disease; and the epidemiological and other evidence is not reviewed here. What is of relevance are reports of changes in dietary fat, both quantitatively and qualitatively over time, and the likely effect of such changes on serum cholesterol and of possible reductions in the incidence of heart disease.

1. *Trends in fat intake*

Within the Western diet there have been major changes in fat consumption over the past 25 years. The proportion of energy from fat has increased from 37 to 42% pari passu with a decrease in that from carbohydrates (Fig. 25.2). Total fat consumption over the same period has altered little and remains about 106 g/person/day (Ministry of Agriculture, Fisheries and Food Reports 1957–1982). The sources of the fat consumed are shown in Table 25.3 and, as can be seen, meat contributes 27% of total fat, dairy products (excluding butter) 19%, butter, margarine and other fats 36%. Dairy products and meat provide the bulk of saturated fatty acids whereas oils and margarines together again with meat provide the polyunsaturates. Over the past 25 years, butter intake increased initially but is now falling, whereas the pattern for margarine is the opposite. Meat and cheese consumption have increased by some 50%.

2. *Fat intake and blood lipids*

It is known that regression of atherosclerosis occurs with wasting diseases (Wilens, 1978). The Oslo Heart study showed that in men with an initially raised serum cholesterol, a polyunsaturated fat diet reduced the serum cholesterol by about 12% (Hjermann *et al.*, 1980). The Finnish Mental Hospital study obtained a difference in serum cholesterol of 15%, those who ate a diet with a polyunsaturated/saturated fatty acid ratio (P/S ratio) of 1.42 to 1.78 had a lower serum cholesterol than those with the "normal" ratio of around 0.25 (Miettinen *et al.*, 1972). A result of similar magnitude with similar dietary changes was observed in other studies (Rinzler, 1968; Dayton *et al.*, 1969). The diet used in the Oslo study succeeded in reducing the total calorie intake from fats to 28% from 44% with a halving in saturated fatty acids (SFA) and a slight increase in polyunsaturates (PUFA) based on an increase in PUFA margarines and oils (Hjermann *et al.*, 1981). Oliver (1981), after reviewing the evidence, suggested a diet containing no more than 30% of the calories from fat with only one-third coming from SFA. Such a diet is unlikely to be acceptable (Marr and Morris, 1982) as it would involve a reduction by half in the consumption of SFA: Without replacement by other foods of minimal fat (especially SFA) content, it was argued that there would be a "loss" in daily energy intake of 1.2 MJ (550 kcal). A more useful approach would be to reduce SFA by one-quarter to about 36 g/day (13–14% of total energy intake), but making this reduction acceptable by increasing PUFA by half, i.e. from the current intake of 11 to 18 g/day. This would give a SFA/PUFA ratio of 0.5, which is similar to the ratio found in southern European countries, where rates of coronary artery disease are low (Keys, 1980). Such a diet would be expected to reduce average serum cholesterol by 6% which potentially could lead to a modest reduction in the incidence of coronary heart disease (Shaper and Marr, 1977).

B. Protein

The intake of protein in the current Western diet of approximately 85.9 g/day is in considerable excess of normal physiological requirements. This excess *per se* has no demonstrable hazard to health but neither has an excess of intake been shown to be of benefit to health. Protein contributes approximately 12% of the total energy intake (National Food Survey), a figure that has changed little over the past 25 years. What has changed is the increase in the proportion of total protein from animal sources, which has increased from 49 to 64% over this period. Within this total figure for meat, however, there has been a change in the source of meat with a decline in carcase meat (beef, lamb, pork) relative to an increase in poultry (Table 25.4). The health consequences of these changes can be considered. Approximately 25% of saturated and 17% of polyunsaturated fatty acids come from meat and thus changes in the source of protein have implications for fat intake. Grimble *et al.* (1979) pointed out that a change of protein from animal sources to vegetable proteins present in pulses would reduce fat intake leaving protein intake un-

TABLE 25.4. Changes in source of total "meats" in the diet:
1955–1957, 1966–1968 and 1978–1980

	1955–1957	1966–1968	1978–1980
Carcass meat	54.0	43.8	40.6
Poultry	1.8	11.2	16.5
Other meats and meat products	44.2	45.0	42.9
	100	100	100

[a] Data from Ministry of Agriculture, Fisheries and Food Reports, 1957–1982.

altered. Ovo–lacto-vegetarians do not suffer ill effects from a lack of animal protein (Passmore et al., 1979). These authors also suggested ecologically in terms of world food supplies that protein from plant sources is a more attractive proposition than that from animal sources. Meat protein provides substantial supplies of iron and the B group vitamins so that a reduction in meat intake would need to be compensated. Recently it has been suggested that the consumption of red meat may be associated with breast cancer, but this is not seen with chicken (Lubin et al., 1981). Though this is unproven and the relative risks are low it only explains a small proportion of the variance.

Total protein intake from meat seems to be determined by income both within a country and between countries (Périssé et al., 1969) and is a reflection of the relative cost of the commodity. There is no indication that a change is necessary in total protein intake.

One other side issue about the source of protein is based on the hypothesis postulated by Sinclair (1977). He observed that Eskimos have a high fat intake which comes from meat as opposed to dairy foods. The former provide large quantities of essential fatty acids, one possible explanation for the low levels of heart disease seen in that population.

C. Sodium

There is evidence from within-population studies of a direct association between sodium intake and hypertension (Gleiberman, 1973). In northern Japan, where the habitual diet is high in salt, the prevalence of hypertension is higher than in southern Japan where a low-sodium diet is consumed (Sasaki, 1962). Within-population studies in Western countries have failed to show a consistent relationship between salt intake and blood pressure (Tuomilheto et al., 1980) though this may be due to a threshold effect, i.e. even those at the extreme left of the distribution for sodium intake consume an excess quantity of sodium (Editorial, 1978). There is evidence, though, that for patients who have an elevated blood pressure, a reduction in sodium intake may reduce blood pressure (Morgan et al., 1978) but as has been pointed out the reduction may not be due to sodium restriction alone (Silman *et al.*, 1983). There is no evidence though, and such would be difficult to obtain, of a reduction in the *incidence* of hypertension, i.e. primary prevention, in those who reduce their sodium intake. It would appear, however, that the physiological requirement is between 20 and 60 mmol/day. Current intakes are of the order of 5 to 10 times this quantity. Therefore, it would appear that a reduction of this magnitude may be effective and should be without harm, apart from conditions where there is an increased requirement, for example, diarrhoea and vomiting. Such a reduction would be partially achieved by not adding salt at the table and in cooking and relying only on the natural sodium content of food. A reduction to the physiological requirements is difficult because salt has been added during bread-making and in food processing and confers palatability. A slow reduction is possible and, eventually, heavily salted foods will be disliked.

VI.   Summary

There is little hard evidence that alteration to the current Western diet would achieve a significant improvement in health. Such hard evidence may never be obtainable, and thus dietary advice has to be based on the balance of probabilities, weighing the benefits and hazards of a proposed dietary change. Dietary changes that are not acceptable to large sections of the population will not, by definition, be acceptable. Thus the ideal needs to be substituted by the "attainable". This, in turn, has as its basis the current dietary habits and the potential basic changes that can evolve from them. If expectations and goals are realistic then there is a real possibility of nutritional change.

References

AHRENS, E. H. (1979). *Lancet* **2**, 1345–1348.

BAIRD, J. D. (1972). *Acta Diabetol. Lat., Suppl.* **1**, 621–624.

BINGHAM, S., CUMMINGS, J. H. and MCNEIL, N. I. (1979). *Am. J. Clin. Nutr.* **32**, 1313–1319.

Canadian Committee on Diet and Cardiovascular Disease (1977). "Canadian Dietary Guidelines," 2nd edition. Bureau of Nutritional Sciences Health Protection Branch, Department of Health and Welfare, Ottawa.

Comité Francais d'Education (1978). "Pour la Santé." Report of Ministry of Health, Family and Social Security, Paris.

DAYTON, S., PEARCE, M. L., HASIMOTO, S., DIXON, W. J. and TOMIYASU, V. (1969). *Circulation* **40**, (Suppl. II), 1–63.

DEN HARTOG, C., VAN SCHAIK, TH.F.S.M., DALDERVP, L. M., DRION, E. F. and MULDER, T. (1965) *Voeding* **26**, 184–208.

Department of Health and Social Security (DHSS) (1979). "Eating for Health." Her Majesty's Stationery Office, London.

Department of Health and Social Security (DHSS) (1981). "Nutritional Aspects of Bread and Flour." Her Majesty's Stationery Office, London.

Editorial (1978). *Lancet* 1, 1136–1137.

GLEIBERMAN, L. (1973). *Ecol. Food Nutr.* 2, 143–156.

GORDON, T., KAGAN, A., GARCIA-PALMIERI, M., KANNELL, W. B., ZUKEL, W. J., TILLOTSON, J., SORLIE, P. and HJORTLAND, M. (1981). *Circulation* 63, 500–515.

GRIMBLE, R., GIBNEY, M. J. and MORGAN, J. (1979). *Br. Med. J.* 1, 818–819.

GRIMES, D. S. and GORDON, C. (1978). *Lancet* 2, 106.

HEATON, K. W. (1973). *Lancet* 2, 1418–1421.

HELLER, S. N. and HACKLER, L. R. (1978). *Am. J. Clin. Nutr.* 31, 1510–1514.

HJERMANN, I., HEDGELAND, A., HOLME, I., LUND-LARSEN, P. G. and LEREN, P. A. (1980). *In* "Proceedings of the Eighth Congress on Cardiology", pp. 164–171. Karger, Basel.

HJERMAN, I., VELVE BYRE, K., HOLM, I. and LEREN, P. (1981). *Lancet* 2, 1303–1310.

HUBERT, H. B., FEINLIEB, M., McNAMARA, P. M. and CASTELLI, W. P. (1982). *In* "CVD Epidemiology Newsletter" (R. B. Shekelle, ed.), No. 31. American Heart Association, New York.

Irish Agricultural Institute (1977). "Report of the Health Advisory Committee of An Foras Taluntais." Dublin.

ISAKSSON, B. (1978). *Bt. Nutr. Found. Nutr. Bull.* 4, 228–232.

JARRETT, R. J., SHIPLEY, M. J. and ROSE, G. (1982). *Br. Med. J.* 285, 535–537.

KAHN, H. A., HERMAN, J. B., MEDALLIE, J. H., NEUFELD, H. N., RISS, E. and GOLDBOURT, U. (1977). *J. Chronic Dis.* 23,. 617–622.

KANNEL, W. B. and GORDON, T. (eds) (1970). "Framingham Diet Study. Diet and the Regulation of Serum Cholesterol," Sect. 24. U.S. Government Print Office, Washington, D.C.

KEEN, H., THOMAS, B. J., JARRETT, R. J. and FULLER, J. H. (1979). *Br. Med. J.* 1, 655–658.

KEYS, A. (1980). "Seven Countries, a Multivariate Analysis of Death and Coronary Heart Disease." Harvard University Press, Cambridge, Massachusetts.

KING, S. H. M. (1981). "Eating Behaviour and Attitudes to Food, Nutrition and Health." British Nutrition Foundation, London.

LEWIS, B. (1980). *Br. Med. J.* 2, 177–180.

LUBIN, J. H., BLOT, W. J. and BURNS, P. E. (1981). Paper presented at *14th Annu. Meet., Soc. for Epidemiol. Res.,* Snowbird, Utah.

MARR, J. W. and MORRIS, J. N. (1982). *Lancet* 1, 217–218.

MIETTINEN, M., TURPEINEN, O., KARVONEN, M. K., ELOSUO, R. and PAAVILAINEN, E. (1972). *Lancet* 2, 835–838.

Ministry of Agriculture, Fisheries and Food Reports (1957–1982). "Domestic Food Consumption and Expenditure. Annual Reports for 1955–1980 of the National Food Survey Committee." Her Majesty's Stationery Office, London.

MORGAN, T., ADAM, W., GILLIES, A., WILSON, M., MORGAN, G. and CARNEY, S. (1978). *Lancet* 1, 227–230.

MORRIS, J. N., MARR, J. W. and CLAYTON, D. G. (1977). *Br. Med. J.* 2, 1307–1314.

MORRIS, J. N., EVERITE, M. G., POLLARD, R. and CHAVE, S. P. W. (1980). *Lancet* 2, 1207–1210.

MRFIT Research Group (1982). *JAMA, J. Am. Med. Assoc.* 248, 1465–1467.

NEWBRUN, E. (1982). *Science* 217, 418–423.

OLIVER, M. F. (1981). *Lancet* 2, 1090–1095.

PASSMORE, R., HOLLINGSWORTH, D. F. and ROBERTSON, J. (1979). *Br. Med. J.* 1, 527–531.

PÉRISSÉ, J., SIZARET, F. and FRANÇOISE, P. (1969). *FAO Nutr. Newsl.* 7, 31–39.

RINZLER, S. H. (1968). *Bull. N.Y. Acad. Med.* [2] 44, 936–949.

ROBERTSON, J. (1972). *Nature (London)* 238, 290–291.

Rose, G. A., Hamilton, P. J. S., Colwell, L. and Shipley, M. J. (1982). *J. Epidemiol. Commun. Health* **36**, 102–109.

Sasaki, N. (1962). *Jpn. Heart J.* **3**, 313–317.

Shaper, A. G. and Marr, J. W. (1977). *Br. Med. J.* **1**, 867–871.

Silman, A. J. (1979). *Lancet* **2**, 905.

Silman, A. J. (1980). *J. Epidemiol. Commun. Health* **34**, 204–207.

Silman, A. J., Locke, C., Mitchell, P. and Humpherson, P. (1983). *Lancet* **1**, 1179–1182.

Sinclair, M. H. (1977). *Br. Med. J.* **2**, 1602.

Southgate, D. A. T., Bingham, S. and Robertson, J. (1978). *Nature (London)* **274**, 51–52.

Trulson, M. F., Clancy, R. E., Jessop, W. P. E., Childers, R. W. and Stare, F. J. (1964). *J. Am. Diet. Assoc.* **45**, 225–229.

Tuomilheto, J., Karppanen, H., Tanskanen, A., Tikkanen, J. and Vuori, J. (1980). *J. Epidemiol. Commun. Health* **34**, 174–178.

Turner, M. R. (1980). "Nutrition and Lifestyles". Applied Science Publishers, London.

Turner, M. R. and Gray, J. (1982). "Implementation of Dietary Guidelines: Obstacles and Opportunities." British Nutrition Foundation, London.

U.S. Senate Select Committee on Nutrition and Human Needs (1977). "Dietary Goals for the United States", 1st edition. U.S. Government Printing Office, Washington, D.C.

U.S. Department of Agriculture (1980). "Nutrition and Your Health: Dietary Guidelines for Americans." USDA-DHEW, Washington, D.C.

Walker, A. R. P., Segal, I. and Hathorn, S. (1982). *Lancet* **2**, 980.

Wilens, S. L. (1978). *Am. J. Pathol.* **23**, 783–804.

Wright, A., Burstyn, P. G. and Gibney, M. J. (1979). *Br. Med. J.* **2**, 1541–1543.

Yudkin, J. and Roddy, J. (1964). *Lancet* **2**, 6–8.

Chapter 26

Summaries

HUGH TROWELL, DENIS BURKITT and KENNETH HEATON

A few contributors have concluded their chapters with a brief summary. Shortened summaries, prepared by the editors, permit a quick review of the whole subject. [Occasionally suggestions have been added by the editors; these are printed as separate paragraphs enclosed in brackets.]

I.   Summaries of chapters 1–25

Trowell (Chapter 1) has traced the history of the concept of dietary fibre, comparing it to tributaries which eventually formed one river and aroused much interest in a *group* of British doctors in the 1970s. One early tributary stemmed from a study of the laxative action of bran in the United States in the 1930s. Another tributary arose among those who attempted to describe in medical articles or books the diseases of civilization, such as McCarrison in India in the 1920s and a succession of doctors in Africa starting with Walker in South Africa in the 1950s. He considered that fibre might be a protective factor in certain cardiovascular and metabolic diseases. It is possible that the late Surgeon Captain T. L. Cleave heard about the diseases of civilization during some of his naval travels for it was hearsay among the doctors in many British African colonies. In 1956 he began to put forward his stimulating hypothesis that all these diseases were due to refining of the carbohydrates, especially sugar, but also white flour and white rice, with consequent loss of fibre.

In the early 1970s it appeared necessary to define fibre. Trowell, after consulting other doctors in the group, proposed a definition of dietary fibre (Chapter 2). The concept of dietary fibre should be regarded as an example

419

of what Professor Kuhn has called a paradigm: it inaugurated a revolution in medical science.

Definitions are discussed by the three editors in Chapter 2. Dietary fibre has been defined as the substances present in the plant foods of man that are not digested by human alimentary enzymes. Its principal components are cellulose, hemicelluloses and pectic substances, all of which are polysaccharides. They have been called the unavailable carbohydrates. There is also the associated lignin, which is not a carbohydrate.

The term "refined carbohydrates", previously used, is considered unsatisfactory for reasons detailed in Chapter 2. It is therefore proposed to introduce a new term, "fibre-depleted foods", defined to include all the plant foods of man, containing often starch, sugars, protein, fat, oil and other nutrients, *from which the fibre has been partially or completely removed.* This often produces concentrated energy-dense foods such as sucrose and oils; the latter subsequently may be converted to fats. These increase palatability and energy intakes and promote overweight in susceptible persons.

Dietary fibre is derived largely from polysaccharides present in plant cell walls but certain storage polysaccharides are also resistant to digestion by human alimentary enzymes.

Chapters 3 and 4 discuss the definition and analysis of dietary fibre in Britain by Southgate and Englyst, and in the United States by Prosky and Harland. Both groups accept the dietary fibre definition of Trowell and colleagues (1976). Both groups report their methods of analysis of total dietary fibre: the former group also publish preliminary data concerning dietary fibre components (cellulose and the non-cellulosic polysaccharides, previously often called hemicelluloses). They also report a new aspect of a complex problem. Some of the starch, termed "resistant starch" is not hydrolysed by the enzymes used in their method of analysis. Resistant starch is present in significant even large amounts, in cooked cereals and potatoes. They state "it may be argued that it should be included in total dietary fibre" but outline the difficulties that would arise if this occurred.

The United States AOAC Collaborative Study is reported in Chapter 4. It has involved 42 collaborators in 14 countries and preliminary data on total dietary fibre in certain food samples are reported.

[It is hoped that international agreement concerning the preferred method of analysis of total dietary fibre and its component polysaccharides will eventually be reached. The problem raised by resistant starch resisting hydrolysis in certain analytical procedures will doubtless receive further investigation.]

It has recently been reported that from 2 to 20% of dietary starch escape digestion and absorption in the small bowel; it enters the large bowel to provide energy for the growth of the microbial flora. In Western diets it has been estimated that undigested starch probably contributes 40–50 g/day and dietary fibre 20–30 g/day for the formation of large bowel microflora (Stephen *et al.*, 1983). These facts must influence profoundly the whole question of the aetiology of diseases of the large bowel.]

Bingham (Chapter 5) has reported that dietary fibre intakes in Western industrialised affluent communities are in the range of 15 to 30 g/day. In Britain at present the adult average intake is about 23 g/day. The adult cereal dietary fibre intake has fallen from about 30 g/day in 1860 to 8 g/day at present, due largely to decreased consumption of bread. Similar long-term trends have occurred in European countries and the United States, also more recently in Japan, wherein the diet has been westernised and at present contains less starch.

In sub-Saharan African rural communities, adult dietary fibre intakes probably range from 70 to 100 g/day, even more. This is due to a high intake of lightly processed starch foods such as maize, millet, plantains, pulses and vegetables. Intakes of fat and sugar are low.

There are few data concerning dietary fibre intakes in other Third World countries. Many tropical foodstuffs have not yet been analysed for dietary fibre and surveys of food intakes have seldom been performed. Wherever white rice is the staple, cereal dietary fibre intakes in adults around 20 g/day are likely.

Eastwood and Bryden (Chapter 6) discuss the action of dietary fibre on the morphology and function of the *entire* gastrointestinal tract. It is not possible to summarise so comprehensive a review; it serves as an introduction to subsequent chapters.

Stephen (Chapter 7) considers the relationship of the diet, especially the dietary fibre content, to constipation. A fundamental difficulty is that it has proved impossible to define constipation in an objective manner either in terms of the frequency of defaecation, stool weight, consistency or transit times. Probably it is best to recognise that defaecation should be performed easily, without straining or discomfort. It then resembles the evacuation of the urine. Constipation is therefore defined to be present in any person who strains hard to defaecate, or has discomfort, in the absence of local disease. The subjective nature of this definition makes difficult any numerical assessment of the prevalence of constipation.

A low intake of dietary fibre is the major causative factor in the ordinary type of constipation which is so prevalent in Western communities. Faecal weight and bulk, also ease of defaecation, are increased by the ingestion of more fibre. Cereal fibre is degraded but little in the large bowel; it increases considerably faecal bulk. Fibre from vegetables and fruit are also degraded in the large bowel to form microflora, but are not as effective in the treatment of constipation.

Painter (Chapter 8) has summarised much evidence that diverticular disease, almost like appendicitis, is a "new disease" that emerged about the beginning of the present century because the consumption of bread and of cereal fibre had fallen considerably (p. 153). High pressures develop in a narrow colon in order to propel inspissated faecal material, and they exploit weak spots in an ageing wall. This occurs in those who have eaten a low-fibre diet. There is general agreement that treatment by a high-fibre bran and whole cereal products such as wholemeal bread, thereby lowering the pressures, relieves the symptoms, reduces the complications and halts progress. One recent trial of bran, mentioned in this chapter, failed to report any improvement. Many, including Painter, have criticised this trial.

[The average intake of dietary fibre by adults in Britain is about 23 g/day and the range is 15–30 g/day (p. 87). In the aforementioned trial, the average dietary fibre intake prior to the trial had been 15 g/day; it was increased during the trial to 22 g/day, a *totally* inadequate increase.]

Cummings (Chapter 9) has reviewed the hypothesis that dietary fibre is a protective factor in cancer of the large bowel. This is an intriguing one and worthy of consideration in view of the physiological studies that demonstrate that dietary fibre alters large bowel function in a number of ways that could be protective. The absence of a proven mechanism for the cause of large bowel cancer makes it difficult to judge the significance of all studies. In the context of Europe, America, and possibly other industrialised countries a case can be made that dietary fibre is protective. Some epidemiological findings and population studies (e.g. Japan) do not support the fibre hypothesis.

[The editors suggest that westernization of the Japanese diet, which is still low-fat low-fibre, has been confined almost to the last 25 years: any comparison with Europe and America, wherein the diet became high-fat, low-fibre many years ago is probably not valid.]

Walker and Burkitt (Chapter 10) have produced much evidence that appendicitis was rare in Western populations until about 1870. Then the disease "emerged" until at present one-sixth of the adult population have undergone appendicectomy. The frequency of the operation is decreasing, but it is unknown how far this is due to increased accuracy of the diagnosis, increased pathology checks, even the psychological and sometimes the financial background of the operation.

Appendicitis is still virtually absent in rural areas of sub-Saharan Africa in the blacks, but in the cities incidence is rising. In South African cities urban blacks still have only about one-tenth of the incidence encountered among the whites. This cannot be explained by failure of blacks to attend a hospital for there is a high incidence of other acute, painful surgical emergencies. Available evidence suggests that the primary causative factor is the low intake of dietary fibre, especially cereal dietary fibre. Intestinal stasis probably favours the formation of faecoliths within the appendix, with increased pressure due to blockage; this causes devitalization of the whole distal portion. Direct evidence, however, of the mechanisms involved is still lacking.

[One editor (D. B.) has been collecting evidence from surgeons in Western countries; several report palpable faecoliths in about one-third of all routine abdominal operations. He has obtained only one figure from a Third World surgeon (Professor N. Rangabashyam, personal communication, 1979), who at a Madras hospital has found only 5% palpable faecoliths in 500 consecutive laparotomies on Indian patients passing bulky stools of about 400 g/day.]

Heaton has considered Crohn's disease and ulcerative colitis (Chapter 11). Several case–control studies report that patients with Crohn's disease have consummed excessive amounts of sugar for many years before they develop symptoms. No explanation has been put forward and no mechanism can be suggested. The incidence of Crohn's disease has increased markedly in the last 30 years in Europe and North America, but this disease remains extremely rare in India, China and South America. In South Africa, whites suffer as frequently as in Europe, but it remains rare in blacks.

[Ulcerative colitis has a low prevalence in many tropical countries and in southern Europe, but cases may be missed because of the frequency of infective bowel disorders. In contrast to Crohn's disease the incidence of ulcerative colitis does not appear to have risen in recent years. Immunological abnormalities occur in both diseases but do not explain the variations in disease incidence in different communities or at different times. There is no evidence that either disease is related to dietary fibre.]

Harvey (Chapter 12) has reviewed functional gastrointestinal disorders: nearly half the patients referred to a gastroenterological clinic have a functional disorder and do not suffer from organic disease. Of these functional cases, nearly half have classical irritable bowel syndrome (IBS), often called spastic colon, characterised by bouts of abdominal pain usually in the lower abdomen associated with diarrhoea which relieves the pain. It is not possible to state if any of these disorders are more common in those eating fibre-depleted foods. IBS (spastic colon) is usually treated with bran. Many improve, especially those treated with coarse bran, if constipation is relieved.

[However, it is not proven that bran is more effective than a placebo; the definitive trial has not yet been performed.]

Tovey (Chapter 13) has produced epidemiological evidence that duodenal ulceration cannot be related to the consumption of refined carbohydrates, as formerly suggested. He visited many parts of India, Bangladesh, and also Africa, and collected evidence from the opinion of experienced workers and the records of surgical operations, radiologists and necropsies.

Incidence often varies in a patchy manner in these countries. There is strong evidence that dietary protective factors occur in the food of low-incidence areas. Animal models of experimental peptic ulcer have demonstrated that unrefined wheat and rice, also certain pulses, contain a liposoluble protective factor; this is not dietary fibre. This unidentified factor appears to increase mucosal resistance.

Segal (Chapter 14) has reported the low prevalence of hiatal hernia in many developing communities in Africa and Asia. For instance, in a Johannesburg gastrointestinal clinic only 3.3% of 1092 consecutive barium meal examinations of black patients had hiatal hernia, compared with 22% in South African whites. This is not explained by the lower age of the African blacks; even black patients who suffer from diverticular disease have a low incidence of hiatal hernia. Burkitt has postulated that abdominal straining to evacuate hard faeces increases intra-abdominal pressures, thereby forcing the gastro-esophageal junction upwards into the thoracic cavity. Intra-abdominal pressures, measured in the sigmoid, are raised during lifting but are highest during the Valsalva manoeuvre. During defaecation measured intra-abdominal pressures exceed intra-thoracic pressures. Obesity is a risk factor and this is uncommon in developing communities until westernisation of diet and lifestyle occur.

James (Chapter 15) has outlined a new theory of overweight and obesity based on recent studies involving for the first time 24-h measurement in whole-body calorimeters. Lean persons have more active brown fat than overweight persons. In lean persons brown fat aids the combustion of ingested fat so that less is stored in the ordinary body fat. Obese persons have less brown fat; they are unable to metabolise much ingested fat; this is therefore stored as body fat. There are no differences between lean and obese persons in their metabolic response to starch or protein.

[Modern dietary changes have provided energy-dense diets containing more fat and sugar. This dietary pattern encourages overweight and obesity in susceptible persons.]

The aetiological factors of non-insulin-dependent diabetes mellitus (NIDDM) are considered by Mann (Chapter 16). Genetic factors play an important role but its frequency in most populations is determined principally by obesity. In recent years few have produced acceptable evidence that sucrose is a causative factor. Mann stated "there is more evidence for, and less against, the hypothesis that dietary fibre and (fibre-depleted) starchy foods are important nutritional factors in the aetiology and treatment of (NIDDM) diabetes. There is, however, strong circumstantial evidence that diets containing much highly processed fibre-depleted starch foods are associated with an increased risk of developing diabetes. Studies showing that diabetic control is improved by diets that contain much lightly processed, full-fibre starchy foods provide confirmatory evidence". These foods contain much fibre.

Heaton (Chapter 17) has developed and modified his fibre-depleted foods hypothesis of the aetiology of cholesterol gallstones, first proposed by him in 1972. It has not proved possible to demonstrate that the size of the bile acid pool varies significantly with changes in the diet. Numerous studies have pointed to raised levels of biliary deoxycholate as a risk factor; these can be lowered by feeding bran. Obesity is the most important risk factor for gall-stones; likewise probably high energy intakes. In gallstone patients, the avoidance of fibre-depleted carbohydrate foods has consistently led to a fall in the cholesterol saturation of bile. A suggested working hypothesis for the aetiology of gallstones is presented in this chapter.

Kritchevsky (Chapter 18) has summarised an extensive literature concerning the hypolipidaemic effects of bran, and certain components of dietary fibre in animal experiments and in man. Rolled oats, guar gum and legumes are hypocholesterolaemic in man, but most varieties of bran, cellulose and bagasse fibres have no effect. A vegetarian or a high-fibre dietary lifestyle have been associated with a decreased incidence of coronary heart disease, but the mechanisms involved have not been identified.

Burkitt (Chapter 19) reports a group of surgical vascular diseases, which are certainly far less common even in comparable age groups in many developing communities; he has related this low incidence to their high-fibre diet. Haemorrhoids are treated nowadays in Britain and other European countries by increasing the intake of dietary fibre or other bulk-forming agents. These produce soft bulky stools and reduce straining during defaecation. These facts support the hypothesis that straining to pass small, hard faecal masses causes sliding down of the anal cushions, even trauma, thereby causing swollen, protruding, inflamed piles.

Varicose veins are certainly far less common in many developing communities. Recent age-standardised prevalence rates in Polynesian men and women and in their descendents, the Maoris of New Zealand, reported a 10-fold increase. It has been suggested that straining to defaecate raises intra-abdominal pressures which are transmitted to the leg veins wherein dilatation progressively renders the valves incompetent.

Deep vein thrombosis certainly occurs less frequently in many developing communities, even in comparable age groups. More attention should be paid to reports that the consumption of bran has decreased the incidence and severity of post-operative deep vein thrombosis.

Walker and Stein (Chapter 20) examine the question of the influence of diet on the slow growth of Third World children compared to children of Western communities. The latter grow more rapidly and to an increased height at maturity but they develop more obesity, diabetes, coronary heart disease and certain varieties of cancer. Numerous factors, dietary and non-dietary, operate in both groups. In Third World children very slow growth, when associated with both stunting *and* wasting, is undoubtedly linked with increased morbidity and mortality. However, it is concluded that, apart from the aforementioned manifestations of malnutrition, no deleterious effects are apparent in those showing only slower growth because of the traditional high-fibre, high-starch, low-fat diet of the Third World.

Blacklock (Chapter 21) has discussed a subject new to many, namely that the Western diet plays a large part in the pathogenesis of idiopathic kidney stone. This diet increases the likelihood of calcium oxalate crystalization in the urine and reduces the activity of mucopolysaccharide inhibitors. The detection of a subset of stone-formers, whose minimal aberations of metabolism are aggravated by sucrose consumption, suggests that they are poorly adapted to present-day high-sucrose, low-fibre Western diets and are at increased risk of idiopathic renal stone. A recent trial of diet, that applied the lessons of this recent research, has shown lowered saturation indices of calcium oxalate.

Walker (Chapter 22) has reviewed mineral metabolism in relation to recent dietary recommendations that Western populations should increase the consumption of less refined cereal products and an increased intake of dietary fibre. Some, but not all, experimental studies of animals and some short-term studies in man have demonstrated a reduced absorption of calcium, magnesium, iron and zinc by high-fibre diets. Third World populations invariably eat a low-calcium diet associated with a high intake of fibre but there is no evidence of an inferior mineralization of bone or any sign of calcium deficiency, or long-term prejudicial effects in the utilization of iron or zinc.

Fisher (Chapter 23) has reviewed the milling of wheat with special reference to dietary fibre. The whole cereals, wheat, rye, maize and millet have rather a small content of dietary fibre but the bran fractions from maize and sorghum contain more dietary fibre than those of wheat and rye. Particle size distributions of coarse, medium and fine bran fractions and of the coarsest fraction of wholemeal wheat flour have been measured; they show considerable variations. The nutrient composition, including the total dietary fibre, minerals and vitamins of white, brown and wholemeal breads are published.

Consumption of bread has been falling for over 100 years; that of wholemeal bread has risen recently but still provides only a small proportion of the total bread consumption; the latter is still falling.

Heaton (Chapter 24) points out that fibre-depleted foods are changed physically in ways which favour increased intakes of energy. Studies of volunteers who ate *ad libitum* diets rich or poor in fibre-depleted carbohydrates indicate that sucrose, but not starch, inflates energy intake and promotes weight gain. If sucrose inflates energy intakes and obesity then it is a causative factor in NIDDM diabetes, and all other diseases associated with obesity such as gallstones and hypertension. Fibre-depleted foods are also depleted of most vitamins and minerals.

Silman and Marr (Chapter 25) point out that dietary advice must be based on the balance of probabilities; if not acceptable to large sections of the population they will not, by definition, be accepted. The ideal needs to be substituted by the attainable. With regard to total dietary fibre intake they recommend an increase of nearly 50%.

II. Conclusions

There is much evidence that the whole community should change its diet. The Health Education Council (1983) have made proposals for health education in Britain. Their long-term proposals involve multiple dietary changes for the whole community in which dietary fibre increments are only a part. Dietary fibre intakes should increase 50% to 30 g from 20 g/person/day and be derived largely from whole cereals; an increase of vegetables and fruit consumption was also advocated.

The HEC also recommended that fat intakes should be reduced from 38 to 34% energy; sucrose intakes should be reduced from 14 to 12% total energy; starch intakes should increase 6% total energy. Total energy intakes should be maintained because more exercise throughout the population should be encouraged. It was envisaged that these overall changes should be achieved over a period of 15 years to allow sufficient time for industrial adjustments to be made.

[The three editors wish to record their opinion that these recommended dietary changes are inadequate. They recommend much greater reductions in fat and sugar and for that matter greater increases in starch and fibre. They recognise that it will be extremely difficult to make major changes in the national diet, but minimal changes will achieve only minimal results. Enlightened individuals have already made these major changes in their own diet.]

References

Health Education Council (1983). "Proposals for Nutritional Guidelines for Health Education in Britain." Health Education Council, London.
STEPHEN, A. M., HADDAD, A. C. and PHILLIPS, S. F. (1983). *Gastroenterology* **85**, 589–595.

Index